W9-BRI-185

DISEASE PREVENTION
AS SOCIAL CHANGE

DISEASE PREVENTION AS SOCIAL CHANGE

THE STATE, SOCIETY, AND PUBLIC HEALTH IN THE UNITED STATES, FRANCE, GREAT BRITAIN, AND CANADA

CONSTANCE A. NATHANSON

Russell Sage Foundation · New York

The Russell Sage Foundation

The Russell Sage Foundation, one of the oldest of America's general purpose foundations, was established in 1907 by Mrs. Margaret Olivia Sage for "the improvement of social and living conditions in the United States." The Foundation seeks to fulfill this mandate by fostering the development and dissemination of knowledge about the country's political, social, and economic problems. While the Foundation endeavors to assure the accuracy and objectivity of each book it publishes, the conclusions and interpretations in Russell Sage Foundation publications are those of the authors and not of the Foundation, its Trustees, or its staff. Publication by Russell Sage, therefore, does not imply Foundation endorsement.

BOARD OF TRUSTEES
Thomas D. Cook, Chair

Kenneth D. Brody	Jennifer L. Hochschild	Cora B. Marrett
Robert E. Denham	Kathleen Hall Jamieson	Richard H. Thaler
Christopher Edley Jr.	Melvin J. Konner	Eric Wanner
John A. Ferejohn	Alan B. Krueger	Mary C. Waters
Larry V. Hedges		

Library of Congress Cataloging-in-Publication Data

Nathanson, Constance A.
    Disease prevention as social change : the state, society and public health in the United States, France, Great Britain, and Canada / Constance A. Nathanson.
        p. ; cm.
    Includes bibliographical references and index.
    ISBN-13: 978-0-87154-644-9
    ISBN-10: 0-87154-644-2
        1. Health promotion—Cross-cultural studies. 2. Medicine, Preventive—Cross-cultural studies. 3. Preventive health services—Cross-cultural studies. 4. Medical policy—Cross-cultural studies. I. Title.
        [DNLM: 1. Health Policy—trends—Canada. 2. Health Policy—trends—France. 3. Health Policy—trends—Great Britain. 4. Health Policy—trends—United States. 5. Primary Prevention—trends—Canada. 6. Primary Prevention—trends—France. 7. Primary Prevention—trends—Great Britain. 8. Primary Prevention—trends—United States. 9. Public Health—trends—Canada. 10. Public Health—trends—France. 11. Public Health—trends—Great Britain. 12. Public Health—trends—United States. 13. Social Change—Canada. 14. Social Change—France. 15. Social Change—Great Britain. 16. Social Change—United States. WA 108 N275d 2007]
    RA427.8.N3844 2007
    362.1—dc22

2006033287

Copyright © 2007 by Russell Sage Foundation. All rights reserved. Printed in the United States of America. No part of this publication may be reproduced, stored in a retrieval system, or transmitted in any form or by any means, electronic, mechanical, photocopying, recording, or otherwise, without the prior written permission of the publisher.

Reproduction by the United States Government in whole or in part is permitted for any purpose.

The paper used in this publication meets the minimum requirements of American National Standard for Information Sciences—Permanence of Paper for Printed Library Materials. ANSI Z39.48-1992.

Text design by Suzanne Nichols.

RUSSELL SAGE FOUNDATION
112 East 64th Street, New York, New York 10021
10 9 8 7 6 5 4 3 2 1

For my mother, Elizabeth, and my sister, Jane
In loving memory

Contents

About the Author

Constance A. Nathanson is a sociologist and professor of clinical socio-medical sciences in the Columbia University Mailman School of Public Health.

Acknowledgments

THIS BOOK is the outcome of a project not only ambitious—too ambitious, it often seemed—but also very long in the time it took to accomplish. Neither the research nor the writing would have been possible without the financial support—reflecting a belief in the project's ultimate value highly comforting to the author—of generous and patient donors.

In the course of earlier work on the comparative social history and politics of women's adolescence as a public problem in the early and late twentieth century in the United States, I had become convinced of the potential of comparative history and social science for illuminating the sometimes incomprehensible trajectories of contemporary public health policies in this country. I was further impressed with the importance of social movements as policy actors. My first step down the path culminating in this book—a comparative analysis of tobacco and gun control as social movements in the United States—was made possible by a grant from the Association of Schools of Public Health and the U.S. Centers for Disease Control and Prevention. My ability to expand this initial project to include other countries and other issues was entirely due to the wonderful program of Health Policy Research Investigator Awards initiated by the Robert Wood Johnson Foundation only a year before I applied in 1994. Research trips to London and Paris! Who could ask for more? A year as a visiting scholar at the Russell Sage Foundation (of which more below) enabled me to consolidate what I had learned and to embark on the historical (that is, late nineteenth and early twentieth century) pieces of my project. It also made me recognize that I needed an extended period of fieldwork in Canada. A grant from the newly inaugurated Fulbright New Century Scholars Program enabled me to spend two productive months at the McGill Institute for the Study of Canada in Montreal and an additional essential week in Vancouver. Finally, it was my extraordinary good fortune to be given four weeks in the late summer of 2005 as a scholar in residence at the Rockefeller Study and Conference Center in Bellagio, Italy. During that never-to-be-forgotten period of peace and seclusion the manuscript took more or less its final form. For this continuing and nearly seamless support throughout a very long period of gestation I am grateful beyond words.

In equal measure this book owes its being to the many individuals in the United States, France, Britain, and Canada who shared with me their expert knowledge of public health policy formation and implementation and handed me on to others with whom, I was often told, I must speak. They were always right. Such insight as I have gained into the contemporary politics of public health is largely due to the generosity of people on the ground (many of whom were actively engaged in the policy process) with their time, patience, and knowledge. Some of those with whom I spoke were public figures with published views, and I have cited them in the text by name. Others less well known I have identified by position (for example, civil servant). There are people, however, whose contributions to this project extended well beyond that of informant, crossing the boundary into colleague and friend. Special thanks are due to Nicholas Freudenberg, Sam Friedman, John Gagnon, and David Vlahov in the United States; Albert Hirsch, Pascal Mélihan-Chenin, Karen Slama, and Monica Steffen in France; Virginia Berridge, William Bynum, Sue and Sebastian Freudenberg, and Simon Szreter in the United Kingdom; and Norbert Gilmore, Antonia Maioni, and Suzanne Staggenborg in Canada. Insofar as this project was a joy and a pleasure—and it often was—they are responsible.

Neither the external financial support nor the internal energy and conviction required to see this project through would have been possible without the steady friendship and commitment of many colleagues, some long-standing and others I was fortunate to meet along the way. All have been important, but two have been critical, one early in my career and the other more recently. W. Henry Mosley was my department chair during most of my long tenure at the Johns Hopkins School of Hygiene and Public Health. I am indebted to Henry for his conviction that the social sciences are critically important to public health, for his unswerving belief in my capacities as a scholar, and for never discouraging me from thinking big. Ronald Bayer, my colleague in my current academic home at Columbia University, took up that baton from Henry. Since our first meeting in Paris in 1998, Ron has been a constant source of intellectual encouragement. Sharing my comparative interests, he drew me into his own cross-national comparative work and played a critical role in expanding my intellectual community to include a multidisciplinary range of scholars with parallel concerns. Last, but not least—and of inestimable importance both personally and professionally, Ron was instrumental in bringing me to Columbia.

The significance of the financial awards I received far exceeded their monetary value, as exemplified by my encounters with Ron Bayer. With the exception of the first, each of these awards brought with them invaluable opportunities not only to meet but also to develop significant collegial relations with scholars with common intellectual interests from a variety of academic disciplines—political science and history as well as my own discipline, sociology. In particular, my appreciation of political science and such knowledge of its contributions to policy analysis as I have managed to acquire I owe largely to those two consummate, lively, and—above all—intellectually generous scholars, Mark Peterson and James Morone, both of whom I was lucky to have in my Robert Wood Johnson cohort of awardees. Yet another Robert Wood Johnson benefit came through its award to Ron Bayer for his work on tobacco politics (in which I participated): this was my meeting with Canadian political scientist Antonia Maioni, director of the McGill Institute for the Study of Canada. I owe a large part of the pleasure of my stay in Canada to Antonia's generosity in offering me an academic home at the Institute during the three months I spent in Montreal. I have emphasized the spin-offs from the Robert Wood Johnson award, but the others—Russell Sage, Fulbright, and Bellagio—were also important as much for the supportive intellectual communities they created as for their support financially.

Much of the work on this project was carried out while I was still at Johns Hopkins, where I benefited greatly from the support and friendship of Ken Hill, director of the Hopkins Population Center; of my dear friend Young Kim whose untimely death in the fall of 2005 left an immeasurable void; of my colleague (and sister-in-law) Laurie Zabin; and of my students and postdocs, in particular Kirsten Stoebenau and Laura Carpenter. My research assistants at Hopkins, Laurie Oaks and Greg Ruiters, worked tirelessly to pull together the masses of documentary material required for this project. The facilities of the Hopkins Population Center (funded by a grant from the National Institute of Child Health and Development)—in particular the generous assistance of its librarians, Jean Sack and her successor, Sheila Thomas, and Yibing Zhao's patient and professional support for a very amateur computer user—were invaluable. Anique Montambeault did splendid work as my assistant in Montreal, finding not only secondary sources but some wonderful archival materials on infant mortality and tuberculosis in Quebec.

This project brought me to New York City—first as a visiting scholar at the Russell Sage Foundation and a couple of years later as a faculty member in the Department of Sociomedical Sciences in the Mailman School of Public Health at Columbia University. It is hard to imagine an intellectual and academic environment more favorable to the fulfillment of this project: a department founded on the premise that basic scholarship in the social sciences was fundamental to the advancement of public health, home to faculty in each of the three disciplines—sociology, political science, and history—on whose work I have largely drawn, and committed to the fostering of policy-relevant and politically edgy research and writing. I owe an enormous debt to my department chair, Richard Parker, who shepherded my appointment as professor of clinical sociomedical sciences and to the colleagues who welcomed me so warmly, encouraged and appreciated my work on this project, and forbore from asking too many times when it would be finished. I am particularly grateful to Jennifer Hirsch, who went well beyond the demands of colleagueship (and long-standing friendship) to organize a discussion forum on the manuscript in the winter of 2006, and to the SMS department faculty who read the book, attended the forum, and made many helpful comments and suggestions: Ron Bayer, James Colgrove, Diane DiMauro, Amy Fairchild, Kim Hopper, Eugene Litwak, Peter Messeri, Gerry Oppenheimer, and Jo Phelan. I owe further special thanks to Bruce Link and Jo Phelan for helping me out with some sticky questions about the relation between public health policy and the fundamental causes of disease.

My debt to the Russell Sage Foundation goes well beyond the wonderful year I spent there as a visiting scholar. First, and not least important, without that year in New York I would not have made the connections that brought me to Columbia. Second, to my great good fortune, the foundation took up its option to consider my work for publication. Surely no more patient and understanding publisher exists. No deadline was suggested and never once—well, maybe once—did my editor, Suzanne Nichols, ask me when the book would be completed. When once I ran into the foundation's president, Eric Wanner, he only wanted to be assured that I was still writing. Far more than more aggressive tactics, this low-key approach made certain that I would—come hell or high water—finish the book. Third, the thoughtful critique (along with generous praise) offered by the Foundation's two anonymous reviewers greatly strengthened the original manuscript, and I am most grateful for their time and patience. Last—but not least—I thank Genna Patacsil for her oversight of the production process, in which thorough professionalism and human understanding for an author's foibles were combined in equal measure.

The manuscript in its final form reflects the combined effort of myself and my in-house editor—formerly the managing editor of *Scientific American*—my husband, Armand Schwab. First in Bellagio and later at home in Gardiner, New York, Armand read every word, parsed every sentence, marginally noted every dash and comma placed and misplaced and then—the best part—we sat together side by side and went over it all again. I enjoy writing, but whatever felicity of expression there may be in this book owes a great deal to the work of a consummate, highly professional, and much beloved editor.

PART I

SETTING THE STAGE

Chapter 1

Introduction

STORIES OF public health are stories about how individuals, communities, and states recognize and respond to the threat of disease. These stories have a dramatic form. Actors—experts, officials, aroused citizens—emerge on the public stage in the first scene, sounding the alarm and demanding action to contain some perceived threat. As the action proceeds, the threat is defined and redefined, its reality contested, and its source disputed. In subsequent scenes, public authorities may or may not respond. Citizens may or may not take matters into their own hands. Dramatic resolution may or may not be achieved. The public's health may or may not be advanced. Tension and struggle—conflicts of power, interest, and ideology—are the hallmarks of the public health drama, just as they are the hallmarks of any circumstance that pits one set of powerful interests, however nobly defined, against another (there is, almost always, another). Dramas of public health presented in narrative form are the raw material for this book. Its subject is the analysis and interpretation of these dramas as forms of struggle for social change.

I define public health as "community action to avoid disease and other threats to the health and welfare of individuals and the community at large" (Duffy 1990, 1). The critical phrases in this definition are "community action"—public health is society's collective response to a perceived common threat—and "avoid disease." This is a book about the vicissitudes of societies' collective struggles to avoid disease. It is not about health-care policy as this phrase is commonly used, to mean policies for the provision of medical care to individuals already ill. Nor is the scope limited to the formal structures in which public health is embodied: health ministries, local health departments, designated public health officials. Action to prevent disease takes many forms, ranging from the charismatic individual on the corner handing out clean needles to injection drug users, through the lawyer spearheading a class action suit against the tobacco industry, to the parliamentary debate pitting proponents of disease prevention against opposing economic and moral interests. Public health policies include

3

any public or publicly advocated policy—ranging from immunization to income redistribution—intended in whole or in part to improve health or prevent disease.

Public health is inherently political. Attributions of disease causation are statements about the location of responsibility for human pain and suffering and, by the same token, about the measures that should be taken to prevent these maladies from occurring. Major sources of variation in these measures are the extent of their challenge to the existing social order and the degree to which they invoke the power of the state. Witness, for example, the nature of debate about the causes of tuberculosis at the beginning of the twentieth century in France (Barnes 1995). The monarchist right gave its etiological preference to the irresponsible and immoral drinking habits of the working class and resisted social reform. Socialists attributed it to unsanitary housing and exposure to the newly recognized tubercle bacillus, downplayed alcoholism, and demanded parliamentary attention to poverty as the ultimate cause. The increasingly influential revolutionary syndicalists rejected mainstream causal theories altogether. Tuberculosis, they maintained, was "inherent in the logic of capitalism." Medical prescriptions, clinics, and sanatoriums were scams intended to deflect real reform and sop the conscience of the "compassionate elite." Defeating tuberculosis required overthrowing the capitalist system. Although this may be an extreme (or just an unusually clear) case, remarkably parallel political commitments continue to be at least implicit, and often explicit, in current intellectual as well as policy debates on disease causation and the role of public health.

The public health stories I have selected to relate and to analyze are infant mortality and tuberculosis at the turn of the nineteenth century and the contemporary dramas of cigarette smoking and HIV/AIDS in injection drug users. The narratives in the first part of this book describe how each of four countries—the United States, Canada, Britain, and France—experienced and responded to these common threats to their publics' health. The goals of the analysis in the second part are to arrive at an understanding of the social and political processes that drive policy making in public health and to explain why countries otherwise comparable in so many respects reacted differently to essentially the same threats.

Background

The idea of public health emerged in Britain and France in the first half of the nineteenth century. It grew from the increased concern of a few physicians and public officials about the devastating health, economic, social, and potential political consequences of urbanization and industrialization, particularly among the urban poor. Its principal investigative tool was the social survey. Its dominant theories were environmental. The unique domain of this new discipline and set of activities was disease as a product of the environment, not sick individuals (who were in the domain of curative medicine).

> Nineteenth-century hygienists emphasized the social and material environments in which disease developed and advocated both sanitary and social reform as the most effective public health measures. (La Berge 1992, 74)

Public health was linked with social reform because disease was attributed to social conditions—from poverty to inadequate sewers and water supply—that, advocates maintained, called for state action. Attention to working class misery and deprivation was triggered in part by labor and social unrest, and public health was advocated as an alternative to social revolution. Referring to the United States, Fee observes:

> Politically, public health reform offered a middle ground between the cutthroat principles of entrepreneurial capitalism and the revolutionary ideas of the socialists, anarchists, and utopian visionaries. [Speaking in 1892, William H. Welch suggested that] sanitary improvement offered the best way of improving the lot of the poor, short of the radical restructuring of society. (1991, 5)

Even during the heyday of environmental theories of disease causation in the nineteenth century, the idea of public health as a rationale for social reform was by no means universally accepted. Advocates confronted ideological opposition to state intervention on behalf of public health—opposition was especially strong in France—as well as ratepayer reluctance to pay for expensive water and sewer projects. And they confronted competing theories—theories of private health—that laid unsanitary conditions, poor health, and excess mortality at the door of the poor themselves: the inevitable consequences of immorality and intemperance. Although the relative salience of each of these strands in opposition to the idea of public health as social reform varied across countries, they were never wholly absent.

The idea of public health as social reform receded in the course of the late nineteenth and early twentieth centuries in the face of new theories of disease causation, shifting attributions of responsibility for disease prevention, and changes in the structure of medical care. The germ theory "drew attention away from the larger and more diffuse problems of water supplies, street cleaning, housing reform, and the living conditions of the poor" (Fee 1991, 7). A "direct appeal from mortality figures to social reform [became] much more difficult" (Lewis 1986, 6). The displacement of social and environmental reform by the control of specific diseases as the preferred solution to public health problems was most noticeable in the United

States. But the accompanying emphasis on individual responsibility—in particular, the responsibility of mothers for the health of children and families—was widespread (Tomes 1990; Klaus 1993; Lewis 1980; Dwork 1987; Meckel 1990).

The exigencies of world wars and depression, though they put new life into the idea of collective *responsibility* for health, failed to revive the idea of public health as social reform. Health was defined as a characteristic of individuals, not of social or physical environments, and health reform became defined as the institution of state-supported arrangements for universal access to individual medical care. Negotiation with respect to the details of these arrangements (or, in the United States, their rejection) was dominated by physicians committed to the individual doctor-patient relationship as the linchpin of population health. In direct confrontation between medical and public health doctors—even in Britain, home to the earliest and best organized corps of local public health officers—public health was hopelessly overmatched (Lewis 1986).

If the idea of public health as a vehicle for societal-level social change had not already disappeared from the ideological armamentarium of the public health establishment, its death knell was sounded in the early 1970s with the popularization of risky lifestyles as the major determinant of disease in the developed world. The risky lifestyle framework—embraced most wholeheartedly in the United States—located both the source of disease and the means of prevention within the individual. Carried to its extreme, this ideology—for ideology it is—relieves the collectivity of any responsibility for population health.

These implications have, of course, been widely contested—from, however, different perspectives in the four countries. And the idea of public health and disease prevention as vehicles for broad social reform has not, in fact, disappeared. The flame has been kept alight by actors, few of whom are public health professionals or even think of their activities as within the domain of public health.

Premises

This book has three premises. The first is that public policies in general, and public health policies in particular, play a critical role in disease prevention and in the decline of mortality. This premise is hardly self-evident. The ideological conflicts described are mirrored in intellectual debate among theories that assign causal priority in accounting for disease prevention to economic development or advances in medical technology and more socially activist theories that emphasize the role of (broadly defined) public health policies and of the social and political context in which they emerge. This debate has generated controversy among scholars for at least the last quarter century.

The debate was initiated in a series of publications by the British epidemiologist Thomas McKeown beginning in the 1950s (McKeown and Brown 1955; McKeown 1965, 1976; McKeown, Record, and Turner 1975). McKeown based his analyses on nineteenth- and twentieth-century mortality declines in England and Wales. Although he did not discount public health altogether, McKeown's principal argument, and the one for which he is most often cited, was that mortality decline was specifically not caused by doctors and hospitals, drugs and therapies, but was the result of an improved standard of living. His thesis left little room for active human agency in the improvement of population health.[1]

Although McKeown's rejection of medical technology is widely accepted, his proposed alternative is not (see, for example, Colgrove 2002). The idea that some combination of greater income and wealth with improved nutrition is responsible for mortality decline has been contested both by British scholars using data from England and Wales (Szreter 1988, 1997; McFarlane 1989; Hardy 1993) and, more broadly, by American scholars, principally Samuel Preston, based on analyses of data from the United States in the first years of the twentieth century and of more recent data from developing countries (Preston 1975, 1985, 1996; Preston and Haines 1991). I summarize these scholars' conclusions in their own words:

> My argument is not that improving nutrition and living standards were entirely unimportant in accounting for the mortality decline (in England and Wales), but that the role of a battling public health ideology, politics and medicine operating of necessity through local government, is more correctly seen as the causal agency involved. (Szreter 1988, 36)

In a later piece on the same theme, Szreter continues:

> A favourable outcome [of economic growth] was in no way inevitable. It had to be devised with the aid of medical science *and fought for politically.* (1997, 696, emphasis added)

Preston makes much the same case for the United States:

> this explanation [of mortality decline] emphasizes a fundamental scientific advance, the germ theory, as implemented by public health officials and, perhaps more importantly, aggressively disseminated by them to an extremely eager audience. (1996, 7)

New analyses of the role played by clean water technologies (that is, water filtration and chlorination) in late nineteenth- and early twentieth-century mortality decline in the United States lend strong support to Preston's and Szreter's conclusions: "clean water was responsible for nearly half the total mortality reduction in major cities, three-quarters of the infant mortality reduction, and nearly two-thirds of the child mortality reduction" (Cutler and Miller 2005, 1). Clean water did not, of course, happen automatically. As with most public health reforms, it had to be fought for politically (Szreter 1988, 1997; Troesken 2004).

Two critical points are contained in these observations. The first, consistent with my initial premise, is that organized human agency as represented by the public health movement has been instrumental in the decline of mortality. I will reexamine that premise in the book's conclusion in light of information from the sixteen country and issue case studies that form the body of my text.

The second point—that this movement reflected social and political developments independent of changes in per capita income—serves to introduce my second premise, that the formation, adoption, and implementation of public health policies are the outcome of social and political processes. These processes were elaborated in the 1980s by demographers working principally in developing country settings (for example, Nag 1985; Palloni 1985; Caldwell 1986; Johansson and Mosk 1987) and by comparative sociologists interested in the determinants of social policies in industrialized countries (Orloff and Skocpol 1984; Skocpol and Amenta 1986). The consensus among these scholars was remarkable. The variables they identified—the characteristics of states and the collective actions of citizens—are central in my conceptual approach to unraveling the politics of public health.

The demographers cited used alternative strategies to determine the causes of mortality decline: comparison of developing countries similar in their income and wealth but with unusually high or low mortality levels, and comparison of industrialized countries with similar mortality levels but—in the late nineteenth century—very different social and economic characteristics. These studies concluded, first, that unexpectedly "low" mortality countries were distinguished by widely distributed public health services (for example, sanitation, immunization, maternal and child health) and, second, that widely distributed public health services resulted, in turn, either from the actions of a strong central government with a reasonably well-educated and cooperative population, or from an organized, politically active population with a reasonably responsive central government.

Along similar lines, Skocpol and colleagues argued that social provision (for example, old-age pensions, health insurance, compulsory unemployment insurance) by industrialized countries cannot be explained by these countries' relative economic growth or their levels of industrialization and urbanization. In common with several of the demographers I have cited, these investigators emphasized "the organizational structures and capacities of states" (Skocpol and Amenta 1986, 147) and, in later work, "the institutional leverage that various social groups have gained, or failed to gain," as the principal shapers of social policy making (Skocpol 1995a, 19).

Comparative demographic research focused primarily on declines in mortality from communicable disease; the public policies at issue were traditional public health policies, clean water, sanitation, immunization, and the like. Public policies are, however, equally relevant to what we may now perceive as the more clear and present dangers of tobacco smoke, breast cancer, HIV/AIDS, and environmental pollution.[2] Changes in public policies to mitigate these dangers come about in large part—if not wholly—through the actions of governments, initiated internally or in response to external popular and political pressure.

Convergence among medical historians, demographers, and comparative sociologists on the importance of government-initiated public policies in the decline of mortality has had little noticeable impact on empirical social research on public health policies or on the conceptual development necessary to guide this research—in part, perhaps, because of a belief that political analysis is not science (see for example, Newman 1999, 279, McKinlay and Marceau 2000, 51). And so, though there is recent recognition, particularly among scholars of public health law, that policies—for example, "[drug laws] and the police practices flowing from them"—are structural factors that influence health (Burris, Strathdee, and Vernick 2003, 881), macro-level theory to guide the identification and analysis of these factors is conspicuous by its absence. As a result, little attention has been paid to specifying the social and political processes that push policy makers toward or away from particular public health policies or shape their implementation. To make change in social policies, the first step must be to understand how these policies came about.

My last premise is methodological: the best strategy to identify the social and political processes that drive change in public health policies is by cross-national comparison. This project is a case-comparative study in the methodological tradition of illustrious forebears past and present, including Max Weber in *The Protestant Ethic and the Spirit of Capitalism* (1904/1949), Barrington Moore in *Social Origins of Dictatorship and Democracy* (1993), Theda Skocpol in *States and Social Revolutions* (1979), and Charles Tilly (whose works are too numerous to list). I mention these scholars not to appropriate their luster but to situate my own more modest effort in a particular methodological fold within sociology, that of case-comparative research (see, for example, Ragin 1987; Ragin and Becker 1992; Mahoney 2004). The advantages of this method for present purposes are that it combines historical specificity—the location of actions and events in specific times and places—with the potential for theoretical generalization.

Selecting Countries and Public Health Issues

The units of analysis for this project—the cases—are sixteen country-and-issue combinations: four countries and four public health issues. I explain my selection of countries and issues below, but let me begin with a reality check: in the practice of case-comparative research "cases are chosen for all sorts of reasons, from convenience and familiarity to fascination and strategy" (Walton 1992, 125). In no sense are these sixteen cases a random sample of countries or of public health issues, nor do I claim that the issues selected are typical of public health issues these four countries faced over the past hundred or so years. My reasons for the selections I made were both pragmatic—convenience, familiarity, and fascination—and strategic in that I attempted to maximize the probability that the social processes in which I was interested—the politics of public health—would be laid bare. In his remarks, Walton went on to say that cases once chosen—for whatever reasons—must be "shown to be a case of something important" (125). I will later return to the questions Walton's observation suggests: what my sixteen cases are cases of and why they are important.

When I embarked on this project, my primary interest was in the social and political dimensions of public health policy making in the contemporary United States. I soon became aware that some of the same public health issues agitating citizens and policy makers in the United States—environmental pollution, smoking, HIV/AIDS—were of equally deep concern in other countries, and that substantial leverage in understanding the American experience might be gained by cross-national comparison. Further, though important comparative work on these issues has been undertaken by scholars from a variety of disciplines, the literature offers little or no systematic cross-national comparative research on the sociology and politics of public health more broadly, in contrast to the large body of comparative research on systems of medical care.[3]

Selecting Countries

I selected Britain, Canada, and France to maximize the leverage from the proposed comparison with the United States. First, these countries are similar in many of the characteristics that might be expected to shape the responses of states to public health problems: the depth and sophistication of their medical and scientific establishments, their economic and political systems, and their economic affluence. Second, though their roles may vary, the actors in the public health drama—physicians, politicians, administrators, advocates of one stripe or another—are essentially the same. Third, these countries were nonetheless quite dissimilar in the timing and character of their response to the public health dangers I have identified. It was not until 1963, for example, that France made tuberculosis reporting mandatory, whereas in New York City reporting was made mandatory in 1897 (with other U.S. municipalities quickly following suit), and in Britain in 1913. Conversely, needle-exchange programs to protect injection drug users from HIV transmission were established in Britain in 1988 with state sponsorship and funding. In the United States, on the other hand, federal funding and sponsorship for these programs have been explicitly rejected and many programs remain underground for fear of police and legal harassment. Not only, then, do these countries react with varying degrees of aggressiveness to the *same* threat, but also there is a good deal of inconsistency in how the same country responds to *different* threats.

In addition to cross-national variation, there is substantial variation within each of these countries in the allocation of formal responsibility for public health between local, regional, and national authorities. I deal with this potential problem by treating the genesis of attention to public health threats and the allocation (or assumption) of responsibility for responding to these threats as empirical questions, not as given by the formal location of responsibility for public health. Starting with an identified public health problem, I trace the major actors regardless of their geographical, bureaucratic, or political location. This location is highly variable across issues, across countries, and across time. For example, in all four countries at the turn of the last century, local public health, medical, and civil authorities played important roles in public health action against tuberculosis and infant mortality. Infant mortality was unique, however, in capturing the attention of the state and of organized women's groups acting nationally as well as at a local level. More recently, predominantly lay grassroots organizations played major roles in the initial response to smoking in the United States but were much less important in Britain and France. These variations result from differences in how the problem is brought to public attention (whether by physicians, civil servants, aggrieved citizens, or someone else), in the location of political power (who is perceived as having authority to do something about the problem), and in citizens' expectations and beliefs concerning the political level at which action should be taken in response to a problem in public health.

Selection of Issues

My choice of public health issues—tuberculosis and infant mortality at the turn of the nineteenth century and, currently, smoking and HIV/AIDS in injection drug users—was driven initially by their public health importance. I measured importance not only by an objective standard—all are major causes of illness and death—but also by the level of medical, public, and policy attention these issues received at the time they emerged on the public stage. Arguably, the sociology and politics of public health are illuminated as much by the problems that are ignored as by those that are engaged. However, apart from the practical obstacles to investigation of problems that failed altogether to attract expert or public attention, the trajectory of issue salience is uneven, so that even dangers highly salient at one time may be largely ignored at another, regardless of their magnitude as reflected in incidence or prevalence rates.

Social movements and other forms of action organized around perceived threats to the life and health of individuals, communities, the nation, even the planet, have been a prominent feature of American life since early in the twentieth century. Recently, cigarette smoking, AIDS, abortion, black lung disease, nuclear power, air and water pollution, breast cancer, drunk driving, and a host of other perceived dangers have engaged politicians and public officials in the United States and have served as catalysts for the formation of groups to challenge accepted definitions of these issues and to demand redress. However, relatively few of these issues received comparable levels of policy or public attention (or both) in more than one or two of the other three countries. A major consideration in the selection of cigarette smoking and HIV/AIDS was that they emerged as significant public health problems in all four countries at about the same time. Each country entered the starting gate with more or less equal inexperience in coping with these particular issues. It was reasonable to anticipate that how they coped would shed light on the social and political processes in which I was most interested (processes I will spell out in the following section).

Cigarette smoking and HIV/AIDS proved, in fact, to be ideal candidates for revealing the roles of ideology and politics in public health. A wide range of actors and forms of action were mobilized in response to these issues, and substantial controversy was generated around the meanings of these problems and how and by whom they should be addressed. Further, it required no more than cursory reading of these countries' national press to become aware of the profound differences between the United States and Canada, Britain, and France in how and by whom these issues were portrayed and addressed. These differences argued strongly for the potential of comparative research to illuminate U.S. policies (and, of course, the policies of these other countries as well). Finally, within the larger problem of HIV/AIDS, I elected to focus on the threat to injection drug users. Although drug users were, in fact, an important part of the AIDS epidemic from the beginning, they have been relatively neglected in the vast literature on the social, political, and ideological dimensions of HIV/AIDS. Further, narcotic drug use is equally stigmatized in all four countries, so that differences in countries' response to the AIDS–drugs nexus could not be attributed to differences in the level of stigma.

To fully understand a country's present public health policies it is essential to know something about its policies in the past. Countries display a substantial degree of continuity across time in their policy-making styles, and attention to the reasons for this continuity is critical to the analysis of policy decisions. By the late nineteenth century, tuberculosis and infant mortality had emerged as significant public health problems in all four countries, and I chose them primarily for that reason. My narratives are cut off at approximately the beginning of World War I not because these conditions were no longer important but to limit the task of reconstruction to a reasonable compass.

Additional reasons emerged in the course of research. Most obvious, perhaps, are the parallels between cigarette smoking and drug injection. Both nicotine and heroin are substances with long histories of medicinal as well as recreational use, and both have moved back and forth over time between the categories of innocuous pleasure and dangerous drug (Berridge and Edwards 1981; Berridge 1997; Goodman 1998). As drugs, however, they carry very different social and cultural baggage, which makes for illuminating comparisons in their treatment within and across countries, both now and in the past. The late nineteenth- and early twentieth-century response to infant mortality is of unique interest because of the degree to which infant mortality was identified with the state and mobilized its energies. Comparison of infant mortality with other public health issues, within countries, across countries, and across time illuminates in particular the circumstances in which states are more or less likely to expend their political capital on public health.

In my selection of cases I have clearly privileged contest and struggle over routine. There are two reasons for this. First is the problem of cross-national comparability. Many routine activities that are considered public health services in the United States—for example, breast cancer screening for poor women—are individual health services in the other countries, provided through their national health-care systems and thus not within the purview of this project. Second, and much more important, the politics of uncontested public health activities were likely to be both well hidden and not terribly revealing about the social and political processes that are the subject of this book.

Casing the Cases

What, then, are my sixteen cases cases of? At the most abstract level, they are cases of struggle over the definition and ownership of public problems (see, for example, Gusfield 1981) and over the power to occupy and dominate the terrain that those problems are claimed to represent. As I pointed out earlier, the cast of characters in these struggles has been remarkably constant across space and time. Their relative success is powerfully shaped by social and political contexts that tend to privilege one category of actors over another, creating the differences in "institutional leverage" that move social policy in one direction or another (Skocpol 1995a). At a slightly less abstract level, each case pits social reformers (who come in many guises, as we shall see) against institutions, groups, and individuals who oppose reform—or at least reform as reformers interpret it. By comparing these cases, mostly across countries but occasionally within a single country, I hope not only to comprehend the particularities of each case—to understand how countries arrive at one set of policies rather than another—but also to build a body of empirical evidence sufficient to support theoretical as well as empirical generalization across cases.

States, Collective Action, and Constructions of Risk

I argued above that specification of the social and political processes that drive policy making in public health is hindered by an absence of macro-level theory to guide identification and analysis of these processes. The volume of data potentially relevant to specification of these processes is enormous. The initial theoretical notions with which I approached this project had two purposes. First, to thread my way through the mass of potentially relevant information, I needed a conceptual map that would tell me—at least preliminarily—where to look and how to sort through the data I accumulated. Second, given my goal of generalization across cases, I needed a set of concepts sufficiently abstract to be applicable to all sixteen country and issue combinations. I developed a conceptual map grounded in work of the demographers and comparative sociologists cited earlier (for a preliminary version, see Nathanson 1996). It has three broad, decidedly macro-level elements: the organization and interests of nation-states, social movements and other forms of collective action outside the state, and ideologies that frame constructions of risk to health. I now briefly introduce each of these elements (for more conceptual detail, analysis, and interpretation, see chapters 7 to 9).

Nation-States

Public policy is powerfully shaped by the actions of nation-states. This assertion—central to the arguments of the scholars cited earlier—sounds like a truism when baldly stated. Nevertheless, the concept of the state as an autonomous actor is of relatively recent vintage in the work of comparative social scientists (see, for example, Evans, Rueschemeyer, and Skocpol 1985). This concept—along with the idea of systematic national variation in what John Peter Nettl called stateness and what later came to be called state strength—was proposed in an influential paper published in 1968 (1968). Nettl's ideas have been elaborated—and critiqued—ever since in publications too numerous to mention. Coming in for particular opprobrium have been "gross characterizations of 'strong' versus 'weak' states" (Evans, Rueschemeyer, and Skocpol 1985, 360). Nevertheless, I have found these characterizations valuable in at least two respects: first, as a reminder to collect ample data on the words and actions of the civil servants, politicians, and other government officials who embody the state in all but its most mythical sense; and second, as a heuristic device, raising questions about why putatively strong states do not act when action seems required and weak states sometimes do. I employ the strong state–weak state dichotomy (explicated briefly below and more fully in chapter 7) as an ideal-type—a logical construct against which empirical reality may be compared (Gerth and Mills 1946).[4] This construct is at best descriptive and in no way explanatory, as the materials that follow will show. It has not been superseded by other and better conceptualizations of state variation, however. Its liveliness is demonstrated by its continuing status as a whipping post for historians and political scientists (for example, Baldwin 2005b).

Adopting the conceptual perspective of Skocpol and other students of social policy, I conceive of nation-states as autonomous actors that "may formulate and pursue goals that are not simply reflective of the demands or interests of social groups, classes, or society" (Skocpol 1985, 9). Weak states are "those unable to formulate policy goals independent of particular groups in their society, to change the behavior of specific groups, or to alter directly the structure of their society—and strong states . . . are able to accomplish each of these objectives" (Vogel 1986, 265). In the ideal typical case, strong states are notable for their capacity to act. Structural characteristics thought to contribute to this capacity are centralization (that is, a unitary rather than a federal structure), concentration of power in the executive branch of government (as opposed to separation of powers, as in the United States), and the presence in the state of politically independent "career officials relatively insulated from ties to currently dominant socioeconomic interests" (Skocpol 1985, 9). In the ideal typical case, officials in a strong state make policy based on their judgment of the greater good, largely insulated from the pressure of private interests (that is, civil society).

Policy innovation and policy implementation may be responsive to different state characteristics. Administrative and financial centralization and government officials' decision-making autonomy (defining characteristics of strong states as noted earlier) are widely held to facilitate implementation. In the ideal typical strong state, execution should go smoothly once policy decisions are made. By the same token, "a complicated division of jurisdiction between a multitude of semi-independent government agencies and a federal stratification of state authority [as in the United States] tends to make policy implementation more cumbersome" (Kitschelt 1986, 63).

States not only are policy actors in their own right but also play a major role in conditioning the opportunities for collective action available to groups outside the formal political and administrative structure (Immergut 1992; Skocpol 1985; Tarrow 1998). Indeed, limits placed on access to policy making by groups outside the formal state structure are a defining characteristic of the ideal typical strong state (Hall 1986; Vogel 1986).

I illustrate the concept of strong and weak states as well as the limitations of this concept for explanatory purposes with a capsule summary of my observations on public health policy making in France and the United States, paradigmatic examples of strong and weak states. If, indeed, strong states were more able policy makers (as I had initially—perhaps naively—hypothesized) then France should have been in the vanguard of action to protect the public's health.

France is a unitary state characterized by cohesion between the executive and legislative branches of government; insulation from the demands of other social actors, such that policy initiatives tend to come from within the state itself; the capacity to implement policy over the demands of other social groups; and an ideological identification of the state with the public interest (Hall 1986; Dobbin 1994). The United States presents a clear contrast, both institutional (as reflected in the separation of powers within the federal government and between the federal government and the states), and ideological, as we are constantly reminded by advocates for the devolution of power from the center to state and local governments. Comparison of these two nations' public health policy making, however, suggests that state strength is as likely to be associated with state paralysis as with effective action. The delayed French response to tuberculosis at the turn of the nineteenth century and more recently to HIV/AIDS can be explained in part by state inaction combined with a weak tradition of local action on the ground. In the United States, on the other hand, relatively weak federal responses to the public health problems presented by cigarettes and by HIV among injection drug users were offset (far more so in the former case than in the latter) by energetic action at the local level. Under circumstances where the central state is unable or unwilling to act, institutional and ideological commitment to centralized power may have the effect of inhibiting *any* action, whereas decentralization may offer a wider range of opportunities.

More generally, I argue in this book that differences among states in how public health policies are made, albeit systematic, are not straightforwardly predictable from their degree of strength or weakness. My research does suggest that national public health policy strategies are remarkably consistent, reflecting each nation's history, social and political institutions, and cultural preferences. For reasons more to do with societal and ideological than with state characteristics, however, the specific policies adopted and whether or how they are implemented vary considerably with the policy issue at hand. Policy strategies premised on a highly centralized state with a monopoly on policy initiative and implementation have worked well in some public health arenas, less well in others. Nor is decentralization synonymous with absent or ineffective public health policies. As Vogel has observed, "instead of seeking to evaluate the relative 'strengths' or 'weaknesses' of particular states, we need to specify those policy areas in which government seems to be capable of asserting its prerogatives vis-à-vis interest groups and those areas in which it is dominated by them" (1986, 268; see also Baldwin 2005b).

Collective Action

Among the most distinctive and enduring features of American society is the perennial mobilization of civil society on behalf of ideologically defined social and political interests and beliefs (for example, Cohen-Tanugi 1987; Clemens 1997). Both today and in the past, this capacity for mobilization is nowhere more evident than in the field of public health. For example, the success of tobacco control policies in the United States is due in large part to the early initiatives of the American Cancer Society in the 1950s and 1960s and of grassroots nonsmokers' rights groups in the 1970s (Nathanson 1999). By contrast, the society's counterparts in Britain and France long remained aloof from the tobacco wars, grassroots groups developed later and their impact has been considerably less. (Although Canadians mobilized against tobacco somewhat later than the United States, the pattern of mobilization there was more akin to that of the United States than of Europe.) Each country's mobilization pattern, though distinctive, is also quite constant across different public health issues.

Collective action on behalf of this or that public health policy appears in many guises, from grassroots social movements to formal organizations. In conceptualizing this variation, I draw primarily on the work of social movement scholars. Among these scholars there is substantial consensus on the categories of variables relevant to the analysis of social movements: political opportunities, mobilizing structures, command of resources, and the construction of supporting ideologies. Let me define briefly each of these constructs. *Political opportunities* are openings exogenous to movement actors themselves that encourage engagement in collective action. "There are two components to such opportunities. One component is openness *within* government to action on a particular set of issues. . . . The second is the prospect for political mobilization *outside* government" (Meyer and Staggenborg 1996, 1633, emphasis added). Further, as Meyer and Staggenborg point out, "political opportunity is not just a fixed external environment that insurgents confront, but also something activists can alter" (1634). The AIDS–drugs nexus, for example, was greeted in some quarters as an opportunity to mobilize against repressive narcotic drugs policies. *Mobilizing structures* are the formal and informal social networks through which individuals with common grievances are brought together.

A classic example of mobilizing structures was turn-of-the-nineteenth century women's clubs in the United States that served as incubators for many
forms of collective action, including against infant mortality (Skocpol 1992;
Clemens 1997). *Resources* critical for social movement emergence and
effectiveness include tangible assets—financing, space, mailing lists—as
well as intangible assets such as organizational experience, social and
political contacts, and, in the case of health-related social movements,
medical expertise (Nathanson 1999). Finally, a major task of social movement entrepreneurs is the *construction of supporting ideologies* or shared
meanings that will inspire people to collective action (Tarrow 1998; Benford
and Snow 2000). Smoking, for example, was redefined from a pleasurable
habit to an assault on the lungs of innocent bystanders.

As Quadagno has recently observed, mobilization of the powerful—
"stakeholder mobilization," in her terminology—"involves the same
processes that social movement theorists usually associate with the
mobilization of politically powerless groups" (2004, 28).

> To be effective in the political arena, stakeholders share with the politically
> powerless a need for leadership, an administrative structure, incentives,
> some mechanisms for garnering resources and marshaling support, a set-
> ting . . . where grassroots activity can be organized. . . . Even though dom-
> inant groups may have privileged and systematic access to politics and to
> elected representatives, they require these same resources to exert political
> influence. (28–29)

Quadagno's perspective is consistent with my own observations of the
policy-making process. The categories developed by social movement
scholars served as guideposts to my collection and analysis of data on the
role of nongovernmental actors—however powerful or powerless—in
advancing or protesting public health policies. The specific form of nongovernmental action—ranging from highly to not at all institutionalized—
is also a variable to be explained. Among the striking facts about collective
action are the degree to which it varies across countries and the degree to
which its forms change and evolve over time.

Ideology: Constructing Risk

Dangers to life and health abound. Whether these dangers will elicit
"community action to avoid disease" depends on relevant actors' perception of a credible and avoidable (or at least controllable) threat. Judgments
of what dangers should be most feared, how to explain them, what to do
about them, and even whether they are in fact public health problems are
the outcome of social processes. In my approach to the analysis of risk
construction, I draw on three theoretical traditions: that of symbolic inter-
actionists who have written about the construction of public problems

(Blumer 1971; Gusfield 1981; Conrad and Schneider 1980); that of the social movement scholars' elaboration of framing processes (Snow et al. 1986; McAdam 1994; Tarrow 1998); and that of Mary Douglas and her colleagues and students, who have studied the impact of political cultures on constructions of risks to the environment (Douglas and Wildavsky 1982; Douglas 1992; Thompson 1983; Wynne 1987).

The first element essential to the construction of a credible risk is the existence of groups or individuals with the authority to define and describe the danger that threatens. Authority in public health is generally presumed to rest with medical and scientific experts. The credibility of medicine and science is, however, highly variable across cultures and political regimes. For example, scientific data on the dangers of cigarette smoking and the health risks of injection drug use as compared with the risks of HIV infection are equally available in all four countries. Neither the French relaxed attitude toward cigarette smoking nor U.S. public officials' rejection of needle-exchange programs to prevent HIV transmission among drug users were due to uneven access to scientific knowledge. They are due to differences in how—and by whom—these issues are initially framed, to the extent of their politicization, and to differences in the cultural authority of experts in addressing public health policy issues.

The second element is the assertion of a causal chain to account for the danger. At the rhetorical extreme, risks are portrayed as hidden, involuntary, and irreversible—as, for example, the risks from fluoridation of public water supplies were portrayed by its opponents when fluoridation was first introduced in the United States (Crain, Katz, and Rosenthal 1969).

The final element is the designation of victims. Risks may be portrayed as universal (we're all at risk) or particular (only they are at risk); victims may be described as innocent or culpable. For example, a major factor in the success of the smoking–tobacco control movement in the United States was the portrayal of nonsmokers as innocent victims (Nathanson 1999).

Although the dimensions along which risks are constructed vary within a limited range, a community's selection of the specific dangers to which it attends and the relative credibility of alternative constructions of danger reflect each community's mode of organization and its valued ideals and institutions. Britain offers a telling example of continuity in both constructions of risk and risk management. Writing about British industrial policy in the nineteenth century, Dobbin observes that it "has been oriented to guarding citizens against harm" (1994, 211). British public health policies that protected the tobacco industry through voluntary agreements between industry and government and that protected injection drug users through state-funded needle-exchange programs were consistent with a policy orientation that privileges the minimization of harm over the political exploitation of risks. Inflammatory rhetoric is decried, conflict among contending parties limited, and policy consensus achieved by gentlemanly negotiation among insiders (see Vogel 1986; Jordan and Richardson 1982). In both the tobacco and the drug arenas, and in other policy-making arenas as well, constructions of risk were less polarized than in the United States, in part because the value attached to consensus makes polarized constructions less effective as counters in the political game.

Contextual Considerations

Of the four countries whose public health policies I consider, only the United States did not by the late twentieth century have some form of universal, state-supported medical care. The different health care systems were associated with differences not only in the scope and activities of public health as an institution but also in the meanings attributed to "public health." For example, in the United States, public health is identified with the poor: "the term *public health* calls up only the picture of a local health department office located downtown filled with poor people" (Beauchamp 1988, 17). In France, by contrast, suspicion is widespread that disease prevention is advocated primarily to protect the public purse (Got 1992). More generally, each country's recognition of and response to new public health threats was conditioned by how it managed routine medical problems.

Further, each country's public health history has been shaped by its most salient social cleavages: in Britain, class; in Canada, language; in the United States, race. In nineteenth-century Britain, public health problems were "understood to be problems of the condition of the working class" (Ramsey 1994, 139); in Britain, far more than in the United States, smoking has been politicized around questions of class (Marsh and McKay 1994). Canadian writing about infant mortality is heavily weighted with concern for differences between English speakers and the historically more deprived French-speaking population. In addition, most of Canada's cigarettes are made in Quebec, so that attacks on the tobacco industry have been portrayed by its supporters as part of ongoing Anglo chauvinism. Social institutions in the United States, particularly institutions for the protection of the socially and economically vulnerable, have been largely shaped by the politics of racial inequality (Quadagno 1994). The consequences of these politics for public health policy responses to the threats of tuberculosis in the early twentieth century and more recently of HIV/AIDS have been profound (for example, McBride 1991; Anderson 1991; Fernando 1993; Cohen 1997; Nathanson 2005).

The boundary-defining role of class, language, or race is played in France by the idea of the citoyen. The literal translation of citoyen is citizen, but the French word has connotations that go far beyond its English meaning. Citizenship in English is a characteristic of the individual; the same word, citoyenneté, in French is a statement about a set of relationships that bind one French citoyen to another (Duchesne 1997). The constellation of ideas that surrounds the French conception of citoyen conditions French response to public health issues in complex ways. French advocates of harm-reduction policies for injection drug users, for example, couch these policies as enabling users to recapture their citoyenneté, that is, as enabling lost sheep to return to the fold. This imagery is absent from the rhetoric of tobacco-control advocates: cigarette smoking in no way compromises citoyenneté. Response to the threats of disease and death, as Rosenberg observes, "lay bare every aspect of the culture in which it occurs" (Rosenberg 1988, 30).

Sources and Methods

The case materials for this project fall into two categories: secondary sources (historical and contemporary research monographs and articles focused on the public health problems at issue as they have been addressed in each of the four countries); and primary sources, including interviews with policy actors, documents (policy, legislative, advocacy, legal) generated in the course of public health action, records of parliamentary-congressional debate on the issues in question, newspaper and other media reports, and electronic listservs for movement participants. Primary source materials are limited to the two contemporary issues; its collection was accomplished in several field trips to each of the three countries outside the United States in addition to field research in the United States.

Secondary Sources

Literature on each of the public health issues I selected was substantial. This depth was of most importance for my narratives of infant mortality and tuberculosis, because primary research on the late nineteenth- and early twentieth-century histories of these issues in each country was well beyond the scope of this project. By limiting the period of primary focus to approximately 1870 to 1915, I was able to include within my purview much if not all of the pertinent work by historians, contributing not only to my command of events in some detail, but also to my ability to cross-check the accounts of different scholars.

Reliance on secondary sources necessarily raises questions about the reliability and validity of both observation and interpretation. This problem is mitigated to some extent when different accounts and interpretations of the same events agree, though even then it is essential to be aware of the selectivity of historical records. For example, nineteenth-century accounts of tuberculosis undoubtedly overrepresent the experience of "interesting" middle-class and literate individuals, and twentieth-century accounts may overrepresent the poor who came to the attention of public clinics, hospitals, and sanatoria. The reliability-validity problem is most serious, however, when accounts disagree, as do scholars' portrayals of the history of tuberculosis at the turn of the last century in France. I am quite sensitive to these disagreements. In addition to acknowledging their existence, I used other strategies to confront them. First, reviews of the work in question by other historians was sometimes helpful in putting disagreements in perspective or suggesting where the weight of evidence lay. Second, I carefully considered the implications of alternative accounts for the story I was telling and for its interpretation: some disagreements were more consequential than others. Although it is important to be constantly aware of the eyes through which historians' accounts are filtered, I believe that these accounts can be valuable sources for the sociologist.

Primary Sources

The sources on which I rely most heavily for my contemporary policy narratives are interviews with participants and observers in each country. I identified key actors initially through contacts at the Centers for Disease Control and Prevention (CDC) in Atlanta, at the Johns Hopkins School of Hygiene and Public Health, at the London School of Hygiene and Tropical Medicine, at Cambridge University, at the Université Pierre Mendès-France in Grenoble, at the University of Toronto, and at McGill University in Montreal. These actors included scholars, health professionals, advocates, and civil servants. I asked each of this first group of informants to identify others with whom I should speak. Consensus was remarkable across the two issues and across countries as to who the key players were, and I was able to interview almost all of these individuals. I completed sixty formal interviews more or less evenly spread across the eight contemporary cases and many more that were informal (for example, I spent two weeks as a participant-observer in the offices of the French Comité nationale contre le tabagisme at Versailles). For the formal interviews, I followed standard sociological practice for open-ended interviews, ensuring that I covered a pre-set list of topics, but with flexibility as to order and with ample allowance for respondents' digression. Almost all interviews in France were conducted in French. The majority of interviews were tape-recorded and professionally transcribed. Where recording was not possible, I made extensive notes and typed up the interview within twenty-four hours.

The purpose of these interviews was to reconstruct, for each country, a detailed account of when, how, by whom, and why a specific public health problem (such as smoking and HIV/AIDS in injection drug users) was or was not identified and was or was not addressed, and, if it was addressed, what form this action took and what accounted for the form that was chosen. Respondents occupied a range of different positions with respect to the events on which they were reporting. From the perspective of my ability to cross-check different accounts this was a major advantage (and, indeed, their accounts agreed substantially). However, it is as important to keep in mind the particular social location from which each of these respondents reports as it is to be aware of historians' filtered accounts.

Interviews were the most important, but only one, and not the most voluminous, of my primary sources. I made extensive use of legislative debates on the issues in question; these are particularly useful in highlighting how issues are framed for public consumption as well as the sources and motives of opposition to public health policy initiatives. Contemporary newspaper and magazine reports and editorial opinions were useful for the same purpose, as well as to keep track of events as they unfolded. Advocacy organizations generate newsletters and other materials; governments generate policy reports; cases brought to court generate legal opinions; participants themselves wrote their own accounts of "what happened." I approached these sources with the same analytic questions and with the same awareness of their potential biases as I brought to the interview data.

Narratives as Data

My data are presented in a series of narratives (or dramas), recounting the time, place, and sequence in which specific public health events unfolded. In adopting this mode of presentation I was guided by a proposition basic to the case-comparative method: "that the time and place in which a structure or process appears make a difference to its character [and] that the sequence in which similar events occur has a substantial impact on their outcome" (Tilly 1984, 79). The narratives are more than stories, however. They have a common structure dictated by the need to ensure that material relevant to each of my three conceptual building blocks—states, collective action, and constructions of risk—was adequately covered. In general—I do not slavishly adhere to an identical outline in each of the sixteen cases—I begin with a more or less chronological account of how a problem emerged and what was done about it. I then describe the cast of characters—who the actors were, how they fit into the larger social and political scene, what accounts they gave of their own and others' actions. The last section of each narrative focuses on attributions of meaning: how a given problem was defined, who was seen as responsible for causing the problem, and who were perceived as its victims. Again, I did not consider this structure a straitjacket. I did not always follow the same order, and some narratives contain more interpretive material or cross-national or within country comparisons than others. Overall, however, I have tried to make the narratives sufficiently complete and sufficiently factual so that readers can arrive at their own interpretations of the data, not necessarily the same as mine.

Finally, the narratives are ordered by public health problem rather than by country primarily to facilitate brief introductions to each problem's history and epidemiology. Should the reader prefer, the narratives may be read by country without doing substantial violence to the text. Because one goal of this work was to highlight other countries' differences from—and similarities to—the United States, each set of narratives begins with the American case, followed by France because it tended to offer the sharpest contrasts with the United States.

Plan of the Book

This is a book about history written by a sociologist. The plan of the book reflects the sociologist's impulse to separate data from interpretation. The book is divided into three parts. The first, this chapter and the next, is intended as introduction and orientation. The next chapter sets the stage, both historically and analytically, for the material that follows. In it, I portray the nineteenth-century settings in which public health as a self-conscious activity was born. Parts II and III of the book, chapters 3 to 6, present my data in the form of narratives. The stories of tuberculosis and infant mortality are told in chapters 3 and 4 and those of smoking and HIV/AIDS in injection drug users in chapters 5 and 6. In part IV, I analyze and interpret the narrative materials. The order of presentation is dictated by the conceptual framework introduced. Chapter 7 examines the roles of the state and civil society in bringing about, or blocking, public health action. It addresses the central question of why these four countries, similar in so many respects, differed in their recognition of and response to the same public health problems. Chapter 8 focuses more narrowly on cross-national variation in forms of collective action—the relative importance of "experts and zealots"—and on interaction effects (in the statistical sense) between actors, countries, and strategies. In chapter 9, I consider how differences in countries' political cultures and in qualities specific to the disease or condition (what was its history, whose interests did it affect, who were its victims) influenced each problem's construction and framing. In the final chapter I summarize and reflect on what I have learned.

Chapter 2

The Nineteenth Century:
From Miasmas to Microbes

P UBLIC HEALTH as an enterprise distinct from curative medicine is a product of the nineteenth century, as are—not coincidentally— nation-states and social movements as we know them today. Through complex and mutually reinforcing processes, industrial and geographic expansion created increased and novel demands on governments, greatly enlarging the reach and capacity first of European and much later of North American states, and offered new opportunities and targets for citizen organization and protest. Confronted with the palpable costs of urbanization—masses huddled together in conditions of appalling brutality—and persuaded not only of the relation between misery and disease but also of the threat this relation posed to public order and the public purse, state and (elite) citizenry became interested in public health. Public health was nonetheless controversial. The principal axes of controversy—the limits of intervention by the state in private property and private affairs, the extent to which individuals bring their misery on themselves, where to draw the line between those who are deserving and undeserving of private or state care—have changed very little between the nineteenth century and the twenty-first. My story begins with a brief account of the social and economic context within which public health was first identified as a significant public problem.

Revolution, War, and Social Change

In the United States, France, Britain, and Canada, the broad parameters of change were much the same: urbanization and industrialization; the large-scale movement of populations from country to town and, in North America, from overseas and across the continent; wars, civil or colonial; and the fear of revolution if not its reality. The pace of change was nonetheless quite different across the four countries, and each country's

25

experience of and response to these changes were shaped by unique historical circumstances.

Industrialization was relatively slow in Britain and even slower in France, the two countries with the earliest start. It was comparatively rapid in the United States, however, and very rapid in Canada, the country that started last. Whereas the process occupied Britain and France during most of the nineteenth century, the United States was transformed from an agricultural to an urban-industrial society in the five decades that followed the end of the Civil War and Reconstruction. The same process was completed in Canada in less than half the time. Industrialization was accompanied by population growth, notably in the United States: by 1900 the U.S. population had grown from the smallest of the (three recorded) populations at the beginning of the century to one and a half times that of Britain or France. The French population, at the other extreme, increased in the same period by less than half.

Of perhaps even greater impact than industrialization or population growth on turn-of-the-century society, politics, and—in particular—the politics of public health, was urbanization, a process that took place under different circumstances and assumed quite different forms in each of the four countries. Presenting "a dramatic contrast with the past and with any other economy" (Matthew 1984, 520), Britain by the middle of the nineteenth century had more people living in towns than in the country. Rapid urban growth far outpaced the availability of housing, and the results were, by all accounts, extremes of overcrowding in conditions of Dickensian squalor (Flinn 1965; Rosen 1993). Urbanization proceeded more slowly in France. Throughout the nineteenth and well into the twentieth century it retained "one of the largest rural populations among the industrialized states" (Stone 1985, 12). The human toll of urbanization and its impact on contemporary observers—largely concentrated in Paris—was nevertheless much the same: "Public health in the early nineteenth century was largely a matter of the sanitary state of [urban] working class dwellings" (Flinn 1965, 3).

The urban populations of Britain and France came from their respective countrysides. In sharp contrast, the urban populations of the United States and Canada were drawn primarily from overseas. Between 1890 and 1910, close to 13 million immigrants entered the United States, amounting to 21 percent of its population in 1890. Canada during the same period received approximately 2 million immigrants, a much smaller number but fully 43 percent of its 1890 population. The bulk of these immigrants settled in cities. By 1900, "60 percent of those who lived in [America's] twelve largest cities were first- or second-generation immigrants, 40 percent came from the nation's smaller towns and the countryside" (Hays 1995, 59).

Economic growth is inherently disruptive, Simon Szreter argues, and the most important dimension of disruption in its potential to influence health outcomes is political: "the scale and nature of political disruption . . .

critically determines the capacity of the society, the state, its citizens, and its various associations and administrative units to manage the disruptions of economic change without incurring [deprivation, disease, and death]" (1997, 697). Although economic, demographic, and urban growth was everywhere accompanied by social and political change, the accompanying disruption varied substantially across each of these four countries.

With perhaps some exaggeration, Britain between the 1850s and the 1890s has been described as "a society of remarkable order and balance, given the extraordinary underlying tensions of industrial and social change" (Matthew 1984, 549). The second half of the Victorian era was characterized by stable and legitimate government, an economic and political ideology of laissez-faire liberalism (belied by remarkable activism in the domain of public health) together with growing economic prosperity, gradual extension of the franchise through a series of reform bills, and—contrary to widespread fears generated by the French Revolution— no revolutionary working class.

The situation in France was very different. Over the course of the nineteenth century, France experienced four governments, oscillating between constitutional monarchy and republic. Fear of revolution was fed by the periodic mass protests of workers in Paris and Lyon, brutally suppressed by armed force. In this context, "the political history of nineteenth-century France can . . . be seen as a continuous search for stability. Eventually this was to be secured only from the 1870s, through the establishment of a strong centralized state, the Third Republic" (Price 1991, 157). In the Third Republic "all those who owned property" came together with the goals of safeguarding what they owned and ending "worker militancy and the dangerous talk of revolution" (Stone 1985, 17).

The United States in the decades around the turn of the century— immediately before and during the Progressive era—has been viewed through many lenses, emphasizing different dimensions of "the response to industrialism" (Hays 1995). Classic accounts such as Richard Hofstadter's *The Age of Reform* (1955) and Robert Wiebe's *The Search for Order* (1967) describe the response of traditional American (Protestant, Yankee) elites displaced on the one hand by urban, big-city political bosses who catered to the new immigrant voters and on the other by newly rich captains of industry. In her book, *The People's Lobby*, Elizabeth Clemens places greater emphasis on the remarkable upsurge of "popular associations" (of industrial workers, farmers, women) organized to advance their particular interests through political means outside of traditional political parties (1997). Common to these various accounts are portrayals of intense dissatisfaction with American society as it was at the time, of a widely diffused impulse—embodied in the incredible range of reform movements—to act on this dissatisfaction, and of a newfound willingness to call on the state for intervention and redress. Among the consequences was an increase in state capacity in the form of a newly created civil service and new federal agencies. Among the things that did not happen in the United States during this period—in contrast to the two European countries—was the emergence of a sustainable working-class political movement. Fears of social conflict and social revolution were not absent from the American response to industrialization—indeed, strikes were often brutally suppressed and federal troops were sent to protect strikebreakers—but these fears were absorbed in and diffused through crusades for social and moral reform.

Canada in the late nineteenth century was a new nation, brought into being by the British North America Act of 1867, and driven by overwhelming pressures—articulated by economic and political elites of all political persuasions—for economic development (McCormack 1977; Avery 1979; McNaught 1982; Penner 1992). These pressures—for coast-to-coast railroad construction, for industrialization protected by high tariffs, for immigration of an "industrial proletariat" to build the railroads, work in the factories, and people the land—were markedly intensified by Canada's proximity to the United States. To survive as a " 'non-American' part of North America," Kenneth McNaught argues, "the Canadas were forced into an intense phase of growth-investment" (1982, 113). Economic growth was unprecedented, its social consequences largely ignored.

An important and highly relevant difference in these four countries was in their late nineteenth-century experience of military conflict. Both France and Britain became embroiled in more or less humiliating and unsuccessful wars, leading to criticism and self-doubt among these countries' social and political elites. France's defeat in the 1870 Franco-Prussian War was instrumental in the overthrow of the Second Empire and the inauguration of the Third Republic. Britain's conflict with the Boers began with a serious defeat in 1895, was renewed in 1899, dragged on far beyond its expected conclusion, and ended with an unsatisfactory peace. The United States, on the other hand, had emerged from the Civil War and, in its first foray into overseas expansion, annexed Hawaii and captured Cuba and the Philippines (all in 1898), proceeding to include these territories within the purview of American zeal for social and political reform. Canada avoided military entanglements altogether. For better or worse, military defeat led British and French elites to an intense concern with the health of their respective populations.

Sanitary Ideas

Disease before the late nineteenth century was a tabula rasa inscribed by physicians, politicians, and other interested actors with explanatory accounts that best accorded with their particular social and political preferences and beliefs. For example, on August 19, 1793, yellow fever returned to Philadelphia for the first time since 1762. Within a month, the disease had become highly politicized. Factions crystallized around alternative causal theories; and not only doctors but also national as well as local politicians (Philadelphia was then the national capital) took sides in the debate (Pernick 1972). The themes around which argument raged would be familiar to observers in Europe and North America for the next hundred years: the disease was local in origin, caused by bad air (miasmas); it was an imported foreign scourge; it was God's punishment for individual or communal sins. The political, social, and economic implications of these positions were considerable. Importationists advocated the quarantine of French ships, which was anathema both to local merchants and to sympathizers with the French Revolution. Proponents of the local miasma theory—the poisonous air of Philadelphia's swamps and unsanitary docks—were accused of conspiring to discredit commercial cities and of lacking patriotism: "Importationists made much of the widely held feeling that independent America was the New Eden," free of the disease and death that plagued old Europe (Pernick 1972, 570). Preachers and the pious among their flocks called attention to French immorality, the pride and vanity of community leaders, and the opening of a new theater as likely causes. The public demanded action to prevent future yellow fever epidemics, but in this fraught environment no single course of action was possible. In the end a compromise—more political than medical— was reached, and Philadelphia as well as other threatened places "undertook *both* quarantine and sanitary reform projects" (570).

Yellow fever was a terrifying disease. It "appeared mysteriously, killed young and old indiscriminately, and disrupted community activities for months at a time" (Duffy, 1990, 38). And, like the other infectious diseases that devastated Europe and North America continuously (tuberculosis) or periodically (smallpox, cholera, typhoid) in the nineteenth century, neither its causes nor its methods of transmission were understood. The latter point is critical. "At a time when diseases could not be attributed to any one specific cause, anything could be potentially hazardous to health" (La Berge 1992, 11). On this essentially empty canvas, as empty in France, Britain, and Canada as it was in the United States, each country's medical, social, and political elites painted their particular pictures of health and disease.[1] These pictures—and their consequences for public policy—reflected, with perhaps more than usual clarity, each country's social and political structure, along with the ideologies of its elites.

New Edens: The United States and Canada

In the eyes of their nineteenth-century inhabitants, the United States and Canada—new countries with seemingly unlimited frontiers—were intrinsically healthy, particularly compared with "decadent Europe."

Contrasting the approaches to the politics of health taken by the United States and France, Roy Porter cites Thomas Jefferson's belief that the New World would be free of the health problems of the Old: "life, liberty, and the pursuit of happiness would foster a healthy nation" (1997, 405). Carrying this perspective to its extreme, a proponent of the foreign origins of disease asserted that to suggest otherwise was " 'treason,' perhaps hoping that the Alien and Sedition acts gave the Federalists the power to deport foreign diseases along with foreign agitators" (Pernick 1972, 570). For much of the nineteenth century, the intrinsic health and virtue of these countries' imagined communities argued against any assertion of collective responsibility for public health.

Writing shortly after Canadian confederation in 1867, Canadians pointed to their bracing northern climate both as the basis of common identity and as a source of mental and physical strength: "The very atmosphere of her northern latitude, the breath of life that rose from lake and forest, prairie and mountain, was fast developing a race of men with bodies enduring as iron and minds as highly tempered as steel" (cited in Berger 1986, 217). Conviction of national hardiness was associated with other characteristics the two countries had in common: first, a response to public health problems limited to times of crisis and, second, a reluctance either to spend public funds or to interfere with private property interests for the sake of the public's health. In the United States, "the endemic disorders responsible for the high morbidity and mortality rates were all too familiar, and without the stimulus provided by a strange and highly fatal pestilence, the average citizen had little interest in—and even less inclination to spend money for—public health" (Duffy 1990, 79). Similarly, in Canada, "the tendency to avoid doing something explicit about health was only broken by a spectacular indication of the need for action—epidemics." Preoccupied with economic development, Canadian elites "did not think in terms of collective social welfare. . . . In general there was a reluctance to raise taxation, so local governments were troubled by a shortage of money" (Cassel 1994, 280).

A salient difference between the United States and Canada (and, indeed, between the United States and both France and Great Britain) was the association in America of health with virtue, of disease with sin, and of sin with poverty and foreign extraction. Depicting America's response to the cholera outbreak of 1849, Charles Rosenberg remarks that "the connection between cholera and vice had become almost a verbal reflex. The relationship between vice and poverty was a mental reflex even more firmly established" (1987, 120). The New York Medical Society's analysis of the 1832 cholera epidemic in that city was predicated on these assumptions:

> Expressing the accepted belief that poverty and disease arose from vice, intemperance, and laziness, the Special Medical Council (of the Society)

proclaimed that "the disease in the city is confined to the imprudent, the intemperate, and to those who injure themselves with improper medicines." Acting on this assumption, the board of health promptly began a campaign to raise the moral standards and personal hygiene of the poorer classes. (Duffy 1990, 81)

Disease, from this perspective, was a form of retribution for man's violation of God's or (depending on one's theological leanings) nature's laws. The moral, the pious, and the hardworking were spared. The appearance of cholera among "respectable" members of society was attributed to "hidden vice or unaccustomed imprudence," the outward sign of inward sin (Rosenberg 1987, 135). It was not until the late nineteenth century that industrialization and—more important because more visible—the exponential growth of cities forced American elites to recognize that "poverty and disease could no longer be treated simply as individual failings; they were becoming social and political problems of massive proportions" (Fee 1994, 232).

Dangerous Precincts: Britain and France

By the middle of the nineteenth century, Great Britain's transformation to an urban industrialized country was well under way, considerably in advance of the parallel transformation in France, as I have indicated. Nevertheless, it was in France that hygiène publique—public health— made its debut as a scientific endeavor and, even earlier, as a responsibility of the state. The authors of the French Revolution had intended that "the new state would inaugurate the reign of virtue, to which health and hygiene were integral" and proposed a comprehensive system that encompassed health surveillance, epidemic monitoring, and vaccination as well as medical services for "citizen-patients" (Porter 1997, 405–6). "Such hopes," Porter observes, "were scuppered by war and the Terror" (405–6), but hygiènisme was revived in the late 1820s, less as an activity than as a science, organized around the first public health journal, *Annales d'hygiène publique et médecine légale.*

France's intellectual precedence aside, there can be no question that the health and sanitary consequences of urbanization confronted urban elites earlier and with greater intensity in France and Britain than in Canada and the United States. Neither European country had the safety valve, symbolic as well as real, of open frontiers. There was essentially nowhere to run from the sights, sounds, and smells of the big city, and it was in the big cities Paris and London that most early public health reformers lived, and so it was that in those two cities the formal study and practice of public health began. The primary focus of experts in both countries, though not always of their governments, was on dangers inherent in the physical and social environment. Included among those dangers were not only disease but also social revolution: the fear that workers would be goaded to rebellion by intolerable living conditions. Working-class riots in the 1830s lent reality to these fears. "By the 1830s and 1840s [in both England and France] the 'laboring and dangerous classes' were considered both a foyer of infection and the seat of insurrection and revolution" (La Berge, 1992, 40–41); and in both countries a large part of the public health mission was seen as the preservation or restoration of social and political order.[2]

There is a striking contrast between the faith of New World inhabitants in the inherent salubrity of their open spaces and the repeated references of early British observers to the problems generated by confined space:

> Disease [said physician John Heysham] "is the offspring of filth, nastiness, and confined air, in rooms crowded with many inhabitants. . . . I think we may without much hesitation pronounce that the occasional cause of it is *human effluvia,* which has been generated in some little dirty confined place, of which there are great numbers in Carlisle [the subject of Heysham's study] and every other large manufacturing town." (cited in Flinn 1965, 25, emphasis in original)

Christopher Hamlin suggests that the late eighteenth-century metaphor of the prison as a confined space in which physical and moral influences were transmitted through the air by a process of contagion (for example, from the master criminal to the innocent youth) was transferred in the early nineteenth century to the urban slum: "Both slum and prison were confined communities; in either the incidence of disease both signaled the social malignancy that was its cause and exacerbated that malignancy as well" (1994, 137).

Because "the pure was corrupted by contact with impurity," the solution advocated by British sanitarians—among whom were counted such major figures in the history of public health as Edwin Chadwick, William Farr, and John Simon—was removal of impurities, namely, "filth." The "natural" purity enjoyed by Canada and the United States would in England, argued Farr, be achieved by state action: "Some of the sunshine, pure water, fresh air, and health of the country, may be given to the grateful inhabitants of towns by the . . . voice of the Legislature" (cited in Flinn 1965, 29). Problems of public health in Victorian England were, as in the other three countries, "understood to be problems of the condition of the working class" (Hamlin 1994, 139). But nowhere else were there higher expectations for the beneficent effects of urban infrastructure—water and sewers: "drive out dirt and you drive out drunkenness, depravity, and despair" (Hamlin 1994, 146). Prevention not only of disease but also of social and moral degradation and even revolution was reduced to questions of high-pressure water supplies and egg-shaped sewer lines.

Overlap between British and French constructions of disease causation was substantial, and experts in each country were aware of the others' work. However, the causal model adopted by leading French hygienists of the early nineteenth century went far beyond hydraulics. The founding editors of the *Annales d'hygiène publique* announced a "programme sociologique, that included within its compass not just the physical, but the social, moral, and economic dimensions of society" (Lecuyer 1986, 100). Based on a remarkable series of empirical investigations, these hygienists concluded that "the variable . . . most closely correlated with incidence of disease and premature death was poverty—a salary inadequate to supply basic needs" (La Berge 1992, 96). Despite the sophistication of this social analysis, few concrete public health measures were taken. Threats to public health were overwhelmed by ideologically more resonant threats to private property. The context within which French public health developed was one of profound ideological conflict surrounding the role of the state in public health management and reform. This conflict was clearly reflected in the views of hygienists themselves who, though radical in recognizing poverty's role in disease, were highly conservative in rejecting state intervention to accomplish large-scale social reform. They relied instead on "the progress of civilization" and the "moralization" of the urban poor to enable them to adopt healthful middle-class habits (La Berge 1992). Even modest efforts in the form of city clean-up campaigns—assainissement—came into direct conflict with ideologies of individual liberty and private property that were extremely powerful in nineteenth-century France: "For many in the ruling classes the right of all to public health was secondary to the rights of a few to liberty and property" (La Berge 1992, 124). This conflict was one of several factors that contributed to France's failure to create a public health system in the nineteenth century comparable to that of Great Britain.

The British were far from immune to conflicts between private property and public health. Szreter argues that municipal improvements were stymied from the mid-1830s through the late 1860s by the emergence "in most towns" of "the petty capitalist class, with their ratepayers' associations and obsessive concerns for economy" who "could not be induced to vote for, still less campaign for, the expensive municipal measures that might have saved their own lives" (1997, 705). This logjam was broken in the second half of the nineteenth century in part by necessity—"the need for the town to survive the health hazards associated with rapid urban development" (Wohl 1983, 175)—but also by "a new civic ethos, a desire for municipal improvement, a competitive spirit with other towns, a growing shame at high death rates or insanitary conditions, an increasing embarrassment at exposures and (literally) muck-raking revelations, and lastly, a growing sense of pride and accomplishment when improvements were effected" (175). What Szreter describes as a "social movement in the town halls of Britain's new industrial cities" (1997, 709) was led and inspired by urban churches and their charismatic ministers.[3] Public health in Great Britain became infused with evangelical zeal:

> with "public health" came legacies of eighteenth century philanthropy as well as more recent evangelism. Thus, to represent improvement [of drains, sewage, streets] as "sanitary improvement" was to infuse it with righteousness . . . a contribution to the physical, mental and moral health of civilization and a sign manifest of the heroism of its builders. To be involved in such a crusade was holy, to oppose it sin. (Hamlin 1994, 145)

Toward the end of the nineteenth century, some semblance of comparable public health reform movements appeared in the United States and France. In neither country, however, did these movements reach the level not only of enthusiasm but of enthusiasm tied to good works apparent in Great Britain where "evangelical justification by conduct, as well as by faith, took on a pragmatism that 'emphasized effectiveness in contrast to good intentions' " (R. Morris, cited in Wohl 1983, 175).

Sanitary Practices

Early Risers: Britain and France

There is a stark contrast between the fainéante quality of nineteenth-century public health practice in France—"most hygienists . . . believed that after they had investigated a public health problem and identified its causes, their work was over" (La Berge 1992, 3)—and the conviction of their British counterparts that investigation was only the beginning. "The end, to which [investigation] was a principal, but certainly not the only means, was a substantial measure of public health legislation" (Flinn 1965, 54). Progress was halting and piecemeal (see, for example, Laxton 2000; Kearns 2000), but by the last quarter of the nineteenth century this purpose had in remarkable measure been achieved. Great Britain had created a public health system that balanced centralized supervisory controls with local implementation and a high degree of deference to local circumstances and constraints.[4] Central to this system was the local medical officer of health.

> The establishment of local sanitary departments, spearheaded by medical officers of health [MOHs], marks the beginning of serious preventive medicine in England. Medical officers of health had been appointed by various local authorities, notably Liverpool and the City of London, since 1847, but it was not until 1856 that they existed in sufficient numbers to form a regular sanitary organization. Under the Metropolis Local Management Act 1855, London's new civil vestries were each required to appoint a medical officer.

In 1856 forty-eight officers took up appointments in the city, forming a unique specialist body with responsibility for, and interest in, infectious disease. (Hardy 1993, 4)

Sixteen years later, under the Public Health Act of 1872, appointment of medical officers of health became compulsory throughout the country, and half of their salaries were—in principle at least—met by the Local Government Board.[5] The act created over a thousand new posts, "extending preventive authority throughout the country" (Hardy 1993, 4). Although the activity and effectiveness of the Local Government Board diminished in the late nineteenth and early twentieth centuries, "a mass of newly hatched public health professionals, the most visible of whom were local medical officers of health, was finding much to do in individual communities" (Hamlin 1994, 151).[6]

Despite the pioneering role of French hygiènistes in laying the intellectual groundwork for public health, no public health system comparable to that of Great Britain emerged in France: "hygienic expertise, one of the great social acquisitions of the pre-1848 era" had surprisingly little impact on public policy (Coleman 1982, 283). Arguably the critical difference was Chadwick's politically astute representation of the health condition of the urban poor as a manageable engineering problem—one of "places and structures—pipes, streets, houses" (Hamlin, 144)—rather than one of poverty, a problem that neither conservative hygiènistes nor the French government was prepared to address.[7]

The primary concern of French governments in the early nineteenth century was to prevent the importation of disease—"foreign scourges" from outside the borders of France (Ramsey 1994, 61)—and the hygiènistes themselves were at best ambivalent about the role of the state in public health, as I have observed. French public health was reenergized in the late nineteenth century, due in large part to the extraordinary impact of Pasteur on French medicine and science (70). Nevertheless, apart from the campaign against infant mortality, which had relatively little to do with Pasteur, the consequences on the ground were minimal. This failure is all the more astonishing given the magnitude of the opportunity presented. The hygiènistes of the late nineteenth century were among the most prominent and politically well-connected physicians of the day. Further, under the Third Republic, "political concerns and social ideology were [for the first time], favorable to legislation [to create a public health system] which would intervene into areas formerly left to the family and local society. In addition, hygienists possessed a scientific theory which could be experimentally validated and which offered specific solutions to disease" (Hildreth 1987, 107). No legislation resulted, however. It was not until 1902 that a much watered-down version of the hygienists' original proposals became law.

French public health reformers active in the late nineteenth century were perfectly aware of France's position as a public health laggard relative to

Great Britain. Henri Monod, the director of assistance and public health within the Ministry of the Interior—the "primary engine of [public health] reform at the national level"—"liked to call attention to the disparity between the English service, with its large central administration and network of health officers, and his own tiny staff" (Ramsey 1994, 74). France's laggard position is counterintuitive in two respects.

First, it is strikingly inconsistent with the picture of the nineteenth-century French state painted in other contexts. Railway policy, for example, was characterized by "state concertation of private activity" in the service of collective goals (Dobbin 1994, 96). The libertarian concerns that agitated nineteenth-century hygiènistes were absent when it came to railways. Comparing British and French approaches, Dobbin observes that "[the British] parliament was particularly concerned to avoid using public powers to expropriate private lands, and thereby abridge property rights" whereas "French bureaucrats were not similarly concerned with protecting landowners against undue state expropriation" (115). Ramsey describes this paradox succinctly: "In France, whose name is virtually synonymous with centralization and the strong state, the central government long played a surprisingly limited role in public health. Far from subordinating the individual relentlessly to the public interest [as it did in the case of railway policy], France was one of the countries in which classic liberalism [in the realm of public health] was most pervasive and persisted the longest" (Ramsey 1994, 45).

Second is an apparent role reversal between Britain and France. In nineteenth-century Britain, "property rights" and aversion to state intervention in local affairs might have been expected to preclude a state role in public health that was considerably stronger than the role of the state in France. Further, in policy arenas where its interests were clearly involved, such as railway construction, France was more likely than Britain to engage in centrally orchestrated state action. Neither an ideological commitment to classic liberalism, which the countries shared, nor differences in political structure are adequate to explain the strong aversion of French authorities to state intervention in public health as compared with Great Britain. To understand this aversion, we must look elsewhere—at doctors and the politics of medicine and public health.

In Britain and France, physicians throughout the nineteenth century enjoyed a level of professional status and access to centers of political power that far exceeded their counterparts in the United States and Canada. In both European countries, medically trained hygienists and sanitary reformers made major contributions to understanding relations between the social and economic environment and social inequalities in patterns of disease, and elite physicians played significant roles as consultants to the government and as members of medical and scientific advisory bodies. Yet only in Britain was the expert power of these professional elites successfully translated into effective political action on behalf of public health. Although ideological differences may have played some role (British sanitary reformers were far more willing than their French counterparts to invoke the power of the state), the more important distinction between the two countries was the sharp social cleavage in France between medicine and public health.

Since the early nineteenth century, the French medical elite has consisted of hospital physicians and professors of medicine attached to universities (Pinell and Steffen 1994). These state-supported institutions were "foreign to the majority of practitioners," local doctors working out of their private offices with little or no institutional protection or support (46). By the late nineteenth century, the growth in both the number and power of health insurance societies (*mutualités*) and the expansion of the state's role in support of medical assistance to the poor had markedly changed local doctors' conditions of practice. Faced with the need to bargain with these entities over fees and other conditions and resentful of "the aristocrats of the profession [who were] indifferent to the issues of insurance societies, medical assistance, and conflicts over fees",[8] local practitioners resolved to protect their social and economic interests by forming medical *syndicats*, or unions. Public health measures supported by "the aristocrats of the profession" were strongly opposed by the *syndicats*. French medical practitioners "were quite willing to call themselves hygienists, basking in the reflected glory of Pasteur and other great scientists of the age, but they were not willing to countenance any public health reform which involved the intervention of the state into the private practice of medicine" (Hildreth 1987, 146).

In sharp contrast to the situation in France, British practitioners (as reflected in the statements and actions of their representatives and in the pages of the *BMJ* and *The Lancet*) not only supported legislation consolidating and expanding the authority of public health but also were influential in bringing that legislation about. As a telling example, the appointment in 1869 of the Royal Sanitary Commission, "whose recommendations had a profound affect [sic] on sanitary legislation of the next decade [the acts of 1871, 1872, and 1875 creating and consolidating the powers of the Local Government Board], was directly attributable to medical men," most immediately to "members of the medical profession outside Whitehall [that is, outside the government]" (Brand 1965, 8, 10). The *BMJ* and *The Lancet* routinely published not only scientific papers from medical officers of health but also annual reports of their public health activities. Although there were areas of disagreement, nothing compared with French practitioners' open hostility to public health.[9] Writing about Britain in the early twentieth century, Daniel Fox observes that "debates about [health] policy . . . occurred among people who, despite frequent disagreements, had a great deal in common" (1986, 3). I would speculate that leaders of these two branches of the larger medical profession (medicine and public health) were drawn from the same stratum of British society, went to the same schools and universities, and were part of overlapping "old boy" networks. Their predilection would have been, then as now, toward the achievement of policy consensus behind closed doors, not in open confrontation (Wynne 1987, 421; Godt 1987, 474).

Not so in France. Ordinary private practitioners "distrusted the medical elites who dominated the public health movement" (Ramsey 1994, 76), and *syndicat* leaders (as demonstrated by remarks of the Rhône physician cited earlier) had no hesitation in giving voice to their members' antagonism, often in harsh terms. The gap between elites who "enjoyed high prestige and wealth from their academic and bureaucratic positions and were able to attract a profitable clientele from among the haute-bourgeoisie" (Hildreth 1987, 5) and doctors in the provinces and poor urban *quartiers* was substantial and long-standing. "The average doctor occupied a humble place among the French bourgeoisie through most of the nineteenth century. . . . [D]octors struggled economically, rarely enjoyed the medical confidence of their local society, and competed with a wide range of traditional healers and practitioners" (3). They openly envied and sought to emulate the benefits enjoyed by the academic and hospital elites. They were powerfully opposed to the appointment of doctors (*fonctionnaires*) salaried by the state (comparable, for example, to the British medical officers of health). In the formation of *syndicats*, they saw their opportunity both to gain some of the benefits they sought and to stave off the threat of becoming no better than civil servants. These concerns found little sympathy, or even recognition, among the alliance of elite physicians promoting the cause of state responsibility for public health.

The *syndicats* were powerful: "in medical legislation in [the late nineteenth century], the support or opposition of doctors in the union movement was critical" (Hildreth 1987, 147). Moreover, they were able to take advantage of physicians' remarkably high level of insertion into local and national politics. "Doctors were present on almost every municipal council in the nation, and served as mayors of hundreds of villages, towns, and cities. . . . This visibility of doctors in the political assemblies of France had few counterparts in other societies" (Ellis 1990, 3,5) and, along with the *syndicats,* was critical to the demise of any possibility for a centralized public health bureaucracy in France comparable to what had existed in England since the mid-1870s.

Among the most consistent observations about French political structure is the weakness of interest groups outside the state. Railways were able to go forward, expropriating property with little more than a by-your-leave, not only because an efficient transport system was seen to be of vital interest to the French state (whereas public health, with the single exception of infant mortality, was not) but also because there was no organized opposition. In this context, the *syndicats* represent an anomaly. This anomaly was a major contributor to the early weakness of French public health, both in relation to the state's activity in other arenas and in comparison with Great Britain.

Latecomers: United States and Canada

The emergence of "community action to avoid disease" (Duffy 1990, 1) in nineteenth-century America differed sharply from the European pattern. First, almost without exception, action was triggered by epidemic crises: the threat of cholera, yellow fever, plague, or smallpox. Second, action was not only local but was limited for much of the century to the port cities of the northeast and middle Atlantic (and later New Orleans) where the epidemic threat was greatest. Third, though physicians played a role—they were among the earliest sanitary reformers—they did not dominate the reform movement as they did in Britain and France. Finally, Americans' embrace of environmental reform as the key to public health was relatively short-lived, beginning around 1880 and extending to the end of the century, when it was rapidly displaced by a new laboratory-driven public health focused on individual-level prevention of specific diseases (Duffy 1990; Fee 1994; Fee and Porter 1991; Rosenberg 1987).

Given local officials' belief that disease was an aberration, the result of personal moral failings or of epidemics and plagues external to the country itself, and given the penury they shared with city fathers everywhere, only the presence or rumor of an epidemic threat to large sections of a city's population was sufficient to galvanize preventive action. And action, when it occurred, was temporary, the impetus expiring with the threat. City boards of health were created and then disbanded as soon as the epidemic disappeared. The National Board of Health, for example, formed in 1879 in response to a widespread yellow fever epidemic originating in New Orleans, lasted only four years, the victim of battles over states' rights, internal squabbling, and congressional disinterest in health, as well as the end of the epidemic. The boards that did exist—almost wholly subject to the vicissitudes of local politics—had little independent power. John Duffy cited the case of the mid-nineteenth century physician reformer John Griscom, the only result of whose Chadwick-inspired report on the *Sanitary Condition of the Laboring Population of New York* was to be fired from his position as city inspector (1990, 96).[10]

Nineteenth-century America has been described as a nation of "island communities" (Wiebe 1967), politically and economically self-sufficient, dependent on the federal government for little more than mail delivery. Public health was construed as a local responsibility. Big cities initiated measures for disease prevention—which expanded over time from street-cleaning and the control of domestic animals to include the staples of nineteenth-century public health, clean water and sewers—less because their public health problems were most severe (as they were) but in response to fear, first of epidemic disease and later of a discontented and restless working class. It may have been the threat of Asiatic cholera that persuaded city politicians to create the New York Metropolitan Board of Health—"the first effective municipal health department in a major city" (Duffy 1990, 120)—in 1866, but Duffy suggested that it was the hundreds of people killed in the Draft Riot of 1863 that convinced civic leaders of the need for social reform.

Among the most significant differences between the nineteenth-century evolution of public health in Europe and in the United States was the role of physicians in the former as compared with the latter.

> Until the early years of the twentieth century, United States public health reform had been directed largely by lay, non-professional personnel, a mixture of lawyers, philanthropists, and some concerned doctors. In Europe, the medical profession dominated events, and started to do so from a much earlier date. Virchow in Germany and Villermé in France were leading scientists and qualified physicians. In Britain, the engineering and legalistic orthodoxies of the sanitary movement declined [in mid-century]. . . . The "sanitary idea" was replaced by the rise of state medicine [exemplified by John Simon and the medical officers of health] during the mid-Victorian period. (Fee and Porter 1991, 28)

The concerned doctors to whom Fee and Porter refer were—much as in France—among the professional elite—wealthy, well educated, and well connected, with established private practices. The enthusiasm for public health of leading physicians in the latter part of the nineteenth century was reflected in—among other things—the fact that the first presidents of the American Public Health Association (founded in 1872) were also active members of the American Medical Association. This enthusiasm was not shared by struggling local doctors, who were at this period not so much hostile to public health as uninterested, regarding it as the province of women and social reformers and of little relevance to their everyday concerns.

Nineteenth-century Americans were heavily involved in social reform movements—abolition, temperance, antiprostitution. Not until late in the century, however, far later than in Britain and France, did they develop a sustained interest in public health. Yet, as Duffy argued, "most of the social evils that horrified British reformers were present in major American cities [before the Civil War]" (1990, 66). Some explanation is required. Among several hypotheses, the most intriguing points to differences in the meaning and place of religion—in particular, of the evangelical movements both Britain and the United States experienced in the nineteenth century.[11] "For the Victorians, public health, like so many other social reforms and endeavours, took on the form of a moral crusade. To most Victorians, epidemics were not scourges sent by God to punish man for his sins but were the consequences of man's sinful neglect of God's earth and of His injunction to care for the sick and the weak" (Wohl 1983, 6). Many Americans of this period believed—and were encouraged by their pastors to believe—that epidemics *were* "scourges sent by God to punish man for his sins" and were urged to seek salvation in personal confession and repentance, not in practical good works (Young 2002). Certainly, there was no religiously inspired "[public health] social movement in the town halls" of the United States comparable to what took place in Britain (Szreter 1997, 709), nor were religious leaders in the forefront of the sanitary movement.[12]

The advent of bacteriology at the end of the century transformed public health more rapidly and decisively in America than in Britain and France and brought American public health into direct conflict with practicing physicians.

> Bacteriology introduced the principle of specificity into understanding disease processes, and it also presented a powerful new way of differentiating scientific experts from mere social reformers. . . . Bacteriology thus became an ideological marker, sharply differentiating the "old" public health, mainly the province of untrained amateurs, from the "new" public health, which belonged to scientifically trained professionals. (Fee and Porter 1991, 33)

However, as they forsook environmental reform and sanitary engineering for the more "elegant and efficient" methods of laboratory science, public health doctors began to encroach on territory jealously guarded by their physician colleagues.

> The relationship between the emerging profession of public health and the well-established profession of medicine [became] problematic and controversial. The increased activity of health departments in the identification and control of infectious diseases tended to bring health officers into conflict with private practitioners . . . [and] the medical profession moved from a position of strong support for public health activities to a cautious, and sometimes suspicious ambivalence. (Fee 1991, 9)

Ambivalence merged into open hostility in the early years of the twentieth century. It was not until the time of World War I, however, that physicians became sufficiently well organized to translate this hostility into effective opposition. Opposition by private physicians to the new public health measures was not, of course, unique to the United States. It emerged earlier and was better organized in France, and was considerably more muted in Great Britain. In all four countries, the long-term outcome of these conflicts has been the marginalization of public health relative to private medicine, but this was by no means a foregone conclusion.

I conclude with a series of observations about public health in nineteenth- and early twentieth-century Canada. I have pointed out that Canada's early years of independence (that is, from 1867) were dominated by what the country's economic and political elites saw as the overwhelming need for economic development. In this context, the social concomitants of rapid industrialization—"slum cities, harsh working conditions, child and female sweated labour, unemployment, and extremes of rich and poor" (Penner 1992, 22) and, of course, contagious disease—were of little interest to the governments in power. Describing federal policy in the 1890s, McNaught points out that "neither party paid much attention to problems other than those of economic growth . . . practically no plans were made or even advocated to assist immigrants to adjust to a new environment in the event of the expected influx; and . . . labour and social legislation was largely distinguished by its absence" (1982, 172). Neither socialism nor organized labor nor even anything comparable to the Progressive movement in the United States had a serious political presence in Canada: "the values of a market economy went virtually unchallenged" (173).[13]

Even had there been the political will to address social, including public health, problems—and Jay Cassel argues that the European idea "that health was a right of citizenship and health preservation was an obligation of the state was quite literally foreign to Canadians" (1994, 281)—allocation of responsibility for public health between the federal government, the provinces, and municipalities was, at the very least, contested. Meeting immediately after the end of America's Civil War, Canada's founding fathers were determined to avoid what they saw as the weaknesses of the American constitution:

> to avoid a "states rights" opening to the provinces, the central government was very purposefully strengthened by giving to it "all the great subjects of legislation", and declaring that any un-named or residual powers should reside in the central government. The provinces were given only specific jurisdictions such as roads, direct taxation, municipal institutions, legislation concerning "property and civil rights", and education. (McNaught 1982, 135)

In Canada in the 1860s "all the great subjects of legislation" did not include public, or private, health. And "in 1894 the British North America Act was interpreted [by the Canadian Supreme Court] as giving the majority of the various responsibilities for citizens' health to the provinces" (Cassel 1994, 287).[14] How this allocation of responsibilities would—or would not—be translated into an attack on problems of public health became apparent as Canadian cities confronted—somewhat later than in Europe and the United States—the disease, disruption, and death associated with urbanization.

A Tale of Two Cities: Toronto and Montreal

The role of human agency—"a battling public health ideology, politics and medicine operating of necessity through local government" (Szreter 1988, 36)—in turn-of-the-century urban mortality is nowhere better illustrated than in the contrast between Toronto and Montreal.

The two cities were comparable in many respects. Toronto in 1880 was "second only to Montreal in terms of population and economic importance" (MacDougall 1990, 10). Port cities, immigrant gateways, centers of industry and commerce, both grew rapidly in the late nineteenth and early twentieth centuries. Moreover, in both cities the dominant commercial class was anglophone and Protestant, this despite large francophone and Roman Catholic majorities in Montreal and in the province of Quebec. Herein, however, lay the critical difference. Montreal was divided by ethnicity, wealth, and power into a majority of poor French-Canadians and a minority of wealthy and powerful Anglophones. Toronto, on the other hand, "with its mixture of native born and British immigrants . . . was proudly Tory and Protestant: a bastion of [British] Empire in the New World" (MacDougall 1990, 10). Montreal labored under what was already a long history of real and perceived inequities in the distribution of wealth and power between French- and English-speakers. Toronto did not. These contrasting circumstances played a powerful role in shaping each city's capacity to take action in response to the threats of disease and death.

Montreal's high mortality rates relative to other large cities in the industrialized world of the time were no secret to contemporaries: a civic-minded resident wrote in 1897 that "the citizens of Montreal should . . . cease discussing the slums of London, the beggars of Paris and the tenement house evils of New York and endeavour to learn something about themselves and to understand more perfectly the conditions present in their midst" (cited in Copp 1974, 15). Nevertheless, the gap between recognition of these conditions and action to address them proved unbridgeable. In its response to the evils in its own backyards, "Montréal probably exhibited municipal irresponsibility and callous indifference at its very worst" (McQuaig 1979, 125).

Toronto's death rates were high as well (though not so high as Montreal's). In its response, however, it occupied the other end of the public health spectrum: "By 1915, Toronto had an international reputation as an innovative leader in modern public health administration" (MacDougall 1990, 17). Indeed, the city's health department was such a model that the Rockefeller Foundation sent international students to the University of Toronto "so [that] they would be eligible to do field work with the city department" (28). How to account for this remarkable difference between two otherwise rather similar cities in the same country? Let me begin with Toronto.[15]

Toronto's city fathers shared the devotion to economic development and the aversion to spending money on anything so economically unproductive (in their view) as public health that were common to municipalities of the period. Their aversion was compounded by the fact that funds for public health came entirely out of local taxes. The first medical officer of health (MOH) was appointed in 1883, not in response to an epidemic outbreak (as often the case elsewhere) or as a result of public demand, but because the government in Ottawa offered a carrot in the form of a grant for the collection of mortality statistics to all cities over a certain size with a permanently salaried medical health officer. The aldermen's disinterest in sanitation and disease control was reflected in the limitation of the MOH's powers to "offering advice to the mayor" (MacDougall 1990, 17). Between 1883 and 1910, two officers resigned in disgust (unable, it appears, to stomach unending battles with politicians), and one was fired. In 1910, however, with the appointment as MOH of Charles Hastings, a prominent obstetrician and public health activist (he was a founding member of the Canadian Public Health Association and was elected president of the American Public Health Association in 1918), the balance of power between the MOH and the city fathers shifted. Hastings was the fortunate beneficiary of several advantages that his predecessors lacked. First, the provincial (Ontario) Public Health Act of 1912 made dismissal of local health officers a provincial (not a local) prerogative. This change substantially increased Hastings' freedom of action: no longer did he have to negotiate every request for expansion of his activities with municipal officials, who often opposed these activities and could fire him at will. Second, Hastings had the good fortune during the first decade of his administration to serve under two reform mayors who "shared his views and supported his efforts" (28). Building on these initial advantages, Hastings created a forceful, active health department, highly centralized, with minimal dependence on the work of voluntary groups.[16]

The contrast with Montreal is very sharp.[17] Although organized public health services—the Bureau de santé de la cité de Montréal—had existed in Montreal since at least 1876, the bureau was denounced virtually from its inception as "badly organized, inadequately financed, and without competent staff" (Pierre-Deschênes 1981, 362).[18] "Societies of hygiene" that grouped primarily Francophone physicians but also some businessmen and political figures demanded reform. The city fathers' first reaction was to abolish the Bureau de santé altogether. Under intense medical pressure, however, it was reestablished, and in 1886—pushed this time by a devastating smallpox epidemic—a provincial law (the Quebec Public Health Act) was passed requiring municipalities across the province to establish local health boards and creating at the same time a provincial board (the Conseil d'hygiène) charged with research and regulatory functions. This law, Terry Copp observes, "was unfortunately a very defective piece of legislation" (1974, 91)—a classic unfunded mandate, to which no money or powers of enforcement were attached: "Municipalities would have to raise the money for such expenditures from their own tax resources and public health, except in time of epidemics, proved to have a low priority" (1974, 92–3).

In 1885, just before the passage of the Quebec Public Health Act, a new director of Montreal's Bureau de santé, Louis Laberge, was appointed. His tenure lasted twenty-eight years—nine more than that of Charles Hastings in Toronto. Unlike Hastings, however, Laberge found himself in continuous battle with the city's politicians for sufficient resources to maintain, let alone expand, public health services (Pierre-Deschênes 1981, 363). Municipal elections in 1910 and 1914 brought no improvement. Indeed, the 1914 election "marked the beginning of a period in municipal politics during which issues were defined rhetorically in terms of language and class," pitting French Canadians against English businessmen and the (wealthy) west end (Copp 1974, 147).

Montreal's incapacity was not due to lack either of medical expertise or of medical interest in public health. Montreal's physicians, anglophone and francophone, not only were among the country's best but also were well aware of developments in modern bacteriology and were energetic advocates of public health reform (Pierre-Deschênes 1981; Copp 1981). In practice, however, these advantages were more than outweighed by the countervailing politics of language and religion. The medical community was plagued by individual and institutional conflicts largely along linguistic lines; the powerful French-Catholic clergy were antagonistic to secular public health activities they saw as competitive with their own interests; and the voluntary sector was weak and itself divided by language and religion (Copp 1981; Pierre-Deschênes 1981; McQuaig 1979). These barriers to concerted action were compounded by the geographic-political separation between wealthy hilltop enclaves (that is, anglophone Westmount and francophone Outremont) with excellent services and the urban flatlands.

> The political separation of these communities coincided with the withdrawal of their upper class populations from involvement in Montréal civic affairs. . . . [Furthermore, after 1910,] politics increasingly tended to focus on emotionally charged nationalist issues which, however important in the larger sense, militated against the development of strong public interest in municipal affairs. (Copp 1974, 147)[19]

In his article examining the politics of public health in late Victorian Britain, Szreter observes that

> from the mid-1830s through the late 1860s, local politics in the provincial, industrial towns was in fact predominantly characterized by debilitating

internal divisions, cross-cutting interests, shifting alliances, and stymied initiatives. As a result stalemate ensued, in terms of the capacities of cities and their governments to respond to the environmental and health problems that they faced as their populations grew rapidly. (1997, 705)

These observations apply without amendment and with equal force to Montreal in the early twentieth century. In Britain's industrial cities, Szreter argues, stalemate was broken in the 1870s by the rise of the civic gospel, the evangelically based social movement that combined belief in social progress with the religious duty to undertake public good works on behalf of the urban poor (709). No such resolution occurred—or, perhaps, was even possible—in Montreal.

The importance of this comparison—and the reason I have dwelt on it at some length—is that it highlights in stark relief critical elements of the politics of public health to which I will continually return in the narratives that follow: the emergent role of the state, the variable interest and capacity of relevant governing bodies; the presence or absence of influential social movements, along with medical, economic, religious, and other actors external to the government, and the impact on policy making and policy implementation of ethnic, racial, and class divisions.

PART II

THE TURN OF THE NINETEENTH CENTURY

Chapter 3

Infant Mortality

INFANT MORTALITY—the number of babies who die in the first year of
life—had been identified by the middle of the nineteenth century as a
"particularly sensitive index of community health and well-being and
of the effectiveness of existing public health measures" (Meckel 1990, 5).
John Simon, then medical officer of health for the City of London, noted
in 1851 that "there was no better index of sanitary condition than the
infant mortality rate" (Lambert 1963, 165). Further, as Richard Meckel
observes and as the narratives that follow will show, infant mortality
"also came to be seen and employed as an emotionally and politically
powerful issue strategically useful in securing government funding for
related health and social assistance measures" (1990, 5). During the last
quarter of the nineteenth century, the so-called massacre of the innocents[1]
became a full-blown public problem—complete with dramatic newspaper headlines, parliamentary reports, and the formation of concerned citizens' groups—in much of the industrialized West (Rollet 1997, 41).

There are few reliable data on infant mortality rates (number of deaths
of infants under one year of age for every thousand live births) at the
national level for the United States before the 1920s (Preston and Haines
1991) and essentially no data for Canada (McInnis 1997). Figure 3.1 compares the infant mortality rates of England and Wales (UK), France and, as
an imperfect proxy for the United States, Massachusetts, from 1870
through 1920.[2] Although there were differences across countries (France's
infant mortality rate was more or less consistently above the other two and
declined more slowly), the most striking aspect of this figure is not the differences but the similarities. Infant mortality rates were high and stable,
hovering above 150:1,000 and spiking in individual years, until around
1900, when they began a long and, again with the exception of individual
years, continuous decline to their present levels of under 10:1,000.

Infant mortality in the nineteenth century was mainly postneonatal—
that is, concentrated in the period between one month and one year of
age—and was due mainly to infectious disease, primarily gastrointestinal

Figure 3.1   Infant Mortality, 1870 to 1920

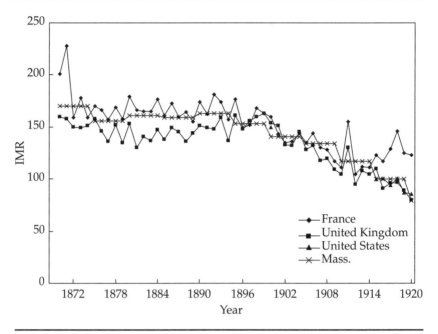

Sources: Mitchell (1992), table A7; U.S. Bureau of the Census (1975) 57.

and respiratory conditions. The pattern of infant deaths in England and Wales has been analyzed in detail by Woods and colleagues and will serve to exemplify the major sources of variation during the latter part of the century (Woods, Watterson, and Woodward 1988, 1989; Woods 1997). Following a brief review of these authors' account, I will indicate where the British pattern appears to have differed from that of the United States, France, and Canada.

The major source of variation in infant mortality in the latter half of the nineteenth century "lies with the urban post-neonatal mortality rate" (Woods, Watterson, and Woodward 1988, 352). Urban rates could be double those in rural areas depending on the year and the specific geographical areas covered and were substantially higher throughout the period in question: "In many rural registration districts [the infant mortality rate] was less than 0.100 [100:1,000] even in 1861, while in certain urban districts it was still in excess of 0.150 [150:1,000] even in 1911" (353). Woods and his colleagues explain this "urban effect" by the interaction of "climatic conditions, especially during the third quarter of the year [that is, dry and hot summers] with poor urban sanitary environments [that] resulted in high levels of diarrhoea and dysentery among infants, particularly those aged between 1–11 months" (360).[3] How, then, do Woods and colleagues account for the rapid decline of infant mortality in the UK beginning in 1900, and how do they explain the relatively good performance of the UK compared to other industrialized countries given its high level of urbanization?

In answer to the first question, they advance four hypotheses. First, fertility decline from the 1870s "served to reduce the level of infant mortality by affecting both the number of pregnancies a woman experienced, and by increasing intervals between successive births" (Woods, Watterson, and Woodward 1989, 130). Second, improvements in women's education increased the likelihood of birth control in some form and had other positive consequences for women's health and that of their babies. Third, late nineteenth-century social movements to improve the health of towns made sanitary advances possible. Finally, improvements in supply and quality of milk and food as well as in maternal and infant care "were all of special significance . . . but usually they served to reinforce an existing trend by focusing attention on those children most at risk in areas with the highest infant mortality" (130).[4] A virtually identical set of factors have been advanced to account for the decline of infant mortality in the United States (CDC 1999, 822).

On the question of why infant mortality in the UK was more or less consistently lower than that of many western European countries, Robert Woods and his colleagues suggest that the explanation lies in British women's relatively high level of breastfeeding. Contemporaries (for example, Arthur Newsholme, medical officer of the Local Government Board from 1909 to 1919) noted that breastfeeding was widespread among urban working-class mothers. Woods and colleagues present data from a variety of sources tending to confirm this observation (1989, 117). In a period when any other source of milk was likely to be highly contaminated, breastfeeding was critical to preventing infection.

The pattern of high urban relative to rural infant mortality was consistent across the four countries though there were substantial differences in rates. Although infant mortality was higher in Paris than in London, Paris was by no means the most lethal of French cities. The highest rates during the last two decades of the nineteenth century were observed in Rouen (more than 300:1,000) and Rheims (250–300:1,000). Rollet and Patrice Bourdelais attribute these high rates to unsterilized milk and—consistent with Woods and colleagues—connect elevated French infant mortality rates in the latter part of the nineteenth century with "the spread of artificial feeding" (1993, 58) and declines in the early twentieth century with "better infant feeding practices" (1993, 62).

Contrary to the nineteenth-century image of the United States and Canada as healthy new Edens, infant mortality in New York, Toronto, and Montreal was substantially higher than in London and Paris. The most detailed relevant analysis for the United States is the work of Samuel Preston and Michael Haines on child mortality in the late nineteenth and early twentieth centuries (1991). Although their study does not distinguish infant mortality from the mortality of children from one to five, the data presented are adequate for present purposes. Based on multivariate analysis of a 1 in 750 subsample from the U.S. Census of 1900, Preston and Haines conclude that the variable most predictive of the child's death was the mother's race. In the United States in 1900, "being black . . . denoted a set of economic and social conditions that powerfully affected child mortality and that was not adequately captured by other variables that may have been associated with race" (171).[5] Size of place, which dominates analyses of late nineteenth- and early twentieth-century infant mortality in England, takes second place in the United States to race.[6]

In Canada, for race read language. Data collected by the Montreal Health Department during the late nineteenth- and early twentieth-century period under review testify clearly to the markedly high mortality rate among French Canadian infants (Copp 1981).[7] Based on his detailed analysis of 1901 death registration and census data for Quebec and Ontario, Marvin McInnis describes "a dual regime of infant mortality, one in Québec (or more precisely in French Canada) and the other in Ontario (essentially English Canada)" (1997, 265). Whereas infant mortality in Ontario (115:1,000) was about the same as that Preston and Haines estimated for the white population of the United States, the rate for Quebec (190:1,000) is higher than that for France and higher than Preston and Haines's estimate for American blacks. McInnis argues that the difference between Ontario and Quebec—the Quebec rate is two-thirds higher than that of Ontario—cannot be accounted for by differences in income, crowding, or literacy. There were the expected urban-rural differences within each province, but "the big difference between Quebec and Ontario was in the rural populations, not in the cities" (266). "Several wholly rural counties of French Canadian Quebec had higher rates of infant mortality than Toronto, the largest city of anglophone Canada" (272). McInnis infers that these differences "must have had a lot to do with feeding practices" namely absence of breastfeeding or early weaning (266). However, beyond accusations of maternal neglect voiced by contemporary physicians, there is little evidence on this point, one way or the other. The infant mortality rate in Montreal continued far above that of other large North American cities, including New York as well as Toronto, well into the first quarter of the twentieth century.

It was not until the last half of the nineteenth century that infant deaths were identified as a serious public problem, and in none of these four countries was this recognition triggered by a sudden increase in the infant death rate. Nevertheless, by the early 1900s—somewhat later in Canada and earlier by several decades in France—the toll exacted by infant deaths had become a (if not the) principal rallying cry of public health and social reformers. There was broad convergence in the solutions reformers proposed: almost all variations on the themes of clean milk and the education of "ignorant" mothers. There was substantial cross-national variation, however, in the triggering conditions or events that brought infant mortality to the fore, in how it was framed as a matter of public concern, and in the institutional responses of governments and private citizens, as the narratives that follow will show.

United States

In his book *In the Shadow of the Poorhouse,* Michael Katz writes that 1890 marked "the start of a new era in the history of social welfare" in the United States (1996, 119): an era of "child-saving" that lasted into the 1920s: "Deployed at a time of great conflict in American life, child-saving was one key strategy for stemming the slide of the poor in great cities into savagery, hostility, and socialism" (120). The campaign to reduce infant mortality was an integral part of that strategy. Infant mortality did decline, and it declined most where the campaign was most "actively supported and pursued" (Meckel 1990, 180). Whether and to what extent the specific policies pursued were in fact responsible for the observed decline are, nevertheless, open questions.

The policies advocated by U.S. reformers had much in common with those of their counterparts elsewhere: regulating milk supplies, educating mothers, setting up well-baby clinics. Many of the major players—physicians, women, and the state—were the same.[8] But the relative importance of these groups, their relations to one another, their roles in framing infant mortality as a policy issue, and the parts they played in devising solutions were very different, in part because of differences in the social and political context in which infant mortality emerged as a public problem.

America at the turn of the twentieth century had no recent experience of defeat in foreign wars to arouse national anxiety about the quantity and quality of her young men, and the state of the country's vital statistics was such as to render any decline in the birth rate largely invisible and, in any case, of little (initial) concern given the massive influx of immigrants. The United States was not threatened with depopulation, nor was its national survival at stake. Meckel suggests that infant mortality's debut in the post–Civil War period was due primarily to its dramatic value: public health officials confronted with penurious taxpayers and skinflint politicians were "well aware that citing mortality levels among the young would generate more public and official support for their programs than would illustrating the more generalized consequences of urban insanitation" (31). Emulating their counterparts in Britain, these officials used infant mortality rates both to justify sanitary reform and as a measure of reform's success.[9]

Not until the late nineteenth century were isolated protests against the nation's high rates of infant mortality transformed into a crusade. The struggles for social and political reform that emerged in response to massive social change (described in chapter 2) found expression in—among other places—public health. Hermann Biggs, among the most influential public health officials of his day, wrote in his (1882) undergraduate thesis for Cornell University that "as the density of population increases and great cities spring up, where vast numbers from the lowest grades of society are crowded together in small areas, which become the breeding places and hotbeds of disease," the observance of state-enforced "hygienic laws" is particularly necessary (cited in Winslow 1929, 40). The observance of hygienic laws became construed as intrinsic to a process whereby "the lowest grades of society" would be weaned from their alien customs and made into good—nonthreatening—Americans.

Claims-Making

In the late nineteenth century, "the annual slaughter of little children" in American cities (*The New York Times*, July 19, 1876, cited in Meckel 1990, 11) metamorphosed from a rhetorical device to loosen the purse strings of city councils reluctant to underwrite tenement house and other environmental reforms to a problem, first, of improper infant feeding and, second (growing out of and overlapping the feeding question), of ignorant mothers.[10] The shift in emphasis from environmental reform to nutrition was due in part to the influence on American doctors and public health officials of European (in particular British and German) medicine. It was further driven by frustration with continued high infant death rates and the perceived difficulty of broader social and economic reforms.[11] In this context—and given these experts' near cynicism regarding the modern American woman's ability and willingness to breastfeed—improving the artificial milk supply appeared as something of a medical magic bullet.

Turn-of-the-century campaigns against infant mortality were, however, driven by more than the discovery of new "solutions" to a longstanding problem. In the United States, in contrast to Britain and France, there was neither a strong central government nor a well-established and state-sponsored medical profession. The fluidity of these institutions created political opportunities both for ambitious medical professionals and for white middle-class women, already well organized through women's clubs and associations such as the Women's Christian Temperance Union (WCTU). Engaged at one time or another with the problem of infant deaths were the newly assertive medical specialties of pediatrics and obstetrics, local and national public health officials, and the American Medical Association, along with politically active women's organizations and the federal Children's Bureau. As causal attributions changed and new strategies were deployed, so leadership and influence in the campaign against infant mortality moved back and forth between experts (primarily physicians, primarily men) and the laity (primarily organized, middle-class white women). Meckel dates the shift in leadership from experts to women ("social welfare and charity workers," in his words) to somewhere between 1900 and 1910 (1990, 79).[12] Women's dominance was, however, both contested and short-lived. By the mid-1920s, experts had reoccupied their turf.

Pediatrics, Public Health, and the Question of Milk   Pediatrics in late nineteenth-century America was an emerging specialty in search of a reason for being. Leading pediatricians staked their claim to recognition on the need for "scientific management" of infant feeding, encompassing the search for acceptable alternatives to breast milk. They emphasized the potential dangers of breastfeeding and the indigestibility of improperly prepared substitutes, highlighting the need for medical supervision of babies and their mothers. Not until considerably later was the potential for bacterial contamination of cow's milk perceived as a serious problem; indeed, most pediatricians opposed pasteurization as altering the chemical composition of milk.

The construction of infant mortality as a problem of bad milk was attractive to public health officials as well, for somewhat different reasons: it promised a simple prophylactic against infant deaths, obviating the need for the fundamental environmental and behavioral reforms that had proved so difficult to accomplish. The pediatric solution, however—which involved carefully supervised dairies and complex formulas—was unaffordable for these officials' principal clients, the urban poor. The strategies that eventually emerged in response to this problem were, first, the establishment of milk depots in tenement districts during the summer months and, second, city-mandated pasteurization of milk.

Milk stations providing free or subsidized milk to poor mothers were inaugurated in the United States in 1893, in New York City on the Lower East Side, funded by a philanthropist Nathan Straus.[13] Straus, much like Léon Dufour, the French physician who originated the Goutte de Lait, was an enthusiastic publicist: by 1910 there were 297 such stations in thirty-eight cities, privately funded by a wide range of charitable agencies. These agencies—settlement houses, women's clubs, children's aid societies—were a major entry point for women into the campaign to reduce infant mortality. Straus's milk depots were also the first building blocks of an at least partially state-supported administrative and clinical infrastructure devoted to infant health. Still, the stations reached only a small fraction of the urban poor. The alternative, advocated and acted on by public health reformers, was to clean up the milk supply coming into large cities.

The years from the turn of the century until the first world war were arguably the period of urban public health officials' greatest influence in the United States. The boundaries that were to separate curative medicine from its stepchild public health had yet to be sharply drawn (see, for example, Starr 1982).[14] "The physicians who promoted public health and served in health departments represented the elite of the [medical] profession. Most came from middle- or upper-class backgrounds and had no financial worries" (Duffy 1990, 196). They were socially and politically well-connected, and they lived and worked at a time of uncharacteristic belief (for Americans) in the power and responsibility of government to rectify social ills. This pattern was exemplified by Hermann Biggs and his associates in New York City, and nowhere were public health reformers more aggressive in pursuit of pure milk, and of other equally or even more controversial public health measures (see, for example, Fairchild et al. 2007). Throughout his career with the New York City Health Department— from 1892 until 1913—Biggs continued his private practice among the city's elite along with his teaching appointments at Cornell University Medical College.[15] Among his grateful patients was the head of Tammany Hall, then the dominant organization in New York City politics: "Tammany gave its full and complete support to all Dr. Biggs's constructive plans for the development of city health work" (Winslow 1929, 188; see also Fox 1975).

Big-city health departments' drive for pure milk brought them into direct confrontation not only with physicians suspicious of pasteurization, but also with a chain of vendors—from dairy farmers to retailers— having strong vested interests in the business of selling milk. The draconian measures taken by the New York City Health Department would almost certainly have been impossible without strong support from the city's politicians and its elites in business and journalism. In 1902 Biggs had the entire milk supply of several large firms "poured into the street gutters" (Winslow 1929, 194). In 1912 he obtained a city ordinance mandating pasteurization of all milk coming into the city, well in advance of comparable measures in the rest of the world.

Historians have emphasized the uniqueness in the United States of the advances in public health pioneered by New York City (Meckel 1990; Starr 1982).[16] Three elements of the New York story are, however, quite generalizable: first, the importance of highly placed political patronage to the cause of public health; second, the presence of politically savvy public health entrepreneurs positioned to seize political opportunities when they arose; and, third, strong media support for public health action.

Enter the Women   Recent scholarship on the development of maternalist policies—policies for the protection of maternal and infant health—in Europe and America in the late nineteenth and early twentieth centuries has strongly emphasized the part of women in this development: "It was in this area, closely linked to the traditional female sphere, that women first claimed new roles for themselves and transformed their emphasis on motherhood into public policy" (Koven and Michel 1990, 1077). Women were at the forefront of maternalist politics in all four countries, but nowhere more so than in the United States:

> In the United States the limited nature of the state created opportunities for women. The power of the evangelical religious tradition, the disestablishment of religion, and the inability of the formal polity to address the problems associated with industrialization all worked to empower voluntary associations. Women's access to higher education and the politicization of domestic life through the ideology of republican motherhood helped to empower women's voluntarism in particular. (Klaus 1993, 137)

Nowhere were women more influential in the creation of administrative structures and in the passage of laws to benefit mothers and children— and nowhere was the structure these women created more fragile.[17]

Women's appearance as major players in the campaign against infant mortality coincided with a reconceptualization of the campaign's objective "from milk reform to maternal reform" (Meckel 1990, 93). Frustrated, again, by the seeming intractability of infant deaths, and attentive to the work of their counterparts abroad, erstwhile milk reformers eagerly followed in the footsteps of Britain and France and refocused their efforts on the education of "ignorant" (largely immigrant) mothers. Milk stations were expanded (initially in New York City) "to encourage breastfeeding, provide medical exams, and dispense information on infant hygiene along with milk" (93). By 1912, mothers had displaced milk as the prime target of organized reform: "the reduction of infant mortality" asserted the infant mortality committee of the National Conference on Charities and Corrections depends "not on the state, the municipality, or the philanthropic agency, 'but upon the health, the intelligence, the devotion and the maternal instinct of the mother' " (121).[18] Unwilling, however, to rely on maternal instinct alone, the many voluntary societies and reform organizations organized in the 1900s to promote infant welfare now embarked on a massive effort to educate mothers in the proper care of their babies.[19]

Richard Meckel is properly skeptical of reformers' belief (or, at least, hope) that prevention of infant mortality could be accomplished by change at the individual level—imparting new skills to mothers—in the absence of fundamental social or environmental reform. "Perhaps the major benefit of the maternal education campaign," he argues, "was that it mobilized American women as a potent political force behind infant welfare" (157). Although the new focus on maternal education was not unique to the United States, American (white, middle-class) women were uniquely positioned—both organizationally and in their relation to the central state—to take advantage of the political opportunities this strategy offered. This summary gives some indication of their response:

> Women in the United States actively influenced [infant health] policy at all levels as professionals and often as public officials. They had a significant voice in the American Association for the Study and Prevention of Infant Mortality, chaired sessions at the annual meetings, and were among its officers. For a few years they ran a committee of the American Medical Association devoted to the welfare of women and children. Women headed many municipal and state divisions of child hygiene and, perhaps most important, organized, administered, and staffed the U.S. Children's Bureau. These professional women saw themselves as the leaders of a massive popular movement whose rank-and-file were the members of women's clubs and mothers' congresses. (Klaus 1993, 91).

"Nowhere else," Kathryn Sklar points out, "did women reformers design and administer a major government bureau [the Children's Bureau, created by Congress in 1912] responsible for the health and welfare of the nation's infants and children" (1993, 44). Women's accomplishments included not only the Children's Bureau, but also the passage in 1921 of the "first explicit federal welfare legislation, the Federal Act for the Promotion of the Welfare and Hygiene of Maternity and Infancy, commonly known as the Sheppard-Towner Act" (Skocpol 1992, 481).[20] Theda Skocpol describes these "state-building successes" for policies to benefit mothers and infants as "the joint political achievements of women reformers and widespread associations of married women" (481), a judgment shared by other historians (Rothman 1978; Koven and Michel 1990; Klaus 1993).

Yet women's successes were more apparent than real. First, women's associations largely excluded representation from that segment of the population with the highest rates of infant mortality, American blacks. Black women organized, particularly in the South, but their influence was minimal:

> Southern black women confronted a state that did not act in the interest of mothers, their children, or family life as a whole. They pursued their social reform through institutions of their own making. So did white women. But white activist women were able to transfer their programs to the state, becoming the administrators of new state agencies dedicated to maternal and child welfare. Black women, in contrast, gained few benefits from the emerging welfare state. (Boris 1993, 215)

Second, women's dominance of the maternal and infant health arena proved unsustainable. Once Sheppard-Towner had been passed, due in part to congressional uncertainty about the political impact of newly enfranchised women, a combination of unfavorable circumstances—the increasing power and hostility of the organized medical profession, fragmentation within the executive branch of the federal government, and emerging weaknesses of women's movements themselves—conspired to undermine women's power as well as national political support for the institutions they had created. Third, such programs as did exist were poorly funded, heavily dependent on private charity, and served low-income, immigrant, and black populations with little political clout. Finally, in contrast to each of the other three countries, these programs did not evolve into broader state-supported benefits for mothers and children.[21] Ironically, among the many reasons for this failure may be, as Sue Tolleson Rinehart has suggested, that the legitimacy of infant and maternal health programs in the United States was undermined because these programs were identified with upstart women, not—as in the European countries and Canada—with the male establishment of doctors and politicians (1987).

France

Infant mortality emerged as a matter of intense concern to France's ruling elites in the second half of the nineteenth century not as an indicator of the public's health but for the perceived contribution of infant deaths to the "depopulation" of the state.[22] Numbers equaled power, and as France's population failed to keep pace with that of its European neighbors—Germany, in particular—its power must decline. Fertility in France had begun to fall before the end of the eighteenth century and continued to decline steadily throughout the nineteenth century and beyond (Bourgeois-Pichat 1965). However, it was not until after mid-century that the dimensions of decline—and its implications for population growth—were fully recognized and the connection to infant mortality was made. These developments can be explained in part by the new availability of census data documenting the steady drop in French birthrates together with published exposures of the terrible toll on infant lives taken by the practice of wet-nursing (Sussman 1982; Cole 1996; Klaus 1993). Data, however, do not speak for themselves. Spurred on by government officials, physicians of the French Academy of Medicine seized on France's high infant mortality rate, framed in the context of its low birthrate, "to create a crisis of national proportions where previously none had been perceived" (Cole 1996, 433).

In framing this crisis, politicians and physicians spoke with one voice because—more often than not—they were one voice. With few exceptions, the major architects of French policy in response to infant mortality were physician-politicians—members of Parliament and cabinet officials.[23] When, in 1869, the government appointed a commission to study the question of wet nursing, four of its members belonged to the Academy of Medicine. By the end of the nineteenth century, the academy had become virtually a branch of government, heavily involved in all legislative activity that concerned les petits enfants (Rollet-Echalier 1990): the boundary between medicine and the state as actors in the campaign against infant mortality was virtually indistinguishable. French physicians were almost entirely men. In sharp contrast to the United States (and, in lesser degree, to Britain and Canada), women's voices in this campaign were marginalized.

Causes and Cures

Much as in other countries, causal responsibility for infant mortality was laid at the door of mothers. "Deprivation of maternal care" (Fuchs 1997, 93) encompassed abortion, abandonment, neglect, and, above all, failure to breastfeed. Policy responses were, however, rather different, for reasons economic as well as political and ideological. The French pattern of industrialization was associated with uniquely high employment of married women—higher than in Canada or Great Britain and much higher than in the United States. When the family's economic survival required that mothers go out to work and there were few safe alternatives for the care of newborns, babies had a high probably of being sent away from home to be nursed.[24] It was this practice of wet nursing and the high infant mortality associated with it that captured national attention in the late 1860s and triggered France's campaign against infant mortality.[25]

Catherine Rollet (1990) has usefully divided this campaign into two phases. One was a period of "intense legislative activity" from 1865 to 1889 that reflected the state's assumption of responsibility for addressing the problem of infant mortality. The second, from 1890 to 1914, was "the era of Pasteur" that saw the invention of the Goutte de Lait and other programs for the distribution of sterilized milk along with advice on child-rearing.[26]

Over a period of four years from 1866 to 1870, the Academy of Medicine devoted thirty-four sessions to study of the wet nursing business and the development of proposals for its regulation. Action on these proposals was interrupted by the Franco-Prussian War and the political upheaval associated with France's defeat, but in 1874 Théophile Roussel, Republican deputy and himself a member of the academy, introduced legislation based on the academy's work. His bill was supported by the new government and—despite its unprecedented interference with parental prerogatives—passed "unanimously and without debate" (Klaus 1993, 56). The loi Roussel created a national bureaucratic structure for the regulation of the wet nursing industry, including registration and medical supervision of wet nurses and the infants they had in charge. It laid out a program of systematic monthly visits by a médecin-inspecteur to all newborns sent from their homes, most often in Paris or other large cities, to the country to be nursed. At one time or another as many as one-third of all French physicians were involved in this activity (Rollet-Echalier 1990, 352). The law was never fully implemented in the form envisioned by its creators, and its impact on infant mortality is questionable (Sussman 1982). Its significance lay as a marker of the entry of the French state as a major player in the protection of infant lives.[27]

The loi Roussel was the first in a long spate of legislation for the protection of mothers and children enacted by parliament between 1874 and 1914. Based on the premises that babies belonged to the state and that women in their capacities as mothers were a "national resource" (it was argued that mothers were equal to soldiers in their service to the state), gender-specific laws were passed regulating women's conditions of work, their pregnancies and births and their methods of child care. Paul Strauss—one of the major architects of this legislation—wrote of his approach that "the national collectivity [had] the right and the duty to exercise . . . suitable protection, and enforce coercion if people fail[ed] to recognize the rules of hygiene" (cited in Fuchs 1997, 103).[28] He and his cohort of reformers believed—and acted on their belief—that infant mortality could be prevented by a combination of bureaucratic surveillance with financial and material aid to needy mothers conditioned on good (that is, hygienic) behavior. Consideration of the most immediate causes of infant mortality (for example, summer diarrhea) was largely absent from discussion of these legislative proposals.

A further striking aspect of these laws was that, though they were addressed primarily to the circumstances of women with few financial resources, they made no distinction between single (fille-mères) and married mothers. This was controversial, but the state's need for babies successfully overrode concerns about the moral status of the single mother. The state and, by extension, the bureaucrats, medical and otherwise, charged with oversight of vulnerable women—and of the many small charitable organizations designed to serve these women—were construed as benevolent patriarchs or as physicians to the French family, acting in the place of absent or incapable fathers.

By the end of the nineteenth century, twenty-six years after the loi Roussel, French infant mortality rates showed no evidence of decline, and individual physicians with practices among poor urban women (the wet-nursing business was largely carried on by poor rural women) turned their attention more directly to the promotion of breastfeeding by the mothers themselves and, when that was impossible, the provision of sterilized milk.[29] In 1892, twelve years after Pasteur had described the technique, the Academy of Medicine gave its stamp of approval to sterilization. The medical profession at large had been powerfully opposed on the grounds that sterilized milk was not only "unnatural" but also "immoral" because it would discourage breastfeeding. This controversy continued through much of the early twentieth century (Rollet 1990, 170–72). Nevertheless, in 1894 the first Goutte de Lait for the provision of sterilized milk to mothers unwilling or unable to nurse was established in Fécamp, Brittany, by a local physician, Léon Dufour.[30] Due in part to his own enthusiastic proselytizing, Dufour's innovation spread rapidly throughout France (and beyond, though without the coercive features to be noted later). In their early days, Gouttes de Lait were privately organized and funded by charitable groups or—not unusually—by the commercial and industrial enterprises that employed married women. In 1903 the French Senate passed a resolution encouraging the formation of Gouttes de Lait and, in recognition not only of their value but also of their relatively low cost, public funds quickly followed.

Rollet describes the period from 1890 to 1914 as characterized by physicians' volonté d'instruire (eagerness to instruct) and women's eagerness to learn (1997, 588). All that was necessary to set up a clinic was a scale to record the baby's weight, milk, and a doctor.[31] Milk and other benefits were not however distributed unconditionally: "Following certain rules of hygiene or attending infant health consultations . . . became a condition for a variety of material assistance and services: free meals, crêches, clean milk, and maternity benefits" (Klaus 1993, 62). In France—as elsewhere—mothers were deemed ignorant of proper methods of baby care; milk depots doubled as "schools for mothers" where they could be educated not only by the staff but also by each other (Fuchs 1997; Rollet-Echalier 1990). So determined were physicians to ensure regular attendance that it was not unusual for mothers to receive compensation for their time, in kind or even in cash (Rollet-Echalier 1990, 368).

France may have basked in the glory of Pasteur, but "very few laws or regulations resulted directly from [his] discoveries" (Rollet-Echalier 1990, 156). In the mid-1890s, responding to medical and political pressure, the Paris municipal council appointed a milk commission to study and report on the milk supply and to make recommendations for its improvement, with particular attention to sterilization. Despite the commission's elite membership—it included many of the major figures in France's campaign against infant mortality—and its devastating and well-publicized findings, nothing was done (180). A few years later the Paris council's circulation of a pamphlet of instruction to mothers on infant feeding that warned against the quality of store-bought milk met with violent protests from the union of milk distributors (181). In 1935, fifty-five years after Pasteur had invented sterilization, a law to control the French milk supply was enacted by parliament, but implementing regulations were never published.

Milk distribution in France was highly localized, sometimes under private and sometimes under community auspices. Whether and how it was regulated varied by city, town, and department. By the eve of World War II, only one city, Strasbourg, had made pasteurization obligatory (Rollet-Echalier 1990, 183). Among developed countries, France—the country of Pasteur—was the latest of the four countries dealt with here to adopt pasteurization. To account for this paradox, Rollet advances the perhaps overly cynical hypothesis that only those public health innovations (for example, diphtheria vaccination) that directly benefited the French "ruling class" were adopted rapidly, whereas new technologies that benefited primarily the poor (for example, pasteurization) lagged: bottle-feeding was largely confined to working-class women, whereas any child could get diphtheria (156). Less than wholehearted support of pasteurization by practicing physicians, together with organized opposition to almost any form of regulation by dairymen and commercial milk suppliers, were probably at least as important as ruling class disinterest in delaying action at the national level.

The Players

Actions taken by French authorities in the name of combating infant mortality—ranging from regulation of wet nursing to provision of maternity benefits—were the outcome of a remarkable convergence of interests between the medical profession and the state: "In seeking to protect child life as part of its efforts to counter the nation's population and social crises, the French government called heavily upon the medical profession. In turn, physicians had a significant voice in the framing of maternal and infant health policy" (Klaus 1993, 45). French physicians' authority derived from their early (since 1803) state-sanctioned monopoly of the practice of medicine, from their long-standing role as agents of the state in disease prevention, and from the aura and prestige conferred on medicine in the last half of the century by the discoveries of Pasteur. These men were also, as I have mentioned, quite literally politicians:

> Doctors were present on almost every municipal council in the nation, and served as mayors of hundreds of villages, towns and cities. . . . They often headed the Municipal Council of Paris and as a group formed 8.6 percent of its membership between 1870 and 1914. The same pattern applied to the conseils généraux or departmental legislatures. (Ellis 1990, 3)

Nationally, physicians were heavily represented in parliament and as cabinet members. They used their political voice to define infant mortality as a medical problem and to solidly entrench their positions in the political and bureaucratic structures created to combat it.

Elite physicians—Roussel and others—played leading roles as legislators on behalf of infants at risk, as innovators in the development of milk depots and infant health clinics, and as founders of voluntary associations to prevent infant mortality (for example, the Societé protectrice de l'enfance, founded in 1866, the Ligue contre la mortalité infantile, founded in 1902). Their success was not uniform, however—as, for example, in the case of the Paris milk commission, just described—and depended heavily on the support of the larger corps médical, the bulk of practicing doctors. The latter—in sharp contrast to their counterparts in the United States—supported the government's maternal and infant health programs, first, because these programs contributed to their authority as family medical advisers and, second, because they needed the money: the loi Roussel was virtually a full-employment measure for physicians. On the other hand, French practitioners failed to support broader public health legislation, including notification of infectious disease, proposed in 1903 and backed by the Parisian medical elite. Indeed, they contributed significantly to this legislation's defeat. These physicians' support for public health measures was highly selective, and depended heavily on the issues at stake.

The role of the French state itself in the campaign against infant mortality is far more difficult to characterize. There was consensus among the parties concerned (physicians, politicians and those who were both) as to where political responsibility to address the problem of infant mortality was located. "Defense of the family . . . [was] one of the functions of the state" (Fuchs 1997, 84), and interests of state—whether that meant having a few more children or complying with physician-enunciated rules of infant feeding—were held to override the private interests of individuals (in particular, of mothers). This consensus was more than rhetorical: laws were passed—intrusive at least in form—for the protection of mothers and children. Nevertheless, beyond accession to the passage of relatively noncontroversial legislation the state's commitment to the campaign against infant mortality was tepid at best. Not only was there a lag of ten to twenty years in implementation of the loi Roussel but the percentage of the French budget devoted to petite enfance was also, as Rollet puts it, dérisoire (a joke), accounting in 1902 for about .2 percent of the budget overall (Rollet-Echalier 1990, 277). The most striking aspect of the French state's action around infant mortality, however, was its selective attention to the behavior and circumstances of mothers and its inattention—indeed, rejection—of measures, such as pasteurization or the notification of births to local health authorities, that in the other countries were deemed essential to the reduction of infant mortality. Debate on these questions was dominated by physicians both as legislative architects and as lobbyists, and the paradoxical elements I have described are in large part a reflection of organized medicine's power to shape the state's agenda in ways consistent with its professional interests.

Among the many paradoxical dimensions of the French policy debate on infant mortality was the limited participation of women. Reform movements existed—tied to the Catholic church or, less frequently, of a more feminist "republican" cast—but these movements were relatively weak and socially and politically fragmented. Even if women had been unified in their political aims, the French political system offered few opportunities for women to translate their voluntary reform activities into political power. Alisa Klaus summarizes French women's position:

> Centralized state structures and a tradition of social intervention effectively excluded French women from policy making . . . The specific political conditions under which women organized for "maternalist" goals [that is, in aid of public policies on behalf of mothers and children] in France prevented them from becoming a distinctive female political force. Not only did the ongoing struggle between anticlerical Republicans and the Catholic church and other conservative forces engage women on both sides, but the depopulation crisis provided fuel for antifeminist rhetoric and policies. (1993, 93)

Routes to influencing maternal and infant health policies through the medical profession were effectively closed to women; their private charitable organizations were often co-opted by the state to further its own maternal and child welfare agenda. And so, although grassroots women's organizations existed, structural limitations on women's access to political power together with the strong pronatalist slant of maternalist ideology in France, seriously limited the influence of these organizations on either the formation or implementation of policies to reduce infant mortality. Certainly in France, if less persuasively elsewhere, the power of women's movements was inversely related to the extent of state action on behalf of mothers and children (see note 17).

Mothers, Science, and the State

The construction of infant mortality as a threat to national survival was driven by intense nationalism together with fears—fanned by popular Darwinism and exacerbated by military defeat—of "degeneration," depopulation, and ultimate extinction. The policy response to these concerns in the period before the first world war, however, had more complex political and ideological underpinnings, inseparable, first, from a gender ideology that subordinated women and, second, from a politics of social reform aimed at securing "social peace"—that is, the end of class warfare—through legislation to improve the condition of the working class (Stone 1985; 1997). In the face of concerted libertarian opposition, republican politicians were ultimately unable to legislate protection for the working man. Women, however, were another story: "gender-specific legislation was enacted because it used the rhetoric of domesticity and natalism, it strengthened gender segregation in the labor market and the factory, and it did not protect men" (Stone 1997, 48).

"The theory and practice of republicanism that shaped politics after 1870 [that is, during the period of the Third Republic] were highly gendered" (Accampo 1997, 3). Republicans embraced an ideology of republican motherhood under which "women were assigned to the domestic sphere, were given the responsibility to rear republican citizens, and were to defer to male authority" (Stone 1997, 30). This ideology acquired new meaning and emphasis in the light of threatened population decline. Women's bodies were not their own; they existed for the sake of the child and in service to the state; the state, in consequence, had the duty to intervene to protect the woman and her child. This interventionist role was further legitimized by the philosophy of solidarité—the mutual dependence that existed among individuals and social classes—elaborated by the politician Léon Bourgeois in support of republican proposals for social reform (Accampo 1997). The paradigm of mutual dependence was the patriarchal family: "the family was often the metaphor used by solidarists to represent the state," its officials and politicians taking the role of "bon père de famille" (49). Within this framework, state assumption of responsibility for regulating many aspects of women's lives—women who were, after all, subordinate within the family, unable to vote, indeed not quite citizens—seemed to republican politicians of the period both necessary and justifiable.

Finally, mothers—ignorant of the new microbiology—could no longer be trusted to know what they were doing.

> Reading the work of contemporaries, one becomes aware of the extent to which [maternal] "ignorance" was relative, of the extent to which it depended on the recent progress, in particular, of microbiology. This was in some sense a modern, post-pasteurian, "ignorance," that could, by definition, only be revealed if one knew something about microbes. (Rollet-Echalier 1990, 364)

That knowledge was, of course, the special province of physicians, at least by attribution if not in fact. In their capacity as targets of the campaign against infant mortality, women were doubly subordinated, to the patriarchal state and to the authority of physicians.

Britain

Britain's high rates of infant mortality were no secret to the great innovators of nineteenth century public health—Edwin Chadwick, William Farr, John Simon.[32] Indeed, Farr suggested in 1841 that the deaths of children younger than five could be the "formula for [triggering state] intervention" in local sanitary conditions (Lewis 1952, 170). It took the disastrous Boer War (1899 to 1902) to concentrate public attention, however.[33] Existing fears of imperial decline were exacerbated by the "appalling" percentage of military recruits rejected for service on medical grounds, and infant mortality was reinvented as a threat to the British empire (Speck 1993, 116). Babies were the future of the race, and the Interdepartmental Committee on Physical Deterioration, appointed in 1904 in response to the recruitment statistics, focused its recommendations on improving the health of infants and children. It may be unnecessary to say that it was with the health of infants and children of the working class poor—from whose ranks ordinary soldiers were drawn—that the committee was primarily concerned.

The committee's report was greeted enthusiastically by the public health and medical communities:

> concern about national degeneration . . . validated infant and child welfare work and it validated an enlarged role for the physician to play in this issue of national importance. "It is not only the right but the duty of the State to watch over the development of its future citizens," the BMJ [British Medical Journal] maintained. "But it is a duty which it persistently neglects. The future of the race, therefore, rests largely with the medical profession." (Dwork 1987, 21)

In its comment on state neglect, the BMJ accurately reflected the retreat of the Local Government Board from its earlier position (under John Simon) as a major actor in the field of public health. From the 1870s until just before World War I, the bulk of public health action—including, despite the imperial rhetoric, action to combat infant mortality—was at the local level, the work of medical officers of health, town councillors, and women organized in voluntary associations. It was these sets of actors—about whom I have more to say later—who were largely responsible for identifying the "causes" of infant mortality and devising strategies to combat it.

Causes and Cures

The most dramatic preventable cause of infant mortality was diarrhea (variously labeled infant diarrhea, epidemic diarrhea, and cholera infantum)— "the disease process was visible: healthy children suddenly sickened violently and all too frequently died" (Dwork 1987, 26)—and it was to the prevention of diarrhea that the energy of public health campaigners was primarily directed. Their focus was hardly new. In 1860 John Simon had completed a survey of infant diarrhea in large towns, concluding with an emphasis, first, on its preventability and, second, on "impure water and tainted atmosphere" as the primary causes (Lambert 1963, 320). By the beginning of the twentieth century, the balance had shifted: water and air over which mothers had little control were increasingly displaced in the causal frameworks of the day by factors more closely tied to the actions of mothers themselves.

By late in the nineteenth century, artificial feeding (that is, feeding a baby with anything other than breast milk) had been firmly identified by British physicians as a principal cause of death from diarrhea. At the same time, evidence on the threat posed by bacterial contamination of the milk supply was accumulating rapidly. For example, "The Great Bacterial Contamination of the Milk of Cities," written by an American bacteriologist was published in England in 1901 (Dwork 1987, 52). Although they exhorted mothers to breastfeed, physicians and MOHs also campaigned actively—with meager success—to ensure that bottle-fed babies received clean milk.[34] This campaign took two forms. First was a movement to clean up the milk supply through the regulation of dairies and commercial distributors. Second was creating what were called milk depots, where milk produced under medically supervised conditions would be given to mothers individually.

There had been scattered local efforts to deal with the sorry state of Britain's milk supply well before the crisis atmosphere engendered by the Boer War (see, for example, Thompson 1984). The issue had been addressed in two pieces of national legislation: the Dairies, Cowsheds, and Milkshops Order in 1885 and the Infectious Diseases (Prevention) Act in 1890. The purpose of these bills was to prevent milk contamination at its source. Their terms were weak, implementation depended on local initiative, and there were no provisions for enforcement. In 1898 a royal commission described the bills as "a dead letter in many places" (Dwork 1987, 71). A few energetic MOHs persuaded their local authorities to obtain special powers of control (called Milk Clauses) through private Acts of Parliament, but affected dairymen simply sent their milk elsewhere.

Based on a survey of local MOHs, the editors of the *British Medical Journal* in 1903 concluded that "throughout England and Wales the conditions under which milk is obtained and dispatched in towns are exceedingly unsatisfactory, and that law and regulations are alike, to a very large extent, [still] dead letters" (cited in Dwork 1987, 86). Notwithstanding a barrage of medically authoritative calls for action coupled with much patriotic flag-waving, no effective action on a national level to control the milk supply was taken until after World War I.

There were two broad reasons for the British government's inaction. The first was scientific uncertainty about the risk from milk. A major impetus for legislation had been the work of British scientists published as early as 1888 and reiterated in reports of two royal commissions that cows' milk was a vehicle for transmission of tuberculosis to humans.[35] This belief was shattered in 1901 when Robert Koch—the world's authority on tuberculosis at the time—announced before the British Congress on Tuberculosis that "the extent of the infection by the milk and flesh of tuberculous cattle [is] hardly greater than that of hereditary transmission . . . and I therefore do not deem it advisable to take any measures against it" (cited in Dwork 1987, 74). Koch's statement proved to be a major roadblock in the way of national legislation to prevent disease transmission through the country's milk supply.

The second set of obstacles was political. From the time of its first appearance in the late nineteenth century, legislation to control the milk supply was opposed by the vested interests of farmers, dairymen, and milk suppliers. Writing in 1895, a British pathologist who had studied the milk question observed,

> when a truth, whether scientific or other, goes against the interests of a large and powerful class of the community, it is generally ignored or resisted until a more powerful class enforces its recognition. For the last 30 years farmers and butchers have been roughly disturbed by mere scientists, medical observers and veterinary surgeons, who have come to the conclusion that it is not safe for man or beast to feed on tuberculous products. (Cited in Dwork 1987, 65)

Pasteurization was opposed not only by farmers and small milk dealers who were well represented in a British parliament dominated by members from rural districts but also, and surprisingly, by the leadership of the National Association for the Prevention of Tuberculosis: pasteurization was a threat to their investment in dispensaries and sanatoria as the "solution" to tuberculosis (Smith 1988, 192). Opposed by entrenched and powerful political interests, pasteurization did not become law in Britain until 1948!

An alternative strategy for getting clean milk to bottle-fed babies was the establishment of milk depots consciously patterned after the French Gouttes de Lait. The first of these was opened in 1899 by a provincial MOH but its resemblance to the French model was, Deborah Dwork suggests, that of "a baguette and stick bread" (1987, 103). In this and the other milk depots opened in England over the next decade, clean milk was supplied to the mothers who attended. Unlike the French model, however, the milk was not free and medical supervision was minimal at best. The experiment was short-lived in Britain and not particularly successful for reasons both pragmatic and, Jane Lewis argues, philosophical. Pragmatically, the depots were expensive to run and mothers did not come, at least not in sufficiently large numbers, either because of cost, or because of the unavailability of medical treatment, or because in Britain, unlike France, most working class mothers breast-fed their babies (Dwork 1987; Lewis 1980).

Lewis suggests further that at least some MOHs "believed that [mothers'] ignorance not milk was the fundamental problem" (1980, 75). The new visibility of infant mortality statistics in the mid-nineteenth century had almost immediately given rise to speculation about the role of what was termed maternal neglect (that is, employment away from home) and other defects of baby care. However, not until the early twentieth century did the attention of MOHs and other campaigners for infant welfare begin to focus almost exclusively on, to use the phrase of the day, mothers' ignorance—of proper feeding methods, of domestic hygiene—and, concomitantly, on education as the remedy. In a 1904 article on the causes of infant diarrhea, the editors of The Lancet made passing reference to microbes and went on to assert that "one of the most important aetiologic factors concerned in this affection is undoubtedly the ignorance of the mothers. A very large number of women, more especially among the poorer classes, have not the least idea of the proper management of children." And though the editors advocated greater attention to the milk supply and wrote in praise of milk depots, "nevertheless, in their opinion 'the most important matter . . . is to try to adopt some means by which instructions could be given to women as to the proper management of children' " (cited in Dwork 1987, 131). Dwork does mention evidence for at least some MOHs' and lay workers' belief that the poverty of women "among the poorer classes," not their ignorance, was the principal cause of infant mortality (133). Nevertheless, education—supported by the public, the press, medical practitioners, and women's groups—carried the day—more specifically, education by female "health visitors" who would take the messages of hygiene and correct feeding to mothers in their own homes.

Health visiting was—and is—a peculiarly British institution. Its origins lay in the work of mid-nineteenth century women's sanitary associations, an outgrowth of Bible mission societies "that stressed house visits. [Sanitary association] workers were well versed in the rudiments of domestic hygiene and . . . did much to bring the gospel of soap and water into the homes of the masses" (Wohl 1983, 37). Although a Victorian concept, as Wohl observes, one that will surely be associated by readers of Trollope or Eliot with visits by the lady of the manor or the vicar's wife to the cottages of poor and, usually, ailing tenants, "the system of lady health visitors did not really catch fire until the Edwardian period" (37). The Interdepartmental Committee on Physical Deterioration in 1903 urged the formation of "health societies" all over the country, with the object of bringing sanitary education "into the homes of the masses" along the lines pioneered in the nineteenth century. By the second decade of the twentieth century a health visit immediately after birth and periodically thereafter had become the strategy of choice for combating infant mortality. Over time—particularly after the 1907 and 1914 Notification of Birth Acts requiring that the local MOH be notified of a birth within forty-eight hours—health visits from appropriately trained women (always women!) became a routine function of the local health authority and eventually covered all births, not just those of the poor. Among the more striking aspects of this system was its widespread acceptance by physicians: "The transition from voluntary lady worker to paid professional accepted as a part of the public health system was . . . relatively easy and unproblematic." Physicians opposed, unsuccessfully, the 1907 Notification of Birth Act, but showed "surprisingly little resistance to health visitors" (Dwork 1987, 158).[36]

The decrease in infant mortality that had begun in 1900, or earlier, some scholars (for example, Woods, Watterson, and Woodward 1989) now contend, had become evident to British activists by the early 1920s (Dwork 1987, 215). Although more sophisticated observers recognized that the reasons for the decline were complex and multifactorial, most child and welfare workers "had no hesitation in attributing it to the education of the mother" (Lewis 1980, 107). Dwork argues that confronted with the failure of alternative strategies, these workers saw education as a last resort—the only way to ensure that mothers were prepared for the "plethora of dangers to which [their] infants were exposed" (1987, 219).

The Players

The principal players in Britain's campaign against infant mortality were central and local government authorities, medical experts, and voluntary organizations of lay women. The marked expansion of the central government's role in public health during the nineteenth century was described in chapter 2: appointment of local medical officers of health was made compulsory; loans for sanitary improvement were used by the central government as carrots and sticks to promote reform; and centrally-employed inspectors went out from London to the provinces to ensure that public health laws were implemented. "It was not until the advent of compulsory education late in the century that the daily lives of Victorians were as widely affected by any government action as by state medicine" (Wohl 1983, 142). During the period in question here, however, from around 1890 to 1914, the central government was less actively engaged. Relatively little pertinent legislation was passed and what did pass depended heavily on local government initiative for adoption and implementation.[37] The reasons were in part organizational. Following the Local Government Board's assumption of responsibility for public health in 1871 and the subsequent resignation of John Simon, the board became dominated by politicians and civil servants with little interest in or sympathy for public health activities. The reasons were also philosophical: a longstanding aversion—overcome only periodically and under well-defined circumstances—to central government "interference" in private interests. In the context of early legislative efforts to protect the babies of working mothers, one speaker to the Social Science Association allowed that he "would rather see even a higher rate of infant mortality . . . than intrude one iota farther on the sanctity of the domestic hearth and the decent seclusion of private life" (quoted in Wohl 1983, 32).[38]

Into this vacuum stepped the local authorities and their energetic medical officers of health. Szreter has described increased attention to public health after the 1870s as a matter of "civic pride" noting that "positions of public leadership in Britain's provincial cities were increasingly sought by practical men of substance and vision as valued positions of honor. The status of the activities involved in municipal services and administration was commensurately enhanced" (1997, 709). Although Szreter is referring primarily to water supply and sewage removal, actions taken a decade or so later to protect the milk supply and to organize health visits to new mothers were also at the instance of local leadership. Local authorities adopted Milk Clauses, opened milk depots, and petitioned the local government board for authority to appoint lady health visitors. Notification of birth was locally initiated, by a private Act of Parliament for the town of Huddersfield.

Key figures in these actions—indeed, their driving force—were the medical officers of health. By the end of the nineteenth century, the MOHs' position in the structure of British public health was firmly established and their authority as experts in the new field of preventive medicine was secure (see, for example, Fee and Porter 1991; Brand 1965). This position was reflected not only in these physicians' dominance of the country's discourse on infant mortality and the voluntary organizations formed to combat it but also in their high status and the importance accorded to their work. As noted in chapter 2, not only MOHs' research but their more routine activities as well (for example, annual reports) were published on a regular basis by Britain's premier medical journals, *The Lancet* and the *British Medical Journal*. Indeed, these men—and they were all men—have been described as "among the most distinguished public servants of their profession" (Hardy 1993, 26).

Voluntary groups of middle-class lay women—the sanitary associations of the mid- to late-nineteenth century—were earliest to engage in maternal education through home visiting, and Britain's maternal and child welfare programs after 1900 were largely modeled on their activities. These programs continued to depend heavily on women—as volunteers in service provision, as health visitors, as clinic nurses, and as powerful advocates for services to women and children (Marks 1996; Dwork 1987). The extent and significance of these activities were greatest at the local level. Vast numbers of women were "employed" by local government in unpaid voluntary and philanthropic services (Pedersen 1993, 40). Where women were elected to local councils, they were often strong voices for maternal and child health programs (Marks 1996).[39] The importance of policy developments at this level has been strongly emphasized in recent work. Pat Thane, for example, argues that "it is . . . to the level of combined

local authority and voluntary action that we must look for the first sustained policy measures concerning mothers and children" (1991, 102). Lara
Marks asserts that "decisions on welfare taken nationally interacted and
were intrinsically informed by those taken at the local level" (1996, 5).[40]
These scholars' emphasis on local action is intended—at least in part—as
a corrective to work exclusively focused on central government action that
downplays the role of women in the making of British welfare policies
and programs (for example, Skocpol 1995b): to minimize the role of local
government was to minimize the role of women.

British women were active in the cause of infant health through
groups such as the Women's Cooperative Guild and the Women's Labour
League. The latter organization "under the auspices of the Labour
Party set up [in London in 1912] the first baby clinic in the country"
(Marks 1996, 138); and women's groups lobbied local authorities to establish maternity centers and appoint health visitors (Dwork 1987, 218;
Thane 1991, 105). Based on original historical research, Marks argues that
provision of maternal and child health services was, however, "largely
governed by the political outlook and mobilization of each [of the four
London boroughs included in her study]" and only conditionally depended
on "the overall participation of women within the philanthropic and
political arena of each area" (1996, 78). Women's lobbying success was—
with a few individual exceptions—contingent on political party support,
and women most often did their political work within not outside of
political parties.[41]

Those national organizations most directly concerned with infant
mortality—the Association of Infant Consultations and Schools for Mothers, the National Conference on Infantile Mortality, and the National League
for Physical Education and Improvement—were dominated by (almost
entirely male) medical officers of health and local doctors (Dwork 1987, 103).
The National Conference on Infantile Mortality was founded in 1905 by
five men, two of whom were local MOH and two were town officials
(Dwork 1987, 113). The Association of Infant Consultations and Schools
for Mothers was established in 1911 with a prominent pediatrician (male)
as its first chairman (163). (The two groups merged in 1912 to form the
National Association for the Prevention of Infant Mortality.)

Lewis is critical of the displacement of (largely female) voluntary workers by state employees during World War I and even more strongly of
male dominance and its consequences for the campaign against infant
mortality. It is worth noting, though, that among the strongest proponents
of state responsibility for maternal and infant welfare were the women
of the Labour Party: "they believed that the state could provide services
more systematically than the voluntary sector and, even more importantly,
could provide benefits and services as rights, as the voluntary sector
could not" (Thane 1991, 101). The question of male dominance—and its

many implications for the design and implementation of strategies to combat infant mortality—is a matter of considerable scholarly controversy (see, for example, Dwork 1987; Koven and Michel 1990, 1993).

Mothers of the Race

The politicization of infant mortality—and through infant mortality, of motherhood—took place in a demographic context of declining birth rates together with high and stable infant mortality and in a political context of intense anxiety over Britain's present and future place in the world. Feeding this anxiety were the rise of competing industrial powers (Germany and the United States) and the realization that half the country's young men were unfit to fight. If babies mattered politically as future soldiers (compare Pedersen 1993), then it behooved the nation to concern itself with their quantity and quality. British commentators, in contrast to their counterparts in France, focused primarily on quality: healthy babies were equated with national efficiency. Across the political spectrum, and whether the proposed solution was clean milk, health visiting, or the education of mothers, advocates tied their programs to "national devitalization" and the survival of the empire (Dwork 1987, 121).

Although mothers' actions had occasionally been implicated in the death of their babies from the mid-nineteenth century on, it was not until the 1900s that "the mothers of the race," their ignorance, and their need for education became the center of reformers' attention. Advocates for clean milk focused on the irresponsibility of "a large and powerful class of the community," not the irresponsibility of mothers. Dwork argues that physicians "recognized . . . that indigence was a critical and fundamental factor in the health of infants and children" (1987, 229). Nevertheless, during the period in question actions on the ground—of public officials and private voluntary groups—moved away from amelioration of the mother's environment to change in the behaviors of mothers themselves. Interpretations of this shift are sharply disputed. Jane Lewis sees it, first, as blaming the victim and, second, as an effort to stop infant mortality on the cheap:

> medical officers of health, physicians and Local Government Board officials skirted, and even denied, the influence of factors such as low incomes, poor housing conditions and sanitation, and contaminated milk. Those involved in the child and maternal welfare movement held women responsible for all infant deaths that were due to preventable causes. (1980, 81)

> Institutions set up to educate women in infant care were designed for the working class, combining middle-class philanthropy with the state's desire to save lives by the cheapest method. (1980, 61)

Dwork argues that, on the contrary, medical officers of health and local government board officials fully recognized the importance of "low incomes, poor housing conditions and sanitation, and contaminated milk," but as physicians "they were trained to be medical care providers; if they concentrated on the clinical aspects of health problems they were but addressing simply and precisely that which they knew how to do best" (1987, 229–30). Dwork asserts, further, that

> the solution of maternalism was not just a cheap and easy remedy. It is clear that maternal education was not a solution which required or even called for fundamental social change, but it was something more than "a few classes" [as Lewis claims]. The systems which were established provided a number of "social and medical services" in addition to instruction. (230)

The cost of maternal education compared to other remedies for infant mortality is, obviously, difficult if not impossible to determine. Regardless of how this shift is interpreted, however, there is consensus regarding the increased emphasis placed on maternal responsibility. "Maternal and child health services [in the early twentieth century] were aimed at drilling mothers in proper infant care and nutrition, placing the onus [of responsibility for her baby's health and well-being] on each individual mother" (Marks 1996, 25).

Canada

Canadian response to high rates of illness and death in the late nineteenth and early twentieth centuries were shaped by the economic, political, and geographic constraints described in chapter 2: the subordination of public health to economic development and the confusion about—and resulting fragmentation of—state responsibility. It was not until the early 1920s, as I have indicated, that the central government in Ottawa became seriously involved in monitoring and controlling public health. Although organized efforts to prevent disease did begin to emerge in the late nineteenth century, they were sporadic and took place primarily at the municipal level.

The framing of infant mortality as an avoidable catastrophe rather than an act of fate did not make its Canadian debut until the first decade of the twentieth century.[42] In Toronto, recognition was triggered by the publication of new and alarming vital statistics "that shocked Torontonians into the realization that their city had the same problem as London, New York, Milwaukee, and Montreal" (MacDougall 1990, 161). The immediate catalyst in Montreal is less clear. However, mortality rates by age were published by the Montreal Board of Health from at least 1900, and the francophone hygiènistes who led the movement for public health reform were fully aware of the campaign against infant mortality long underway in France (Gagnon 1910).[43] Initially at least, responses in the two cities were broadly parallel: voluntary groups or committed individuals launched "ad hoc experimental measures [for example, milk depots, well-baby clinics, health visitors] borrowed from reformist ideas and practices adopted in Britain, France, and the United States" (Comacchio 1993, 21). The fate of these measures and the ideologies surrounding them were, however, quite different.

The campaign against infant mortality in English Canada was initiated by women's groups (for example, the National Council of Women of Canada, the Imperial Order of Daughters of the Empire). The causes of infant deaths were identified broadly as "poverty, maternal ignorance, and diarrheal disease from improper feeding" (MacDougall 1990, 161). The most visible enemy, however, and one that could be immediately be addressed with models drawn from Britain, France, and the United States, was impure milk. Copying these models, voluntary groups in Toronto

> set up a system of milk depots and well baby clinics [in a number of settlement houses]. Several women's groups, churches, and Women's College Hospital, also joined the Hospital for Sick Children in providing pasteurized milk to less affluent Toronto children. Most of these groups depended on part-time medical staff and philanthropists for funding . . . in 1912–13 [when these efforts were initiated] the basic objective was to provide pasteurized milk and train Toronto's mothers in proper infant feeding techniques. (MacDougall 1990, 162)

Much more striking, however, than women's initiation of milk depots and clinics is how quickly these volunteer efforts were abandoned once there was a viable local government-run and -funded alternative. Within a year or two, the volunteers had—at their request—turned their activities over to the Toronto Health Department, where they were quickly incorporated into a new Division of Child Hygiene, expanding not only the department's staff but also the power and reach of its MOH.[44] At the same time—indeed, in the same year, 1914—Hastings was successful in obtaining a by-law making milk pasteurization compulsory throughout the city, thus largely obviating the need for milk depots.

There was no lack of opposition to Hastings's rapid expansion of his department's functions and powers. Local medical practitioners saw the department's work as infringing on their prerogatives—"they wanted public agencies to relieve them of care for the poor but to leave paying patients to their exclusive ministrations" (MacDougall 1990, 164); dairymen saw pasteurization as an unfamiliar innovation with potentially devastating economic consequences. Hastings was able to surmount these and other sources of opposition to the health department's work for reasons outlined in chapter 2: his own considerable public relations and political skills combined with strong local public and political support.

Events in Montreal took a different path. The city's response to infant mortality was shaped in large part by the francophone medical elite who dominated public health by virtue of their university positions, their active professional organizations and their leadership of provincial and municipal public health bodies (Pierre-Deschênes 1981; Baillargeon 1996, 2002).[45] These physicians were committed Quebec nationalists and were left in no doubt—the city's data made it crystal clear—that the highest infant mortality was among their compatriots.[46] Nationalist sentiment—the threat of French-Canadian infant death to the survival of French-Canada—was a major catalyst for action against infant mortality (not only by physicians, but by women, the clergy, and politicians as well). At the same time, it immensely complicated and in fact may have retarded that action (Baillargeon 1998, 2002).

Although Montreal's physicians—committed sanitarians in the Victorian mold—at first implicated bad water, bad air and in particular bad housing as causes of infant mortality (see, for example, Turmel and Hamelin 1995, 445), their attention—like that of their compatriots in Toronto— soon shifted to the mothers. In contrast to Toronto, however, where bad milk was identified as a primary cause of infant mortality, in Montreal it was secondary to mothers' failure to nurse: "le sevrage prématuré joint à un nourisson défectueux est l'un des principaux facteurs qui contribue à assombrir la statistique des morts par diarrhée [early weaning combined with poor feeding practices is one of the principal factors increasing deaths from diarrhea]" (Gagnon 1910, 716). Not poverty, but the mothers' ignorance, is responsible for mistakes in feeding, Eugène Gagnon went on to say.

To address these problems, gouttes de lait (milk stations) following the French model (along with the French nomenclature) were established on private initiative, the first in 1902 and three more in 1910. Over the next several years, some twenty such stations were set up by "small groups of reformers"—women's groups and physicians, often in association with parish priests (Baillargeon 1996, 33). Of these twenty, fifteen (75 percent) were attached to francophone Catholic parishes located in poor neighborhoods. Their activities appear to have been quite limited: the distribution of specially prepared milk for babies "deprived of the maternal breast" along with educational pamphlets (for example, Hygiène de la première enfance), and little attempt was made to adapt operations to the convenience of mothers.[47] Activities were limited, in part to assuage the hostility of private physicians resentful in Montreal, as elsewhere, of any competition with private practice. Other reasons, however, were more peculiar to Montreal.

In a series of analyses of Montreal's struggle against infant mortality, the French-Canadian historian Denyse Baillargeon makes a strong case that the obstacles to Montreal's mounting a concerted attack on what all agreed was a serious threat to the political future of French Canada arose more from power struggles among the francophone elite—physicians, feminists, and clergy—than from conflict between Francophones and Anglophones (Baillargeon 1996, 1998, 2002). The women's groups were eased out early on, their efforts denigrated by physicians. Concerted municipal action was blocked by authorities' fear of alienating the Catholic clergy. When, in 1919, the city health department decided to establish its own network of child health clinics, new clinics were opened only in parishes without an existing goutte de lait to avoid competition with the local priest, and even then the head of the health department consulted with the archbishop of Montreal before proceeding (Baillargeon 1996, 33). Baillargeon suggests, finally, that the "legendary fertility" of francophone Quebec—in which nationalists took great pride— may have resulted in some complacency about the province's far less enviable rate of infant mortality (2002).

Given that Montreal's public health reformers were preoccupied with the importance of breastfeeding, it is perhaps not surprising that they paid less attention than their counterparts in Toronto to the pasteurization of milk. Rules intended to regulate the conditions under which milk was produced—for example, inspection of dairy farms—were promulgated early in the century (that is, before 1910) by the provincial Quebec government and by the city health department. "The inadequacy of even this limited sanitary inspection was fully revealed in 1914 when the Federal Department of Agriculture published the results of a bacteriological study of the milk supply of Montréal. . . . By the time the milk reached Montréal . . . 90 percent of it was unfit for human consumption" (Copp 1974, 96–97). None of this information was new at the time. Nevertheless, in shocking testimony to the profound effects of the anglophone-francophone gulf I have described, though "pasteurization of milk was begun in the city in the first years of the twentieth century . . . prior to World War I only dairies in the English-speaking west end of the city were supplying pasteurized milk to their customers" (96).

The Canadian state's interest in infant mortality—and in the health of its citizens more generally—was catalyzed by World War I. Before that date, Comacchio argues, child welfare concerns had "derived from the natural impulses of human sympathy." By the war's end, babies had been redefined as national assets, and concern about infant mortality "came to be seen as part of the defensive foresight of citizens who would protect the future of the state" (Comacchio 1993, 59). Baillargeon has a somewhat different take, suggesting that English Canadians' campaign against infant mortality before the war was motivated less by "natural impulses of human sympathy" and more by a fear they shared with their American neighbors to the south that their own "white" population would be submerged by waves of immigrants from Eastern and southern Europe (Baillargeon 1996, 31). Whatever may have been the underlying motives of English Canadians, those of the francophone physicians who drove the response to infant mortality in Montreal and Quebec were crystal clear: the survival of francophone Canada (Gagnon 1910; Baillargeon 1996, 1998). Speaking before the Medical Society of Montreal, Gagnon said,

> Pour nous français d'origine, que l'on voudrait en certains milieux traiter comme les étrangers sur cette terre qui est nôtre pourtant, si nous voulons conserver à notre nation le prestige que lui réserve la destinée, nous devons plus que jamais étudier les moyens qui nous permettrons de diminuer la mortalité dans notre province [For us French by origin, whom some would treat as strangers in this land which is, after all, our own, if we want to retain for our nation the prestige which is its destiny, we must more than ever study the means that will allow us to reduce the mortality in our province]. (1910, 714)

It is ironic, of course, that the same passion moving Gagnon to speak so eloquently of French-Canadians as strangers in their own land made it almost impossible for many years after his talk in 1910 to bring about the mortality reductions he sought.

I have had little to say about campaigns against infant mortality in rural areas or in western Canada, due in part to a dearth of secondary sources but also to the fact that recognition and response came after the time period with which I am primarily concerned. Let me say a word, however, about western Canada, where by 1920 a strong movement on behalf of maternal and infant health had emerged, grounded in organizations of farm women (such as the women's section of the Saskatchewan Grain Growers and the United Farm Women of Alberta) and supported by the Victorian Order of Nurses (Langford 1995). Settlement of the Canadian prairies, largely in the form of isolated homesteads, peaked in 1911. There were few, or no, doctors or health services, and women gave birth at home, often with no trained attendant. Infant mortality was high not so much in the postneonatal period—infection was not the most pressing problem—but in the first week of life, associated with complications of childbirth. In this context, farm women were less concerned with the preventive measures associated with classical public health than with the provision of medical services, if not by physicians then by district nurses trained in obstetrics or by midwives. Responsibility for these services should, they believed, be assumed by the provincial and federal governments, and women lobbied these governments accordingly (Langford 1995, 297). Predictably, professional associations of doctors and nurses were strongly opposed to the farm women's demands. Given this background, it should be no surprise that agitation for government-funded health services in general would later arise first in Saskatchewan.

Chapter 4

Tuberculosis

IN 1815, an English physician, Thomas Young, wrote, "of all hectic affections, by far the most important is pulmonary consumption, a disease so frequent as to carry off prematurely about one-fourth part of the inhabitants of Europe, and so fatal as often to deter the practitioner from attempting a cure" (cited in Dubos and Dubos 1987, 9). About the same time, a French physician, Antoine Portal, observed that "there is no more dangerous disease than pulmonary phthisis [the Greek word for this condition], and no other is so common . . . it destroys a very great part of the human race" (8). A recent U.S. medical textbook on tuberculosis offers the estimate that "at the turn of the nineteenth century, one in every five people developed TB during their lifetime, making TB the number-one killer, the 'captain of all these men of death' " (Braden, Onorato, and Kent 1996, 85). For many reasons these are not particularly reliable estimates; they are as likely to be too low as too high (Dubos and Dubos 1987; Ott 1996). They convey, nonetheless, the overall importance of tuberculosis as a cause of death in nineteenth century Europe and America, its emotional impact, and its medical intractability.

Tuberculosis is a chronic infectious disease that manifests itself in different forms. Respiratory (pulmonary) tuberculosis, also known as phthisis or consumption, is the form we most commonly think of as TB. In addition to being chronic—the time from the disease's first appearance until death was counted in years rather than days or months—tuberculosis was severely debilitating and through much of the nineteenth century its ravages were greatest among young adults.[1] Historians of tuberculosis uniformly emphasize its romantic association with promising youth cut off in their prime (Dubos and Dubos 1952/1987; Guillaume 1986; Smith 1988). Despite its prominence as a cause of death, however, tuberculosis commanded little in the way of public attention in Europe or America until late in the nineteenth century. There was no cure until the discovery of antibiotics in the 1940s, and for much of the nineteenth century there was no agreement on its cause. The stories of how and why the condition known as phthisis moved onto the public stage vary considerably across our four countries. They share, however, a common scientific heritage in the discoveries of a Frenchman, Jean-Antoine Villemin, and a German, Robert Koch.

Villemin's critical findings, presented to the French Academy of Medicine in 1865 and published in 1868, were that tuberculosis is a specific disease and that it is transmissible by inoculation between animals and from man to animals (Haas and Haas 1996, 16). In 1882, Koch announced his isolation of the tuberculosis bacterium, which he identified as the cause of tuberculosis.

The different stories I will tell are composed of common elements.[2] Although Villemin had been ignored, physicians in each country openly confronted the implication of Koch's uncomfortable discovery, that TB was contagious. Reporting of cases, disinfection of victims' possessions and premises, isolation, and quarantine as means of prevention and control were uniformly considered, but not, as we shall see, uniformly adopted.[3] Establishment of sanatoria for the rehabilitation (some said cure, some said isolation) of persons with tuberculosis preceded Koch and became an important part of each country's armamentarium, as did specialized "dispensaries" for tuberculosis patients. And in each country, both governments and voluntary organizations formed around the turn of the century to combat tuberculosis were important players on the TB stage.

Before I turn to each country's story, let me briefly summarize what is known about tuberculosis mortality rates at approximately the turn of the century. The best data are from the UK. However, given the uncertainties of TB diagnosis and reporting in the nineteenth and early twentieth centuries even these data must be treated with a healthy skepticism (Cronje 1984; Smith 1988; Hardy 1993). Thomas McKeown famously argued that mortality from respiratory tuberculosis in England and Wales began to decline early in the nineteenth century, before any of what we would call public health measures had been initiated. This assertion has been widely challenged and, indeed, Ann Hardy suggests the decline may not have begun until the 1870s (1993, 214). In any case, Francis Smith (1988) presents data, based on registrar-general reports and other sources, indicating a rate for England and Wales of 128:100,000 in 1901. Neither the United States nor Canada reported country-level mortality rates with any reliability or consistency until the 1920s. Data for the cities of New York, Toronto, and Montreal all indicate mortality rates in 1900 of between 200 and 300 per 100,000 (Lerner 1993; Wherrett 1977).[4] The highest tuberculosis death rates of any North American city were in Montreal (and remained so for much of the early twentieth century).

Relative to our other three countries the highest rates were in France (Mitchell 1988, 215). Guillaume (1986) cites figures for 1888 to 1897 ranging from 577/100,000 in Paris to 145/100,000 in towns with a population of less than 5,000.

Mortality rates from pulmonary tuberculosis declined markedly in the course of the twentieth century. Despite a large body of historical and demographic as well as medical literature on tuberculosis, the reasons for this decline remain controversial. I return to this issue in the final chapter.

United States

The earliest chapters of the tuberculosis story in the United States are dominated by the rapid and enthusiastic welcome given to the idea of contagion by physicians of the New York City Health Department.[5] In 1889, seven years after Koch's announcement and six years after the first translation of his report to appear in a United States medical journal, Hermann M. Biggs (at the time a pathologist with the City Health Department) and his colleagues reported to the New York City Board of Health that tuberculosis was contagious, "acquired, as a rule, through its communication from man to man" (Teller 1988, 21). Contagion was a medically unpopular hypothesis. Only three years earlier, and two years after Koch's identification of the tubercle bacillus, the Journal of the American Medical Association (JAMA) reported that tuberculosis was not contagious. At stake in this controversy was less the etiology of tuberculosis, however, than the "relative authority of private physicians and the department of health" to oversee the prevention and management of tuberculosis (Fairchild et al. 2007). There was ample precedent for notification of communicable disease. In the last decade of the nineteenth century, in the face of "often pitched battles between physicians and health officials," New York's "municipal authorities embraced notification" of tuberculosis (n.p.).

Public Health Paternalism

Within the year following Biggs's report, the Board of Health issued a circular, "Rules to be Observed for the Prevention of the Spread of Tuberculosis," for distribution to (at the very least) households in which a death from TB had been reported. Reporting of tuberculosis cases (including names and addresses) to the health department by public institutions was made mandatory in 1894, and in 1897 this requirement was extended to all physicians. With this information in hand, the health department "dispatched a sanitary inspector to the home to initiate a program of education and supervision" (Rothman 1994, 187). In practice "education and supervision" targeted the poor: "the non-English-speaking inhabitants of the poorest tenement-house districts" (Biggs and Huddleston 1895, cited in Fairchild et al. 2007). Wealthy private patients were likely to be spared.

The spread of notification across the United States was initially uneven. Philadelphia enacted mandatory physician reporting in 1893 and rescinded it in 1894 under pressure from the Philadelphia College of Physicians. By 1908, however, eighty-four cities required registration of persons with tuberculosis and disinfection of their lodgings. The pattern set by New York City's relatively aggressive response to tuberculosis, which included "forcible detention [in public hospitals]" of "wilfully careless consumptives" (Lerner 1993, 760), characterized other dimensions of the U.S. response as well. Throughout the country, measures to combat tuberculosis were embodied in local ordinances: against public spitting and the common cup; in favor of pasteurization of milk and testing of cattle (Ott 1996; Tomes 1998; Teller 1987).

New York City's approach to tuberculosis—narrowly focused on the individual and the germ as opposed to the "larger and more diffuse problems of water supplies, street cleaning, housing reform and the living conditions of the poor" (Fee 1994, 237)—signified a watershed in American public health. Charles Chapin, commissioner of health for Providence, Rhode Island, and a leading advocate for bacteriologically based public health, made clear his disdain for old-fashioned sanitary reform: "The filth theory erroneously assumed that the infectious diseases were caused by emanations . . . from decaying matter." The public health required scientific laboratories and coordinated epidemiological research. "Instead of an indiscriminate attack on dirt, we must learn the nature and mode of transmission of each infection, and must discover its most vulnerable point of attack" (Chapin 1887, cited in Rothman 1994, 182).

Crowded, unventilated, unsanitary immigrant-occupied tenements had been implicated as a cause of tuberculosis, and a movement to improve tenement house living conditions was active in New York City at the turn of the century. The advantages of a more "discriminate attack" were clearly spelled out by one of Chapin's admirers:

> To control tuberculosis . . . it was hardly necessary to improve the living conditions of the one hundred million people in the United States—only to supervise the 200,000 active tuberculosis cases "merely to the extent of confining their infective discharges. . . . Need any more be said to indicate the superiority of the new principles, as practical business propositions, over the old?" (cited in Fee 1994, 237, italics in original)

"Bacteriology," Elizabeth Fee observes, "became an ideological marker, sharply differentiating the 'old' public health, the province of politicians, physicians, and reformers, from the 'new' public health, which would belong to scientifically trained professionals" (236).[6]

Among the—no doubt intended—effects of New York's approach was to substantially increase the authority of the city health department not only in relation to city residents but also to the city's medical practitioners. Hermann Biggs justified his conception of the department's role:

> The government of the United States is democratic, but the sanitary measures adopted are sometimes autocratic, and the functions performed by sanitary authorities paternal in character. We are prepared, when necessary, to introduce and enforce, and the people are ready to accept, measures which might seem radical and arbitrary, if they were not plainly designed for the public good, and evidently beneficent in their effects (cited in Rothman 1994, 188).[7]

Public good or no, physicians' opposition to the tuberculosis-reporting requirement was intense: "the outcry from doctors was immediate and vigorous" (Teller 1988, 22), but their reasons were mixed. Duffy, for example, points out that "a diagnosis of tuberculosis was viewed by most laypersons as the kiss of death" (1990, 197). Insurance companies often denied coverage in the event of death from tuberculosis, so that patients and their families as well as physicians who depended on the insurance for their fees had reason to conceal the diagnosis. Compliant physicians are said to have feared losing patients to less compliant colleagues or simply to colleagues willing to offer a less fearful diagnosis. And some physicians feared the consequences of public branding for the patient's relationship with family, friends, employers, and landlords (Teller 1988, 22–23). The battle to prevent tuberculosis notification was one that U.S. physicians ultimately lost. Where they succeeded was in shaping a two-tiered system that targeted the poor, the foreign-born, and African Americans, sparing affluent consumptives and their families from the more intrusive forms of surveillance and supervision (Fairchild et al. 2007).

"Zealous Activity for Stamping out the White Plague"

A further highlight of the U.S. response to tuberculosis was its incorporation in a series of crusades bordering on the religious (Tomes 1998).[8] As pointed out by the official historian of the National Tuberculosis Association (NTA), Richard Harrison Shryock, tuberculosis was "the first specific disease against which voluntary efforts were mobilized" (1957, 57). Organization began in 1892 under the leadership of a physician, Lawrence F. Flick, who had himself been diagnosed with tuberculosis in 1875.[9] By 1904, when the National Association for the Study and Prevention of Tuberculosis (later the National Tuberculosis Association) was formed, twenty-three state and local societies were already in existence, dedicated primarily to mass public education to prevent tuberculosis. The NTA had three presidents of the United States as honorary officers, along with the "backing of prominent physicians, philanthropists, and politicians":

At the peak of its influence in the late 1910s, the NTA and its approximately 1300 [largely autonomous] affiliates enlisted thousands of American men, women, and children in the work of preventing tuberculosis. Their methods were so spectacularly successful that they were imitated by subsequent groups organized to combat mental illness, cancer, diabetes, and infantile paralysis. (Tomes 1998, 114)

Among the most spectacularly successful of these methods was the Christmas Seal campaign initiated in 1908 in cooperation with the Red Cross and taken over by the NTA in 1911. Employing the most up-to-date marketing techniques, antituberculosis workers enlisted entire communities in the fight against tuberculosis.[10] The essence of the fight consisted in detailed behavioral prescriptions in the form of "tracts," "catechisms," and "commandments" to protect self, family, and community against germs. "By turning this cosmology of germ dangers into a concrete code of hygienic behavior, tuberculosis workers extended accountability for disease prevention into every nook and cranny of daily life" (Tomes 1998, 125). As Nancy Tomes points out, a striking dimension of the antituberculosis campaign was its amalgam of scientific with Protestant evangelical discourse.

The armamentarium against tuberculosis promoted by the NTA and its local counterparts included many of the same goals advocated in the other three countries: sanatoriums for advanced cases, dispensaries for the ambulatory, fresh air camps for children. What clearly distinguished the American campaign was its character as a social movement. Systematic grassroots mobilization and deliberate exploitation of the mass media aimed at converting the "hygienic heathen"—the American poor—were strategies unique to the United States. Reflecting on the movement's early years, C.E.A. Winslow, the biographer of Hermann Biggs, observed with pardonable hyperbole: "the discovery of the possibilities of wide-spread social organization as a means of controlling disease was one which may almost be placed alongside the discovery of the germ theory of disease itself as a factor in the evolution of the modern public health campaign" (1929, 200).

As in the case of infant mortality, Progressive era mobilization against tuberculosis was overwhelmingly white and middle class, classic examples of organization on behalf of rather than by those persons most affected. Far more than in the case of infant mortality, however, the national leadership of the antituberculosis movement was dominated by male physicians. Although the latter crusade was—much like the crusade against infant mortality—"a vehicle for women's action and organizing" on the state and local level (Feldberg 1995, 119), it played a less important role in nurturing women as a national political force. The balance to be struck between medical and lay leadership was a continuing bone of contention in the antituberculosis movement; the lay leadership in these early years, however, were largely male social workers.

Amy Fairchild and her colleagues characterize community-based initiatives against tuberculosis (and other diseases) in the Progressive era as "the informal state," intending thereby to emphasize the degree to which charitable organizations were "viewed [by the New York City health department] as a vital part of the landscape of TB control" (2007, n.p.; see also Feldberg 1995, 110). As they point out, these initiatives "often ended up leading to the creation of state bureaucracies as the efforts of local reformers became institutionalized within state agencies" (110). The Children's Bureau is a classic example—indeed the period's only example—of a parallel process at the federal level. The boundaries between state and—putatively nonstate—collective action were considerably more blurred in practice than they may have appeared in the abstract.

Victims and Villains

As the label for tuberculosis changed from consumption to phthisis to tuberculosis, so did the social construction of the sufferer (Rothman 1994; Ott 1996).[11] In the nineteenth century consumption was a "romantic, ambiguous affliction" (Ott 1996, 7). Accounts of the disease focus on symbolic figures such as Shelley and Keats (Dubos and Dubos 1987) or on what Sheila Rothman calls "the invalid experience" represented in the diaries and letters of educated men and women (1994). The dominant causal hypothesis accepted by most U.S. physicians was heredity—a family predisposition. This hypothesis, however, left ample room for invocation of more proximate determinants, ranging from a sedentary occupation (writing, the ministry), through an "improper" lifestyle, to the dangers of city air (Rothman 1994; Feldberg 1995). Although heredity was the preferred explanation for consumption, "no one was considered safe from its ravages" (Rothman 1994, 14). The critical turning point in construction of the disease came at the end of the nineteenth century, when physicians began to accept that tuberculosis was contagious, not hereditary, and consequently transmissible from person to person.

Accompanying this shift in understanding were not only a change of name (henceforth the condition would be identified firmly with its causative agent, the tubercle bacillus) but complex and often contradictory changes in definitions of who was at risk. Such evangelists of tuberculosis as Lawrence Flick emphasized that "consumptives are everywhere." They are

> to be found in all our places of industry, in our stores, in our factories, laundries, restaurants, in short everywhere where human effort ministers to the wants of others. In all such places their presence, unless precautions are taken, is a source of danger to fellow employees and to the public at large. (1897, cited in Ott 1996, 114)

Although statements such as these may have generated public support for the necessary "precautions," they also "bred a fear of associating with persons who had tuberculosis" (Rothman 1994, 182).

> Consumptives had to contend with the anger and prejudice of a phobic society. They were shunned, evicted, and refused treatment by doctors and nurses. . . . Consumptives and suspected consumptives alike feared for their jobs. (Ott 1996, 113)

Danger was everywhere, but not everyone was perceived as equally dangerous, nor was everyone equally endangered either by the disease itself or by the measures adopted for its control. From a condition that affected rich and poor alike, the socially prominent as well as the slum-dweller, tuberculosis came to be defined as "a disease of only some, not all, people, essentially the immigrant and the poor, not the middle or upper classes" (Rothman 1994, 181). And so, though danger was everywhere, it was the immigrant and the poor who were most to be feared, most likely to be reported to health authorities, and most likely to be "supervised" and "confined":

> By 1900 the "contagious consumptive" was a highly politicized entity, most often pictured as a menial laborer or a domestic servant, usually a recent immigrant or African-American migrant newly arrived in a city. (Ott 1996, 101)

African Americans figured prominently in early twentieth-century imagery of tuberculosis—"a primary site of meaning for the middle-class white psyche" (Ott 1996, 101)—in part because black mortality from tuberculosis was anywhere from three to four times the mortality of whites.[12] Throughout the Progressive era, the trappings of science were used by white physicians, public health officers, statisticians, and social reformers to portray African Americans either as savages inherently more susceptible to tuberculosis or as rendered more susceptible by ignorance, improvidence, and immorality and, at the same time, as a "deadly conduit of TB into the white community" (McBride 1991, 28). Southern blacks did organize, speaking against the prevailing white wisdom and launching their own antituberculosis campaign parallel to that of the National Tuberculosis Association. Their voices went largely unheard by the country's established medical and public health elites.

Finally, among the dominant themes in the campaign against tuberculosis—just as in the late twentieth-century campaign against smoking—was the protection of innocent bystanders. The adoption of "autocratic measures"—from disinfection of private homes to the prohibition of public spitting—were justified on the grounds that they protected the "innocent and unsuspecting" (Feldberg 1995, 88). "In the new tuberculosis religion spitting constituted the worst of the mortal sins" (Tomes 1998, 124): the spitter exposed not only his neighbors but his family and—worst of all—his children to the dangers of tuberculosis. Could anyone argue, one physician asked (in language almost identical to that used by anti-tobacco activists some sixty years later), "that the adult's right to do as he pleased [that is, spit] was 'greater than the right possessed by every child that is helpless to . . . determine its own surroundings—the right to receive from the community every reasonable chance to bring to its later tasks of life a sane mind in a healthy body' " (cited in Feldberg 1995, 110). *Plus ça change. . . .*

France

Jean-Antoine Villemin's report to the French Academy of Medicine in 1865 that tuberculosis was transmissible from man to rabbit by inoculation was greeted by a resounding silence. Described in a 1996 medical textbook as "the beginning of the modern era—that point at which experimental research finally began to unravel the mystery of the exact nature of tuberculosis" (Haas and Haas 1996, 16), Villemin's conclusions—that phthisis was a contagious disease and that appropriate precautions should be taken—were rejected by the academy not once but repeatedly (Guillaume 1986).[13] Villemin was a highly respected scientist, elected to the academy in recognition of his work. His conclusions were rejected not because his colleagues doubted his science but because they found the implications of his work socially and morally unacceptable.

The French medical elite's discomfort with Villemin foreshadowed a fifty-year history of medical, social, and political paralysis in the face of tuberculosis. Not until World War I called dramatic attention to the high rates of tuberculosis among the military and to the danger returning soldiers presented to the civilian population, the latter danger recognized by foreign observers but largely ignored by French authorities, did this disease begin to engage the interest of the French state (Dessertine and Faure 1988, 27). Concerted efforts to address the problem were not in fact initiated until 1917 and not by the French but instead by the Rockefeller Foundation.[14] Many of the same elements that contributed to the French failure of nerve—and arguably to France's relatively high rates of tuberculosis—reappear in other public health episodes. These elements included a politically influential medical profession with little interest in or commitment to disease prevention; a weak and divided voluntary or "philanthropic" sector; a vocal political left that argued tuberculosis was caused not by germs but by poverty and should be addressed not by dispensaries and sanatoriums but by higher wages and better living conditions; and finally a central government characterized by *prudence extrême*, fearful on the one hand that acknowledging the truth about TB would cause public panic and on the other hand that measures to address TB would be fiscally disastrous (Guillaume 1986, 172).

"If Consumption Is Contagious, We Must Speak It in Whispers"

What horrified the members of the French Academy in 1865 and continued to horrify many French physicians for the next century was not the fact that tuberculosis was contagious, but the implications of that fact for their own actions, the reactions of their patients, and the relation between doctor and patient. If tuberculosis was contagious, then its victims were dangerous to their family and friends and, one physician said in a speech to the Academy of Medicine,

> "What a calamity such a result would be! . . . [P]oor consumptives sequestered like lepers; the tenderness of [their] families at war with fear and selfishness." The possibility was too horrible for him to contemplate. "If consumption is contagious, we must say so in whispers [Si la phthisie est contagieuse, il faut le dire tout bas]." (Hermann Pidoux 1867, cited in Barnes 1995, 46)

As Guillaume observed, "l'opposition aux idées de Villemin sont une attitude de défense professionnelle, qui prend appui sur une contestation scientifique [opposition to Villemin's ideas arose from professional defensiveness that took the form of scientific disagreement]" (Guillaume 1986, 112).

Public declaration of contagion initiated a train of dramatic and unpleasant consequences—segregation, isolation, quarantine, the burning of personal effects—highly familiar to physicians of the nineteenth century from their experience with cholera and yellow fever. It was not only the disruption of victims' family and community relations that French physicians feared but also the threat to traditional relations between doctors and their patients. Particularly in the case of tuberculosis, an incurable disease, the central role of the physician was as comforter to both patient and family. He was not to frighten them, not to abandon them, and not to shatter their hopes of cure (Guillaume 1986, 79).[15] The patient's trust in the doctor was conceived as essential to this relationship. The keystone of trust was the *secret médicale*: the obligation of doctor-patient confidentiality that was almost sacred to French physicians then and now. Notification was supported by "all of France's important hygienists" (Hildreth 1987, 195) and by the health officers of major cities as early as 1894. It was, nevertheless, anathema to France's private doctors and did not become mandatory in France until 1968.

The success of French doctors in derailing notification raises interesting questions. First, medical opposition to mandatory case notification was hardly unique to France; arguments made by French doctors were made by practicing physicians in the other countries as well. Why did the French doctors prevail when doctors in Britain, Canada, and the United States were overruled? Second, if, as has been argued elsewhere, physicians' opposition to notification was part and parcel with Frenchmen's "historically conditioned" resistance to government regulation (Mitchell 1988, 229), why were these same physicians quite willing to countenance government regulation as participants in the campaign against infant mortality? The answers to these two questions are interrelated. I will return to them in the last section of this narrative, where I compare the actions of the medical profession in regard to tuberculosis with its role in combating infant mortality.

Private Action

The French began to organize against tuberculosis in the last decade of the nineteenth century, beginning with local associations to promote sanatoriums for the poor. The rich were treated by private physicians and, if necessary, sent to sanatoriums outside of France (Guillaume 1986, 185). The first such sanatorium in the Paris region was founded by Catholic sisters and opened in 1876. Others followed, organized and led by local political, business, and medical elites. Their efforts—however well intentioned—were wholly inadequate to France's massive tuberculosis problem. Regardless of whether sanatoriums were or were not an appropriate response, the weakness of the sanatorium campaign is reflected in the fact that by 1917 there were still only twelve such institutions in all of France, a total of 1,162 beds.

A second mode of action was the tuberculosis dispensary, an ambulatory service where—depending on local circumstances—persons afflicted might receive anything from medical consultation to nourishing food to home visits, to ensure appropriate sanitary arrangements and the protection of family members. Among the arguments for dispensaries as opposed to sanatoriums was that forcing the poor into sanatoriums was "not in keeping with the French love of individualism and liberty" (Hildreth 1987, 138). Sanatoriums were considered a German invention. The first such dispensary—on the politically and ideologically more acceptable model pioneered by the dean of British antituberculosis campaigners, Sir Robert Philip—was opened by Albert Calmette in 1901 at Lille.[16] Nevertheless, dispensaries did not come into their own until after World War I, largely as a result of the Rockefeller program.

French efforts against tuberculosis were directed at two groups: the poor, for whom sanatoriums and dispensaries were created, and children. And so a third project of various antituberculosis groups was the institution of summer camps where children (of all ages) could be sent for a month or more (sometimes much more) to benefit from sea, mountain, or farm air.[17]

The first national antituberculosis association—la Ligue nationale contre la tuberculose—was formed in 1902 by an eminent Bordeaux physician who was also a member of the Conseil suprême de l'assistance publique [the national council for public assistance], a quasi-public body. In addition to being medically dominated, the Ligue had much else in common with the various local associations that preceded it and with other national associations that followed. In addition to support for the projects I have mentioned, the Ligue mounted educational efforts directed primarily at the medical profession. In its structure and in many of its activities, the Ligue reflected the close association of the French campaign against tuberculosis with its campaign against alcoholism. The latter prefigured the former. The two campaigns employed the same modes of action (public meetings, educational brochures) and used the same rhetoric (patriotism and saving the race). And the same medical and political elites moved back and forth between them, acting sometimes as leaders, sometimes as participants.

Guillaume argues that the actions of the various antituberculosis groups brought tuberculosis in France out of the shadows, forcing recognition of the disease as a public problem and requiring the medical profession and public officials to speak out. The effectiveness of these actions was limited, however, not only because they were sporadic and unsystematic but also because they were highly controversial. Local doctors feared the loss of patients to dispensaries and resented the intrusion into their terrain of the medically elite hygiènistes. Local villagers—persuaded by antituberculosis campaigners that the disease was highly contagious—demanded that facilities for the tubercular be removed from their midst and ostracized urban children sent to benefit from the country air. One community's protest was led by local sanitary commission members who claimed that antituberculosis activists were "trying to convert the healthy village into a 'tuberculosis den' " (Hildreth 1987, 144). It was the multiplication of such events that led public authorities to confront tuberculosis, if at all, with *prudence extrême*. "Their attack on the tuberculosis problem was by means of the most general measures, and they left as much as possible to private initiative, ready to disavow [any action] when reactions against it were too strong" (Guillaume 1986, 172).

Public Action

The actions of the French state were nothing if not contradictory, reflecting at one and the same time anxiety about France's high rate of tuberculosis, especially in comparison with the much lower German rate, and fear of the repercussions that any action might entail. Between 1896 and 1912, no less than four parliamentary commissions were appointed to investigate the problem. Tuberculosis was declared a "grande cause nationale."

The cause was espoused by Leon Bourgeois, the father of solidarisme and among the most famous and influential French political leaders of the period. Bourgeois moved back and forth throughout his career between the presidencies of government-appointed and nongovernmental bodies to combat tuberculosis (Guillaume 1986, 191). Despite all of Bourgeois' eloquence, however, it was not until 1916—when, in the middle of World War I, the fight against tuberculosis could be equated with the fight against the Germans—that anything concrete was done.

On April 15, 1916, the loi Bourgeois creating a national system of dispensaries "d'hygiène social et de préservation antituberculeuse [for public health and protection against tuberculosis]" was passed by the French Assembly almost without debate. There was, however, less there than met the eye. Establishment of a dispensary was not obligatory. The question was left to local initiative and to a large extent to local finances. Further, the law was careful to protect the prerogatives of private physicians. Dispensaries were to provide education and referral, not medical care, and even those services were free only to the indigent. The loi Bourgeois nevertheless represented a first step toward accepting care of the tubercular and the prevention of tuberculosis as responsibilities of the state. The second step was the 1919 loi Honnorat, which defined a sanatorium as a specialized institution for the treatment of tuberculosis and was more exigent than the loi Bourgeois, requiring every département to have established a sanatorium within five years (later extended to ten years). The problem, again, was financing. Exhausted by the demands of World War I, the state was in no position to underwrite construction of sanatoriums to anything like the extent required by the law, and local authorities were in no better circumstances. Only the intervention of the Rockefeller Foundation allowed even a partial fulfillment of the law's intent.

What they perceived as the fainéante behavior of the French state in response to tuberculosis—in particular its eagerness to rely on charitable organizations—was a matter of disgust to elite hygiènistes. In a scathing editorial, the reformer Paul Strauss "blamed an excess of voluntarism for France's inability to cope with the tuberculosis crisis. 'The state does not have the right to be disinterested,' he admonished, and it was therefore up to the current government to give the signal for a general 'crusade' " (1900, cited in Mitchell 1988, 232). This conception of the state—l'État—as a prerequisite for meaningful action is equally present in the reflections of recent French historians of tuberculosis. "Missing from mobilization against tuberculosis was the usual partner in such operations, the State. Despite some important financial efforts, it neither could nor wanted to organize and coordinate the offensive" (Dessertine and Faure 1988, 122). The underlying theme of these observations, omnipresent in French discourse on public health, is that nothing can, will, or even should be done in the absence of leadership by the state.

Competing Voices

Tuberculosis in early twentieth-century France had become highly politicized. Beliefs about etiology and the measures proposed for treatment
and prevention coincided with political divisions between right-wing
defenders of capitalism and private property, the moderate (socialist) left,
and anarcho-syndicalist revolutionaries. The former—dominant in parliament and in the government throughout the period in question—
accepted theories of contagion but blamed high rates of tuberculosis
among the working class on their own bad habits: unsanitary dwellings
and—of even greater importance—alcoholism. "I am convinced," said
Paul Brouardel, dean of the Paris medical faculty, "that alcoholism is the
major factor in the high tuberculosis death rates among men" (cited in
Guillaume 1986, 149). Both victim-blaming rhetoric and proposed solutions that relied on private charity were calculated to accommodate la
morale bourgeois [the bourgeois morality] that dominated French society
and politics of the day. Fear among the propertied classes of "the dis-
gruntled French worker" as a threat to public order reached its peak in
the first years of the twentieth century, coincident with increased public attention to tuberculosis. It would have been politically dangerous,
Guillaume observed, for hygiènistes to assert that the underlying cause
of tuberculosis was poverty (la misère).

The socialist opposition departed from politically received opinions
only in downplaying the importance of "alcoholism and other immoral
behavior" in favor of "the pathogenic role of unsanitary housing and any
exposure whatsoever to the bacillus" (Barnes 1995, 219). Otherwise, there
was little to distinguish the socialist platform from that of the medical and
political establishment.

Of far greater interest is the oppositional critique of mainstream thinking about tuberculosis developed by physicians sympathetic to the anarcho-
syndicalist trade union movement.[18] David Barnes describes the two
decades that preceded World War I as the "heyday of revolutionary syn-
dicalism" in France and argues that tuberculosis as a political issue was
central to the syndicalist program. "What most distinguished the syndicalist perspective on tuberculosis from the others was its complete rejection of the medical establishment's strategy and terms of debate. In place
of slum housing, exposure to the bacillus, and moral depravity, the syndicalists targeted overwork and low wages as the chief causes of the disease"
(Barnes 1995, 230). Opposed to electoral politics and legislative solutions
as well as to private bourgeois charity, syndicalists used tuberculosis as a
recruiting tool, arguing that since unions were the only effective means to
increase wages, union membership was an attack on tuberculosis.

The syndicalist perspective announces a recurring theme in French discourse on public health—voiced by political parties, philosophers, and
some social scientists—that public health measures are at one and the

same time a distraction from the real problems of the poor and the working class and a means of normalizing and controlling their behavior. In the early twentieth century, France was unique as the only one of the four countries to have spawned an organized movement in opposition to the dominant individualist construction of tuberculosis.

Representation of the causes of tuberculosis was, as the foregoing observations make clear, an ideological and political minefield.

> To claim tuberculosis was contagious was to label the victim a danger to others and, in addition, to legitimize the intervention of public authorities, contrary to strict liberal logic. To say it was hereditary was to pillory the family. To hide the risk of contagion when one had every reason to believe in it was to choose security for the sick at their families' expense. To limit causality to heredity and contagion was to deny the importance of individuals' work and home environment (milieux de travail et de vie). At the extreme, to construe tuberculosis as the result of exploitation of man by man [as did the syndicalists] was to court revolution. (Guillaume 1986, 33)

Given these unattractive choices, it is little wonder that French public officials shied away from the topic as long as they could, saying as little as possible and making what they did say as obscure as possible.

Tuberculosis and Infant Mortality: A Digression on Medical Politics

Physicians' reception (enthusiastic or hostile) and interpretation of the scientific discoveries of the late nineteenth century depended heavily on the perceived consequences of these discoveries for the prestige and power of the medical profession in general, and of their own position within the profession in particular. Describing late twentieth-century scientific conflict over the dangers posed by the ozone layer, Karen Litfin remarks that there is no straight path from knowledge to policy consensus. "Information is incorporated into preconceived stories and discourses; it is framed, interpreted, and rhetorically communicated. In policy controversies, information begets counter information. Knowledge is embedded in structures of power: disciplinary power, national power, and socioeconomic power" (1994, 51). Late nineteenth-century bacteriological knowledge was embedded not only in structures of disciplinary and national power, but also in structures of—and struggles over—professional power: the power of medical elites, of physicians in private practice, and of physicians who practiced public health. In broad terms and across all four countries in this study, the new bacteriology was embraced by public health officials and medical elites (often the same individuals), who saw it as a source of increased legitimacy and status for themselves and their profession, but was greeted with suspicion and even hostility by local doctors. This generalization, however, does little justice either to the complexity of the issues involved or to cross-national differences in the strength of the protagonists and in how the pertinent issues were framed and resolved. Let me elaborate beginning with the contrast between French physicians' enthusiastic endorsement of infant mortality as a public danger and their extreme reluctance to similarly characterize the dangers of tuberculosis.

France: Tuberculosis and Infant Mortality   The gulf between France's local doctors who practiced in provincial towns and villages and the poor urban quartiers of Paris and other big cities and the country's hospital-based medical elite was described in chapter 2. Convinced that their social and economic interests were threatened, and that elite physicians were indifferent to the threat, local physicians moved to protect those interests by forming their own *syndicats*. State support for the protection of infant health was consistent with this project: "French medical organizations were among the most vocal supporters of public maternal and infant welfare programs" (Klaus 1993b, 243). State-mandated reporting of contagious disease for the purpose of isolating the sick person was not and was, as I have remarked, vehemently opposed by these same organizations (Latour 1986, 375; Hildreth 1987). The difference appears paradoxical. Among the strongest objections of French physicians to contagious-disease notification was that it made them into servants of the state, obliged to "denounce" their patients to the authorities (Guillaume 1986, 123). At the same time, Alisa Klaus argues, these physicians "depended heavily on the state for their professional legitimacy. They derived much of their authority in maternal and child health through public institutions, as they were called upon to certify, inspect, and supervise in the name of the state" (1993b, 284). The paradox, however, is more apparent than real. Physicians organized into syndicats were able to use their positions of political influence in the Third Republic to ensure that medical assistance to mothers and babies was structured to their liking, preserving the private contract between doctor and patient as the cornerstone of preventive as well as curative medical care. In the same period, and with equal success, they thwarted the passage of any legislation that included mandatory tuberculosis reporting requirements (Hildreth 1987; Ellis 1990; Ramsey 1994). The aim of the syndicats in both cases was the same: to protect the authority and power of individual practitioners against encroachment by the state. The ultimate irony, of course, was that the corps médical did not hesitate to bask in the "favorable reputation created by the work of Pasteur and Lister" even as they actively opposed many of the public health reforms this work implied (Hildreth 1987, 13).

France and New York City: An Instructive Comparison   When it came to tuberculosis reporting, France was an outlier among the four countries.

The sharpest contrast was with New York City, where tuberculosis reporting became mandatory in 1897. Given that private physicians were at this period almost uniformly opposed to notification, what accounts for the cross-national variability in the speed with which reporting was adopted and in the rigor of its enforcement? In sorting out plausible from implausible explanations, it is helpful to focus on the extremes.

There were many similarities in the circumstances that confronted physicians in France and New York City at the end of the nineteenth century. Medical practice was highly competitive (not only with other physicians but with practitioners of alternative therapies), and the majority of local doctors, American and French, struggled to make a living. In both countries, by contrast, not only did "the physicians who promoted public health . . . [represent] the elite of the profession" (Duffy 1990, 196), but in both cases these elites were extremely well connected politically. There were, nevertheless—and, again, in both places—substantial and well-publicized disagreements among elites as to the causes and contagiousness of tuberculosis, aired at length in the French and New York Academies of Medicine (Mitchell 1988; Fox 1975). Uncertainty about its scientific underpinnings was magnified and used by opponents in the academies and among the leaders of organized medicine to undermine the public health argument for tuberculosis reporting.

A critical difference between the two settings—arguably the critical difference—was that in France, but not (at that time) in the United States, organized medicine was a powerful force. "New York medicine on the eve of the twentieth century was fluid, chaotic, and riddled with factions. This disorganization," Daniel Fox argues, "may have been more influential than the mystique of modern science in enabling the innovations in tuberculosis control to occur" (1975, 179). Comparison of New York City with France at the same period lends considerable support to Fox's hypothesis. The two settings were distinguished not by differences in enthusiasm for "the mystique of modern science," not by the prestige and political connections of advocates for public health, by practitioners' concerns for their economic livelihood, not even by the extent of factionalism. What did distinguish them was the presence throughout France of the *syndicats*. Not only were they organized for the specific purpose of protecting the economic interests of local practitioners but also, as noted earlier, the syndicats were able to take advantage of French physicians' remarkably high level of insertion into local and national politics to ensure that those interests were fully represented. American physicians enjoyed no such representation.

In the United States, mandatory reporting of tuberculosis was a question decided at the municipal level, and the speed of adoption was highly dependent on local circumstances. Comparing New York with other U.S. cities, it is difficult not to conclude that the major factors bringing about notification were strong public health leadership, strong local political and media support, and the absence of effective medical or community opposition. The British case—in which notification was delayed but ultimately adopted before World War I—presents a somewhat different set of issues, as we shall see in the narrative that follows.

Britain

Tuberculosis emerged onto the public stage in Britain in the 1880s and 1890s, corresponding to a shift in public consciousness from the idea of TB as solely an "individual concern" of the patient and the family to TB as a "social problem to be tackled by the state on behalf of society" (Hardy 1993, 253). The first TB dispensary opened in 1887 and the first specialized hospital in 1889. Both were founded in Edinburgh by Sir Robert Philip, an Edinburgh physician and "a prominent figure throughout the anti-tuberculosis campaign in Britain until his death in 1939" (Bryder 1988, 19). The major voluntary organization, the National Association for Prevention of Consumption and Other Forms of Tuberculosis (NAPT), was founded in 1898 with royal sponsorship and with leading physicians and government officials in attendance at the inaugural meeting (Bryder 1988, 15). Mandatory reporting came later. Tuberculosis was omitted deliberately from the Infectious Diseases (Notification) Act of 1889; the first locality to institute mandatory notification was Sheffield, in 1904, and case notification did not become compulsory throughout Great Britain until 1913.

What accounted for the changed perception of tuberculosis in the late nineteenth century? British historians of the disease propose several hypotheses (Bryder 1988, Hardy 1993). First, and most obviously, were Koch's revolutionary discoveries that suggested "new possibilities of preventive action" beyond sanitary reform. Second, Hardy suggests that public discussion of the new bacteriology effectively dissolved "private reservations about a socially sensitive disease," making possible, for example, the formation of the National Association for the Prevention of Consumption and Other Forms of Tuberculosis (Hardy 1993, 260). Finally, Linda Bryder argues that "[a] more important factor [than the germ theory]" in the emergence of tuberculosis as a national problem was public attribution of Britain's imperial decline to the poor physical condition of its people: "tuberculosis cannot be viewed in isolation from the general health movement which arose and flourished in the early twentieth century" (1988, 22).

Recent historiography of tuberculosis in Britain has been carried out in the context of scholarly controversy over when and why tuberculosis mortality declined in England and Wales (McKeown 1976; Szreter 1988; Mitchell 1988; Hardy 1993; McFarlane 1989; Cronje 1984). Central to this controversy is Britain's early development of a medically dominated public health infrastructure (Fee and Porter 1991). Disputing McKeown's emphasis on improved nutrition, Hardy, Mitchell, and others argue that social intervention in the guise of sanitary reform spearheaded by the MOHs was of primary importance in the decline of tuberculosis (Hardy 1993; Mitchell 1988; see also Szreter 1988).

> As with typhus, whose etiology appears in many ways to have been similar to that of tuberculosis, the efforts of London's MOHs, in terms of demolishing old housing stock, cleaning houses, improving domestic ventilation, and educating the public, seem to have played a critical role in reducing the impact of [tuberculosis]. (Hardy 1993, 265)

Hardy goes further, suggesting that MOHs were concerned about phthisis from the 1850s onward, a concern they seldom recorded due to the "prevailing social conventions and mythology of tuberculosis" but on which they acted nonetheless (1993, 228). More recently Robert Millward and Frances Bell have identified housing regulation by local government as a major factor in late nineteenth century mortality decline: "the alleviation of living congestion by better town planning and better housing may have reduced exposure to airborne diseases like tuberculosis" (2000, 157).

Tuberculosis was believed by most nineteenth-century British doctors, as well as the general public, to be hereditary. Other causal hypotheses abounded, however, including "impure air" and "culpable deviations from a normal moral healthy state"—for example, sexual indulgence, alcoholism, immodest dress, mental exertion, and so on (Smith 1988, 27). The hereditary hypothesis continued to be preferred, even after Koch, in part because of what British doctors—like the French—saw as the unacceptable consequences of embracing contagion: "A phthisic would have to be treated like a medieval leper 'separated from his family, to be isolated, shut up . . . refused admission into hospitals and asylums . . . his clothes should be destroyed, and whether he die or recover, the home . . . should be burnt' " (Bennet 1884, cited in Smith 1988, 49).

The social and political sensitivity of tuberculosis delayed acceptance of the fact that it was contagious until the end of the nineteenth century and generated substantial resistance to mandatory notification:

> Tuberculosis was no ordinary infectious disease. Many doctors dreaded committing themselves and their patients when diagnosis was peculiarly difficult, prognosis was uncertain and the pattern of infection was unverifiable and ubiquitous. Compulsory notification also daunted local authorities because it entailed isolation hospitals, removal from employment and schools for indefinitely long periods and widespread home fumigation. (Smith 1988, 69)

Given the fear of notification's social consequences together with the active opposition of the Local Government Board, even the most progressive MOHs were unsure that compulsory notification was desirable (Hardy 1993, 262). The MOH for Glasgow, James Russell, wrote in 1896 that "when the issues concern interference with human conduct, and involve the personal liberty of a considerable section of the community, even on the plea of the safety of the remainder, we are bound to ask if the game is worth a candle" (cited in Hardy 1993, 258).[19] Hardy argues that notification and other "preventive" measures were ultimately made possible by a "politically motivated" redefinition of tuberculosis as a disease of poverty:

> If preventive programmes for phthisis were to have a chance of success without disrupting the fabric of society, then the well-to-do classes' frantic fear of infection—"indiscriminating even to absurdity"—must be diffused, and the stigma of infection relieved. The preventive authorities sought to achieve this by emphasis on transmission through dust, but also by stressing the connection of the disease with poor hygiene and poverty. Notification, sputum tests, disinfection, and associated preventive paraphernalia could be disassociated from the better classes by judicious propaganda. (1993, 263)

And so, compulsory notification was introduced gradually, starting "where it was cheapest" by requiring Poor Law medical officers to report their cases beginning in 1908 (Smith 1988, 69).[20] All cases were made notifiable from 1913 on recommendation of the Royal Commission on Tuberculosis.

Returning briefly to the questions raised in this narrative, why did mandatory tuberculosis notification ultimately prevail in Britain and not in France, and why was its enactment delayed until 1913, later certainly than in New York City and later, even, than in many cities, states, and provinces elsewhere in the United States and Canada? Unlike in France, the delay cannot be attributed to the relative political clout of medicine and public health. Great Britain in the late nineteenth century was distinguished not only from France, Canada, and the United States but also from every other Western country in the sweep and power of organized public health and the ability and effectiveness of its often distinguished medical officers of health, located in every city and town throughout the country. Local practitioners, however, were also well represented in the power structures of medicine and public health. The British Medical Association, the BMA's lobby in Parliament, and—of particular importance—the *British Medical Journal* and *The Lancet* were active and vocal advocates of practitioners' interests. Both forms of practice were strongly entrenched and there is little evidence of the antagonism between them that existed in France. Nor were British practitioners opposed to notification as such.

Notification of most contagious diseases—with the striking exception of tuberculosis—was made compulsory by act of Parliament in 1899, and might have happened fifteen years earlier had it not been for the opposition of the Local Government Board (Brand 1965, 60). More important reasons for the delay in Britain were the absence of central government support for tuberculosis notification, together with the extreme social stigma—created in large part by antituberculosis campaigners themselves—that attended this disease.[21]

Tuberculosis dispensaries and sanatoria for the working classes were a prominent dimension of the British response to tuberculosis; indeed, much of the twentieth-century history of tuberculosis in Britain is the history of these institutions (for example, Smith 1988, Bryder 1988). Dispensaries appear to have functioned primarily for record-keeping purposes and as an entrée for "Lady Health Visitors" to inspect the home and conduct a "march-past" of its occupants for signs of tuberculosis (Bryder 1988, 33–34). Francis Smith describes sanatoria as "medically supervised refuges from the bad air, crowded households and wear of industrial life, set in well-drained, breezy but mild countryside" (1988, 97). This attractive picture is somewhat belied by the fact, cited by Linda Bryder, that in 1911 over 60 percent of beds provided for tuberculous patients were in Poor Law institutions (1988, 32). The perceived importance of sanatoria in the management of tuberculosis (and the salience of the disease itself) is attested to by the fact that a "sanatorium benefit" was included in the 1911 National Health Insurance plan, providing, in principle, for the treatment of "every tuberculous man, woman, and child in the country" (McFarlane 1989, 66).[22]

Among the most influential actors in the antituberculosis campaign was the National Association for the Prevention of Consumption and Other Forms of Tuberculosis: "a highly vocal and effective pressure group in advocating sanatoria and disseminating propaganda on the infectious nature of the disease" (McFarlane 1989, 65). In many respects the activities of the NAPT paralleled those of its American counterpart: an antispitting campaign, mass education, and the like. However, the patronizing tenor of its message ("the masses must be instructed") and its composition (which Francis Smith described as "medical panjandrums and aristocratic ladies") suggests a rather different organization. The NAPT was dominated by individuals with a vested interest in dispensaries and sanatoria, and was more markedly class-based than the corresponding association in the United States. Tuberculosis became an "item for fashionable philanthropy" (Smith 1988, 124).[23] The popular Christmas seals that brought tuberculosis into every corner of the United States from as early as 1911 were not adopted by the British until the 1930s. Nor, with the single exception of compulsory notification, did the British follow the U.S. efforts to achieve prevention through local ordinances. "The campaign against the disease was carried out in the twentieth century by diverse means, not least following the NAPT's precept that the force of law should not be used to carry out preventive objects in connection with tuberculosis" (Hardy 1993, 264).

Between the nineteenth and early twentieth centuries, tuberculosis was redefined by anti-tuberculosis campaigners from "being a socially indiscriminate disease transmitted by hereditary tendency and/or adverse environmental circumstances" to "a social disease, determined by poverty and all the unfortunate hygienic habits which poverty induced" (Hardy 1993, 263). Risk among the rich was attributable to the poor: "Tubercle is in truth a coarse, common disease," an NAPT council member said in 1912, "bred in foul breath, in dirt, in squalor. . . . The beautiful and the rich receive it from the unbeautiful poor" (Bryder 1988, 20). Prevention required that "individuals and communities [be] shown that the disease is maintained through ignorance and folly, and its removal lies completely in their hands" (Robert Philip 1912, cited by Bryder 1988, 19), in other words a classic appeal for personal responsibility and lifestyle change.

Among the consequences of the scare tactics employed by the NAPT was a profound fear of tuberculosis and stigmatization of its victims, leading to a phenomenon familiar in the repertory of responses to stigmatized health conditions. "A proposal in 1925 to buy a site in Lincoln Grove, Manchester, for a new dispensary was blocked by local ratepayers who argued that a consumption den in the neighborhood would congregate undesirables and reduce property values" (Smith 1988, 71). Francis Smith raises the question—interesting in part because it is a question not raised by American historians of tuberculosis—of why "respectable lower middle class and working class people" did not rise up in response to a system of prevention and care that was both inadequate and patronizing. In explanation, he cites the "hidden, shameful" nature of tuberculosis "among families with a job or small business to protect," (112) the physical and social weakness of tuberculosis sufferers, and the influence of the "sanatorium benefit" in buying off manual workers protected under the 1911 National Health Insurance plan (245).

Canada

A full translation of Koch's 1882 address to the Physiological Society of Berlin describing his discovery of the tubercle bacillus was published that same year in the *Canadian Medical and Surgical Journal*. Georgina Feldberg argues that "leaders of Canadian medicine easily and publicly accepted Koch's bacillus as the specific cause of tuberculosis and quickly began to formulate programs of disease control predicated on the eradication of this bacterium" (1995, 40). Some leaders—particularly in Ontario—may indeed have begun to "formulate programs," but not all physicians, let alone government officials and the public were on board. Until experiences in the first world war exposed the full dimensions of tuberculosis in Canada and demonstrated governments' capacity for a serious response, mustering the economic, social, and political resources necessary to accomplish these leaders' ambitions was an almost unremittingly uphill battle (McQuaig 1979).

The Canadian response to tuberculosis was shaped by climate and geography, by the overriding concern of political and business elites with economic development and peopling of the country's vast open spaces, by beliefs that targeted immigrants and Canada's native peoples (among whom tuberculosis death rates were starkly high) as the principal vectors of disease, and. by a constitution ambiguous in its allocation of responsibilities between the central government, the provinces, and the municipalities and with "no specific provision for public health" (Cassel 1994, 281).

This ambiguity is starkly reflected in a paper by one Dr. E. J. Barrick, read before the Canadian Medical Association in 1899. Dr. Barrick advocated that a sanatorium be built for "the consumptive poor."

> It is claimed that the Dominion Parliament has "no power," the British North America Act having delegated that power to the provinces. . . . It is claimed that the provinces, having a fixed income and an increasing demand from the existing charities, have "no money" for rural sanatoria. It is claimed by prominent municipal politicians, and I have heard them say, "it is none of our business; it is a national question and should be dealt with by the Government." It is said by philanthropic and charitable people that there is "no use trying to cope with a question of such magnitude unless the three other sources mentioned co-operate." (1899, 3)

Barrick's solution—one that would sound entirely familiar to anyone acquainted with the language of contemporary Canadian health-policy pronouncements—was that the three levels of government, along with "philanthropic and charitable people" should "co-operate" to fund the sanatorium: "I am sure that when a clear, well-defined and workable plan is presented wherein the three other mentioned sources would co-operate, a liberal response would be forthcoming from the charitably-disposed" (1899, 6).

Barrick's cooperative ideal was not realized in his lifetime: "By 1900 [the situation of the 'consumptive'] was indeed desperate—provincial governments refused to act, claiming lack of funds, the federal and municipal governments both denied responsibility and in the latter case pleaded poverty as well" (McQuaig 1979, 12). Into the vacuum created by what they perceived to be a governmental shirking of responsibilities stepped a wide range of voluntary associations "founded by wealthy and middle-class citizens and aided by various women's groups . . . women's institutes, and local councils of women." Local antituberculosis leagues, "fueled with idealism and enthusiasm inspired by the social gospel, were chronically short of funds, and organized on a local, patchwork basis. As one pioneer . . . later reflected, it was 'primarily a humanitarian movement of lay people' " (McQuaig 1979, 17–18).[24] The National Sanatorium Association was formed in Toronto in 1896, and the Canadian Association for the Prevention of Consumption and Other Forms of Tuberculosis had its first meeting in 1901. Their titles notwithstanding, these associations were largely confined to the few large cities of English Canada. They depended heavily on their U.S. counterparts not only for educational materials but also for overall guidance. And, as Katherine McQuaig repeatedly emphasizes, they had very little money. Not until 1927— fourteen years after the United States—was a nationwide Christmas Seal campaign launched in Canada, with help from the United States.

Canadian antituberculosis associations saw health as a government responsibility. They lobbied for legislation against public spitting, for notification of tuberculosis cases to public health authorities and, above all, for the building of sanatoria (McQuaig 1979).[25] The effectiveness of these efforts varied widely. In 1912 the Toronto chapter of the Canadian Association for the Prevention of Tuberculosis considered that its work could now be done by the health department and gave up its charter (110). At about the same time on Prince Edward Island, "pressure from the well-educated segments of society . . . proved unable to convince either municipal or provincial governments to part with the needed funds [to construct a sanatorium]" or, for that matter, to hire a public health officer (Baldwin 1990, 126). The notorious indifference of Montreal's city government to public health and the complex circumstances that gave rise to that indifference were described in the narrative on infant mortality. As noted earlier, Montreal had the highest rates of tuberculosis in North America. "The tuberculosis workers unceasingly both pleaded and demanded more enforced legislation, dispensaries and accommodation for consumptives—to no avail" (McQuaig 1979, 125).

Mandatory notification of tuberculosis cases was slow to be enacted, and "few doctors reported cases of the disease from their practice [voluntarily] because victims were often denied life insurance coverage" (MacDougall 1990, 127). Writing in 1899, Barrick remarked that "public opinion is not and will not for some years be ripe for notification and compulsory isolation in tuberculosis as is now enforced by the Boards of Health in cases of small-pox, diphtheria, and scarlet fever" (Barrick 1899, 7). Notification was made mandatory in Ontario in 1911; nevertheless, "only 40 per cent of the tuberculosis deaths in 1913 had been reported to the authorities prior to death" (McQuaig 1979, 123). Jay Cassel remarks that Ontario's move "immediately prompted protests, but the regulation remained and was soon adopted by other governments" (1994, 294).

The purpose of notification—at least as practiced in New York City in those early years—was the institution of measures to prevent further spread of the disease (Rothman 1994; Lerner 1993). It is an intriguing reflection on the rather different Canadian perspective that (as McQuaig points out) tuberculosis workers in that country began to place less emphasis on notification once they "recognized notification was of little use unless they had facilities [that is, sanatoria] to treat the cases once they were reported" (1979, 123). Canadians have historically, suggests Cassel, paid more attention to treatment than prevention (1994, 276).

Inscribed in the ideology of late nineteenth- and early twentieth-century Canadians, as noted earlier, was belief in the health-giving properties of the Canadian outdoor climate and the attendant resistance to disease of native-born Canadians. The obverse of these beliefs was a conviction that urban life was insalubrious (overcrowded urban slums were breeders of disease) and that tuberculosis was most common among immigrants, except those from Great Britain (McQuaig 1980; Cassel 1994).[26] Tuberculosis was "the inevitable consequence of the rot of urban civilization" exemplified by "low wages, poor working and living conditions, alcoholism, and even eugenics" (McQuaig 1984, 297). The solution was urban reform. " 'Thus, for each municipality tuberculosis becomes a sociological problem. To improve the social conditions of poverty, living conditions and ethics is in great part to overcome this disease' " (Canadian Association for the Prevention of Consumption, 1909, cited in McQuaig 1979, 16). In practice, antituberculosis campaigners' attack on city life was largely rhetorical; their energies were focused instead on schemes to move tuberculosis patients to the country, schemes of dubious value to poor city dwellers.

Imbued with the myth of the healthy Canadian outdoorsman, campaigners against tuberculosis blamed the disease on immigrants: "the evidence would seem to show that this country is simply the dumping ground for those afflicted with tuberculosis and other diseases" (physician-in-chief of the Canadian Association for the Prevention of Consumption, 1907, cited in McQuaig 1979, 54). Tuberculosis workers "were blatant in their preference for the Canadian born, and unshakable in their belief that the native product was better physically and mentally than the imported one. . . . They found it galling that government would spend funds to import these 'inferior' people instead of protecting their own" (McQuaig 1979, 122). Enthusiasm for the native product did not extend to Canada's native (aboriginal) peoples. Indians' high tuberculosis rates were blamed on their racial and moral inferiority, justifying government policies of remarkable cruelty and neglect (Lux 2001). Ironically, the high rates among Indians were a strong "stimulus to the crusade" against TB, "for there was a general fear that the Indians could infect the white settlements" (Wherrett 1977, 14).

Commenting on the early history of the antituberculosis campaign in Canada, Cassel remarks that "the campaign only got up to speed when government stepped in at the end of the 1910s" (1994, 294), that is after World War I. The major accomplishment—if that is the right word—of the voluntary associations I have described was to create awareness, and fear, of tuberculosis and of the tubercular. In brochures, pamphlets, posters and public lectures, they stressed the ubiquity of the germ and the dangers of contagion. "The result of all this discussion," complained Toronto's medical officer of health, "is that matters at the present time [1901] are in a worse condition than they were ten years ago. The dissemination of the knowledge and the fear that the disease is communicable has had the effect of closing the doors of every hospital and home against the unhappy victim, and they are now literally left to die uncared for" (McQuaig 1979, 35). Individuals with tuberculosis "were ostracized unmercifully" and it became extremely difficult to find a site for a sanatorium: " 'In trying to educate the people as to the contagious nature of tuberculosis, it is to be regretted that we have unfortunately created a sort of horror of sanatoria' " (cited in McQuaig 1979, 37). These comments are a measure of the voluntary associations' success in constructing a perceived threat to the public's health. Concerted action in response to that threat would have to wait.

PART III

THE LATE TWENTIETH CENTURY

Chapter 5

Smoking

THE CONNECTION between smoking and lung cancer was established, to all intents and purposes, simultaneously by British and American investigators following virtually identical scientific pathways. An "alarming" rise in death rates attributed to cancer of the lung was observed in both countries in the late 1940s, in England by statisticians employed by the registrar-general's office and in the United States by epidemiologists at the American Cancer Society (Lock, Reynolds, and Tansey 1998; Nathanson 1999; Kluger 1996). In 1950 retrospective case-control studies concluding, in the words of the British study, that "smoking is a factor, and an important factor, in the production of carcinoma of the lung" were published within four months of each other in the *British Medical Journal* and the *Journal of the American Medical Association* (Doll and Hill 1950; Wynder and Graham 1950). Responding in part to the skepticism with which these early studies were received, large-scale population-based prospective studies quickly followed (limited in both countries to men), and, again, the results were reported simultaneously, "on almost the same day" in June of 1954 (Kluger 1996, 168). These results are, of course, no secret. Both the British (Doll and Hill 1954) and the American (Hammond and Horn 1954) studies demonstrated a powerful association between smoking and not only lung cancer but heart disease as well. These associations were accepted as causal by the British Medical Research Council in 1957 (Doll 1998) and by the authors of the first U.S. Surgeon General's Report on Smoking and Health in 1964 (U.S. Department of Health, Education, and Welfare 1964). Not until thirty-five years after the publication of the surgeon general's report were these causal relations publicly acknowledged by the industry itself: "there is 'an overwhelming medical and scientific consensus that cigarette smoking causes' diseases including lung cancer, emphysema, and heart disease" (Meier 1999, A1:4). And thereby, of course, hangs many a tale.[1]

Whereas AIDS burst suddenly upon the world, forcing countries into almost immediate confrontation with this new and exotic threat to their populations, cigarettes and tobacco were old friends, and recognition of the dangers they presented came slowly and unevenly. Tobacco was introduced into Europe by Jean Nicot, the French ambassador to Portugal, who in 1560 sent seeds and plants (originating, most likely, in Brazil) to the French court. Promoted as a "wonder plant"—an herbal remedy for countless ills, from the migraines of the French queen mother to ulcers and epilepsy—and legitimized by its royal and noble associations, tobacco use was rapidly incorporated into European culture, permeating "all European social classes at about the same time" (Goodman 1993, 47).

Tobacco made the transition from herbal remedy to an essential element in the colonial political economy of Europe during the course of the seventeenth century. For the English and French, it became the sine qua non of settlement—grown in the colonies, principally the American colonies, as a cash crop, exported to the mother country, and re-exported to the rest of the world (Goodman 1998). Jordan Goodman makes a useful division of tobacco's history into three periods: first, the seventeenth and eighteenth centuries, when tobacco became a key element in the construction of the European mercantile state; second, the rise of the cigarette as an item of mass consumption in the late nineteenth and early twentieth centuries; and, finally, the late twentieth-century globalization of the tobacco industry in the form of giant multinational cigarette companies (1998, 5). I will return to this history in more detail in the context of each country's tobacco story. The point of these initial comments is to emphasize the massive and well-entrenched economic and political constituencies that tobacco enjoys and has enjoyed for four centuries. Furthermore, though there have long been dissenting voices against tobacco, only in the second half of the twentieth century did these voices become a serious challenge to the tobacco industry.[2]

The gradual discovery of tobacco and smoking as major public health problems over the past fifty years has generated an enormous professional, scholarly, and popular literature, far more, however, in the three Anglo-Saxon countries than in France, and far less contentious in tone than the literature that surrounds AIDS. Here I summarize very briefly the epidemiologic data on smoking and on smoking-related mortality (primarily lung cancer mortality) from each of the four countries, and describe the major strategies for prevention of the diseases associated with smoking.

Prevalence and Mortality

There are two alternative ways of estimating how much a country's population smokes: on the basis of tobacco sales (consumption) and on the basis of population sample surveys (prevalence). Nicolaides-Bouman and colleagues argue that smoking is substantially underreported in prevalence

Figure 5.1   Annual Cigarette Consumption, 1970 to 2000

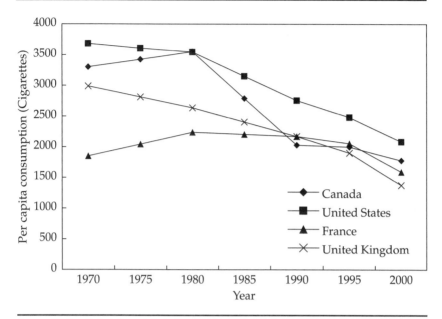

Source: Shafey, Dolwick, and Guindon (2003).

surveys, ranging from 30 to 40 percent in Canada, to 10 to 30 percent in France (1993).[3] Sales data have the additional advantage that they are reported in comparable form over relatively long periods. Data on annual per capita cigarette consumption for the 1970 to 2000 period are shown in figure 5.1. Most striking is the markedly different consumption pattern in France as compared with the other three countries. Consumption in the United States, Canada, and the UK dropped almost continuously beginning in 1980, whereas only in the past decade has French cigarette consumption begun to show signs of decline. This distinctive pattern appears even more clearly in figure 5.2, which shows each country's average consumption over time relative to its position in 1970.

Prevalence data are consistent with these observations. As shown in figure 5.3, self-reported smoking prevalence in 2000 among French men was markedly higher than in the other three countries.[4] French women, on the other hand, appear to smoke no more than women in Canada and the United States and less than those in the UK.[5] Smoking patterns vary markedly by social class both within and between countries. Before it was publicly recognized as a danger to human health, smoking was essentially classless. Everybody smoked. Declines in smoking, however, have

Figure 5.2   Annual per Capita Consumption, Three Year Moving Average, 1970=100

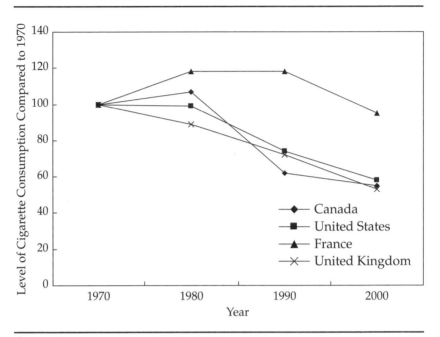

Source: Shafey, Dolwick, and Guindon (2003).

been more pronounced in the middle class and much more pronounced in the upper class, however class is measured (Nathanson 1999; Townsend, Roderick, and Cooper 1994; Health Canada 2005).[6] Again, France is the exception: depending on the population surveyed, social class differences in smoking are much less marked there or absent altogether (Hill 1998; de Peretti et al. 1995). Thirty-four percent of French physicians smoke, for example, compared with 3.3 percent in the United States (Shafey, Dolwick, and Guindon 2003).

In 1996, Cole and Radu (1996) reported the first overall decline of cancer death rates in the United States since 1900 and attributed about half of the decline to reductions in smoking since 1965.[7] Whereas lung cancer mortality rates increased steadily in all industrialized countries during most of the twentieth century, by the mid-1980s male rates had begun to flatten or decline; the turn-around to a declining trend was clearly evident in Britain (Thom and Epstein 1994). Data on lung cancer incidence and mortality reported by Michael Coleman and his colleagues in 1993 are consistent with these observations. With respect to Canada, these authors report that "the trends are qualitatively similar" to those in the United

Figure 5.3   Smoking Prevalence, 2000 to 2002

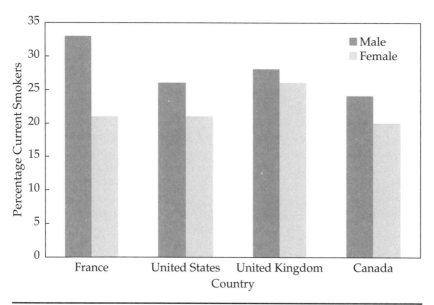

Source: Shafey, Dolwick, and Guindon (2003).

States, though the pattern of decreasing male risk "is considerably more pronounced in the USA" (Coleman et al. 1993, 333). In France, by contrast, men's lung cancer incidence and mortality rates have been increasing since the 1960s. The country-specific trends in lung cancer mortality reported by these authors in 1993 and 1994 are clearly evident in the most recently available data, shown in figure 5.4. Men's lung cancer mortality rates dropped earliest and most sharply in the UK; these rates have begun to drop in the United States and Canada as well, following parallel curves in the two countries; and French male rates have increased to the point that in 2000 they were the highest of the four countries.

In all four countries, the lung cancer rates for women are substantially below the comparable rates for men. The pattern of change in these rates, however, is quite different not only as between women and men but also as between countries. In the United States, Canada, and the UK, women's rates have increased steadily throughout the period of observation, albeit with some slight evidence of flattening in the UK. Rates among French women have remained low and increased slowly since the early 1980s. Both gender and country difference in lung cancer mortality trends are, in large part, a reflection of differences in timing: women in northern Europe and North America did not start smoking

Figure 5.4   Lung Cancer Mortality Rates, 1980 to 2000

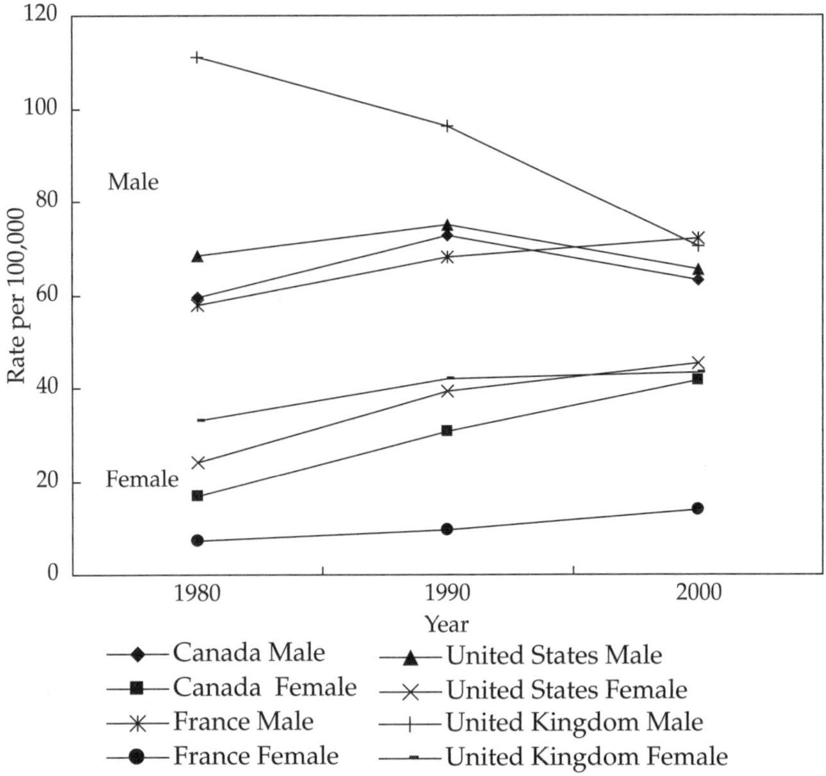

Source: World Health Organization (2005).

in large numbers until immediately before and during World War II, and French women not until the late 1960s (Nathanson 1995; Lopez 1995; Hill 1998).

Prevention

Prevention of the diseases associated with smoking requires reduction or, preferably, elimination of exposure to tobacco smoke. Beyond this simple prescription, though there is relative consensus among public health authorities cross-nationally on a toolkit of desirable prevention strategies, there is little agreement as to which strategies are most effective and for whom. Furthermore, the contents of the toolkit have both multiplied and markedly changed their character over time. The earliest instruments, physician exhortation and health education directed primarily at the individual smoker, though not entirely abandoned, have been largely displaced by strategies (nicotine patches and the like) intended to help the smoker to quit, to create an unfriendly smoking environment (regulations that restrict smoking in an increasing range of public and even relatively private [workplace] spaces; package warnings, advertising bans and other marketing controls; and price manipulation), and to penalize (through litigation) and demonize (through the media) the tobacco industry. The extent to which these strategies have been adopted and implemented is a major source of variation among the four countries.

United States[8]

In 1964, the year of the first U.S. surgeon general's report on smoking and health, over 40 percent of the American population smoked. By 2004—some forty years later—that percentage had been cut in half. Outdoor advertising of cigarettes had virtually disappeared, limited to small placards at the point of sale. Prohibitions of cigarette sales to minors were visibly displayed everywhere cigarettes were sold, taken as much for granted as similar long-standing prohibitions on the sale of beer and alcohol. Smokers had become an endangered species gently ridiculed in cartoons and on *New Yorker* covers, and the industry that continued to feed their habit was reviled. The compelling story—or stories—behind this dramatic social change have been told many times from as many different perspectives. The April 2006 issue of the *Journal of Health Politics, Policy and Law* reviewed seven books, all published since 2000, by no means exhausting the literary store. For reasons that will appear, my story focuses on the emergence of the antismoking movement in the 1970s and 1980s. In the United States for much of that period, this movement was the only antismoking game in town. I come back to the movement—and to the other actors in the tobacco drama—following a chronology of U.S. smoking-tobacco control policy in the forty-two years since the 1964 surgeon general's report.

Fragmented Policymaking

The story behind tobacco policy in the United States is one of almost continuous struggle—for much of the time a very lopsided struggle—between the tobacco industry and its allies on one side and a disparate array of antismoking forces on the other. With a few exceptions to be described, policy making at the federal level was absent or hostile to tobacco control. Action was more meaningful at state and local levels but limited by and large to restrictions on public smoking and to increased taxation. Even these latter actions were generated from the bottom up by a grassroots movement against secondhand smoke. Nationwide restrictions on tobacco advertising—among the first objects of public policy in the other three countries—were imposed only in 1998 and only then as an outcome of litigation.

(In)Action at the Federal Level   In 1959, U.S. Surgeon General Leroy Burney stated in *JAMA (Journal of the American Medical Association)* that "the weight of the evidence at present implicates smoking as the principal factor in the increased incidence of lung cancer" (Burney 1959, 2104). Burney's article, published under the title, "Smoking and lung cancer: a statement of the Public Health Service," followed by the surgeon general's report five years later, officially and publicly labeled cigarettes as a hazard to human health "of sufficient importance in the United States to warrant appropriate remedial action" (U.S. Department of Health, Education, and Welfare 1964, 33). The report said nothing about what that action should be.

Serious congressional attention to smoking and health was triggered less by the surgeon general's report than by its political fallout: actions in several state legislatures to pass package-labeling laws and an initiative taken by the Federal Trade Commission within a week of the report's public unveiling to require package warning labels administratively. With much huffing and puffing about chaos in the states and administrative encroachment on legislative authority, Congress took back its turf and in 1965 passed the Federal Cigarette Labeling and Advertising Act. This bill was regarded by contemporary advocates of smoking–tobacco control as considerably stronger in its protection for the tobacco industry than in the remedial action recommended by the surgeon general (Pertschuk 1986; Fritschler 1989; but see Derthick 2005). The warning label was far milder and less certainly legible than advocates would have preferred. Adding insult to injury, the bill prevented individual states from imposing their own and possibly stricter labeling requirements, a tactic known as preemption and much reviled by tobacco-control advocates. The bill's language mandating annual reports by the surgeon general on the health consequences of smoking was less noted at the time but was of overriding importance in the long run.[9] The continuing drum-roll of these reports throughout the 1970s and 1980s played a critical role in fueling the antismoking movement.

The Public Health Cigarette Smoking Act of 1969 changed the warning label from cigarette smoking *may* be dangerous to *is* dangerous to health, renewed the mandate for annual reports on smoking and health, and continued the preemption of state by federal regulation. It also banned tobacco advertising on radio and television. The consensus of observers was that the advertising ban passed only because of tobacco industry distaste for an earlier, and demonstrably effective, court-imposed requirement of equal time for antismoking messages (Warner 1979).

Federal agencies took action in the early 1970s to restrict smoking in airlines, trains, and buses. No further legislation of significance was passed until the 1980s. On the contrary, Congress took every opportunity to exclude cigarettes from regulation under seemingly applicable statutes. In 1973, for example, the issue arose as to whether the newly created Consumer Product Safety Commission should regulate cigarettes as a dangerous substance. Responding to this controversy, in 1975 Congress passed and President Ford signed legislation specifically exempting cigarettes (along with guns!) from the commission's jurisdiction (Fritschler 1989, 118–19).[10] Not until 1984 did Congress bow to combined pressures from the Federal Trade Commission and a newly politicized group of health organizations to further strengthen the warning labels and to impose a system of rotating labels. The new system was enacted in the Comprehensive Smoking Education Act—again, however, accompanied by significant protection for the tobacco industry. Finally, the single piece of tobacco-control legislation to pass Congress in the 1990s (apart from relatively small cigarette tax increases) was the Synar amendment (1992), named for Representative Mike Synar of Oklahoma, mandating state enforcement of restrictions on cigarette sales to minors under threat of losing federal block-grant funding for mental health and substance abuse services. Implementing regulations at both federal and state levels substantially weakened this legislation, however, and expert consensus described it as ineffective, in part because of its status as an "unfunded federal mandate" and in part because of the low priority given by the police to enforcement of these restrictions (Rigotti 2001, 157).

By the late 1990s, there had been convergence of political opportunities and pressures—massive lawsuits by individual states against the tobacco industry to recover excess Medicaid costs allegedly due to smoking, the presence of an activist FDA commissioner (David Kessler) who asserted FDA authority to regulate tobacco products, and a sympathetic president—that appeared highly favorable to prospects for restrictive antismoking legislation. In the spring of 1998, with considerable fanfare and high hopes, legislation (known as the McCain bill for its chief sponsor, Arizona Senator John McCain) giving the FDA authority over tobacco, imposing substantial restrictions on cigarette advertising and marketing, and authorizing large cigarette tax increases (along with limits on industry liability) was introduced in Congress. Within barely two months, the bill was dead, defeated by (depending on the observer) the tobacco industry's political power or the intransigence of zealous activists unwilling to compromise the perfect for the sake of the good (Pertschuk 2001; Givel and Glantz 2004; Derthick 2005). As if this defeat were not enough, the U.S. Supreme Court ruled in 2000 that the FDA lacked authority to regulate tobacco, effectively sending the issue back to Congress, and in 2001 overturned a Massachusetts advertising ban, arguing that it unduly restricted commercial speech. Legislation that would have regulated tobacco under the FDA was again introduced in Congress in 2004 and again defeated. For the time being at least, legislative action on tobacco control at the federal level was stalled.

Nevertheless, due in part—but only in part—to what Martha Derthick describes as a "dramatic shift in the way governments make policy toward the tobacco industry" (2005, 2), the United States had by the beginning of the twenty-first century acquired a tobacco-control regime that included virtual prohibitions not only of public smoking but also of billboard, mass transit, and other outdoor advertising. This latter change was the result of a master settlement agreement (MSA) settling state claims against the tobacco industry for reimbursement of the health care costs of smoking, not—as in the other three countries—the result of direct action by agencies of government. Let me explain.

States' claims against the industry for recovery of Medicaid costs were settled out of court in 1997, by which time thirty-eight states had joined the suit. In addition to substantial industry payments to each state (amounting to approximately $350 billion over twenty-five years), the settlement had many of the same restrictions on advertising and market-ing that would subsequently be part of the MSA. However, it also included provisions—FDA regulation of tobacco, liability protections for the industry—that could only be enacted by legislation (the McCain bill). With the defeat of this bill, the states' legal team and the tobacco industry returned to the bargaining table and hammered out the Master Settlement Agreement (MSA). It was this scenario—regulation through litigation rather than legislation—that Derthick identified as a "dramatic shift" in the way tobacco policy was made.[11]

Action at the Local Level   On January 11, 1971—the seventh anniversary of the surgeon general's report—U.S. Surgeon General Jesse L. Steinfeld, spoke before the Interagency Council on Smoking and Health.[12] At the end of a speech devoted primarily to the consequences of smoking for women, he said:

> Nonsmokers have as much right to clean air and wholesome air as smokers have to their so-called right to smoke, which I would redefine as a "right to pollute." It is high time to ban smoking from all confined public places such as restaurants, theaters, airplanes, trains, and buses. It is time that we inter-pret the Bill of Rights for the Nonsmoker as well as the smoker. (1258)

By accident or design, Steinfeld thus gave voice to the central idea that would henceforth animate the tobacco-control movement in the United States.[13] Action on this terrain has taken place almost entirely at the state and local level. Within a few weeks of Steinfeld's speech, nonsmokers' rights groups had sprung up across the country. Within a couple of years, Arizona had become the first state to cite the dangers of "involuntary" smoking as a reason to ban smoking in public places. In 1976, Madison, Wisconsin, became the first municipality to restrict smoking in restaurants. Although they vary in scope and restrictiveness, smoking bans in public buildings, workplaces, restaurants, and even—in California and New York City—in bars are now a fact of everyday life throughout the United States, ubiquitous and largely self-enforcing (Jacobson and Zapawa 2001; Jacobson and Wasserman 1999). States and localities have taken other actions as well: mounting educational programs, instituting telephone "quit lines," limiting young people's access to cigarettes, raising cigarette taxes. But bans on smoking indoors and, increasingly, outdoors as well are by far the most visible elements of the U.S. tobacco-control regime.

Actors in the Tobacco Drama

Throughout the seventeenth and eighteenth and well into the nineteenth century, the United States was the world's foremost producer of tobacco (Goodman 1993, 210). Tobacco—in the somewhat overheated words of a sympathetic historian—"originated in America; it was this nation's first business; Americans brought it to its present stage of development" (Heimann 1960, 5).

The Tobacco Industry   By early in the twentieth century, the tobacco industry—encompassing tobacco farming and the manufacture of cigarettes—had assumed more or less its present form. Cultivation of the tobacco leaf was concentrated in the "tobacco states" of Georgia, South Carolina, North Carolina, Tennessee, and Kentucky. James Buchanan Duke, with the help of the newly invented Bonsack cigarette rolling machine, had created the American Tobacco Company and made cigarettes into an item of mass production and—through aggressive nationwide advertising campaigns—mass consumption.[14] Although the American Tobacco Company was declared in 1910 to be in violation of the Sherman Antitrust Act, and its assets distributed among four newly created companies along with several smaller firms (the parents of today's multinationals), concentration of power among relatively few tobacco manufacturers and distributors was undisturbed. Two companies, Philip Morris and R. J. Reynolds, currently account for more than 70 percent of the total U.S. tobacco consumption.

By the time the first intimations of smoking and health as a public problem were heard in the United States, "tobacco power" had been an established force in American politics for more than fifty years (Fritschler 1989, 6). Lee Fritschler describes the cozy relations that characterized the federal "tobacco subsystem" in the period before the deluge: "[Tobacco policy] was made in a spirit of friendly and quiet cooperation between small segments of Congress, the bureaucracy, and the interest group community. . . . [The tobacco subsystem] cuts across institutional lines and includes within it all groups and individuals who are making and influencing government decisions concerning cigarettes and tobacco. . . . This was a small group of people well known to each other and knowledgeable about all aspects of the tobacco industry and its relationship with the government" (4). The cause of smoking and health was placed on the federal government's agenda not by persuading or converting this "small group of people" but by circumventing them.

Agents of Change   In an article published in 1981 in the journal *Science*, the health economist Kenneth Warner analyzed data to account for the steady decline of smoking in the previous decade. Warner used multiple regression techniques to take account of changes in media attention to smoking's health effects and in taxation and concluded that both "declining consumption and growth in legislation [restricting smoking in public places] probably reflect a prevailing nonsmoking ethos" induced by the movement for nonsmokers' rights (1981, 730).

The core of the smoking–tobacco control movement in the United States for at least the first two decades of the movement's existence (approximately 1970 to 1990) consisted of three sets of players: the health voluntaries (American Cancer Society, American Lung Association and American Heart Association); ASH (Action on Smoking and Health), and the nonsmokers' rights groups. They varied in relative importance over time and played different and arguably complementary roles in advancing the tobacco-control agenda. Conspicuously absent from the roster of these early risers were the American Medical Association, the American Public Health Association, and the majority of state and local public health officials. As the movement gained legitimacy in the 1990s, the range of participants expanded markedly to the point where what was once a small sect has become an established church, now including organized medicine and public health along with the legal profession as major players.[15] My primary focus in this account is on what happened in the first phase, when—as Warner's article suggests—the groundwork for change was laid.

The American Cancer Society.   From the perspective of the larger smoking–tobacco control movement, the ACS played its most important role in the 1950s and 1960s, using its resources and authority to help create and then to promote smoking and health as a public problem within and outside the government. In 1948, the ACS annual report noted that lung cancer mortality was increasing; in 1951 a National Lung Cancer Committee was created and the society issued its first public warning of the rise in lung cancer. In 1952 the ACS began its population-based follow-up study of smoking and death rates in "white men between the ages of fifty and sixty-nine" (Hammond and Horn 1954). In an interview published in 1965, E. Cuyler Hammond stated that "only an institution like the American Cancer Society" could have carried out this study (Pfeiffer 1965, 12). The ACS committed its substantial resources to this project despite considerable skittishness on the part of some of the society's officials, who were perfectly aware of the study's potential political sensitivity (Kluger 1996, 146). Many observers have described and commented on ACS's long reluctance to act on the study's striking results (Jacobson, Wasserman, and Raube 1992; Pertschuk 1986; Interview with ACS official, ACS files, 1990), and during the 1970s the society virtually disappeared as a public advocate of the relation between smoking and health (Troyer and Markle 1983, 68). Driven by conservative leadership and an unwillingness to risk other interests for the sake of the smoking–tobacco control movement it did not resurface until the early 1990s (Pertschuk 2001, 54; Jacobson, Wasserman, and Raube 1992).[16]

Action on Smoking and Health.   ASH was founded in 1967 by John Banzhaf, a professor of law at Georgetown University in Washington, D.C., for the sole purpose of engaging in legal action at the federal level. Its initial focus was on cigarette advertising, but it soon branched into additional arenas, including public transportation, warnings on birth control packages, and others. By far the largest part of its activities were actions before the various regulatory commissions involved with tobacco (FCC, FTC, FDA, and the like) as advocate, for example, on behalf of smoking bans on planes, trains, and buses. In no sense was ASH a grassroots organization. It was a small, professionally operated public interest group with a paid staff and no organization or activities at the local and state levels.

Nonsmokers' Rights Movement.   America's "prevailing nonsmoking ethos" first began to take shape in the early 1970s. This ethos was the creation of locally initiated grassroots groups. These groups proliferated across the country with remarkable rapidity, becoming within a few years to all intents and purposes a national social movement. In its scope and intensity this form of action against tobacco was—among the four countries—unique to the United States and accounts for many of the particularities of its tobacco-control regime. (The movement's mobilization and organization strategies are typical for contemporary health-related social movements in this country.)

Grassroots Mobilization Against Smoking: An Illustrative Case of Social Movement Formation   By 1971 deaths of white males from lung cancer had reached a critical threshold of visibility: fathers and uncles of the generation that came of age in the late 1960s and early 1970s—an activist generation profoundly influenced by the example of civil rights, antiwar and environmental movements—were dying of lung cancer.[17] The activists I interviewed identified a latent constituency composed of two groups: individuals who had lost loved ones to smoking and a much larger group who were profoundly irritated by tobacco smoke. The latter could be persuaded to come out of the closet, so to speak, by persuading them first that their irritation was legitimate and, second, that it was shared.

Clara Gouin, the founder of GASP (Group Against Smokers' Pollution), had been active in a local environmental movement. She attributed her father's death from lung cancer at the age of fifty-seven to cigarette smoking, and friends complained to her about the odor of cigarette smoke in their hair and clothes.[18] In her own words, "You suddenly get an inspiration. That's what it was. I convened a meeting of my friends. There were several friends in the neighborhood, and several friends at church, and some mothers of young children my girls' age, and we had a meeting and said let's start this group and see what we can do" (Gouin, interview, November 1995). Gouin contacted local branches of the health voluntaries. The interest of the local lung association's program director made it possible to combine her inspiration with critical resources: space, a mimeograph machine, and—of inestimable importance—a mailing list. The first issue of *The Ventilator*, published in March 1971, went out to local lung associations throughout the country. Buttons (reading "GASP—nonsmokers have rights, too") and posters were offered, plus a subscription to the newsletter for $1 a year. The response was far beyond the group's anticipation. Chapters were quickly formed in Berkeley and San Francisco. By 1974, the newsletter listed fifty-six local chapters in the United States and two in Canada. At least twenty-two (and probably more) of these chapters were unofficially associated with their local lung associations. From the beginning, GASP chapters were locally organized autonomous groups, staffed almost entirely by volunteers.

> Once we got a bunch of chapters going, we organized all the names we had by states and localities and mailed those names out to local lung associations and local GASP groups around the country, saying, "these are people who have written to us from your area. Contact them, get them active in your group." . . . We actually sent them envelopes with just stacks of little mailing labels. (Gouin interview, November 1995)

The group's initial tactics were almost entirely local and on a small scale, focused on getting smoke-free meeting rooms (particularly meeting rooms of obvious groups, like environmental groups and lung association chapters), doctors' offices, hospitals, natural food stores, and the like. Funding requirements for these activities were minimal (Gouin's budget never went above $10,000 per year) and were covered by contributions and by the organizers themselves. Although there was some public hostility to the group's efforts, the media were very interested: "we got a lot of free publicity," at first locally and then nationally and internationally. Exposure brought new recruits.

By the mid-1970s, the focus of nonsmokers' rights activists began to shift from "passing out leaflets and buttons" to passing state and local antismoking regulations (Hanauer, Barr, and Glantz 1986, 2). Seventeen of the fifty-four GASP groups listed in 1974 were in California. These groups, later incorporated as Americans for Nonsmokers' Rights, focused increasingly on regulatory action, first at the state and later, after narrow defeats in 1978 and 1980, at the local level. Minnesota's Association for Nonsmokers' Rights had an unusual early success at the state-level: the Minnesota Clean Indoor Air Act was passed in 1975 (Wolfson 2001). While the Association is given major credit, elite support (physicians, the health voluntaries) and—perhaps more important—the absence of tobacco industry opposition (largely responsible for the defeats in California) were major contributing factors. Minnesota took the industry by surprise. It would not be surprised again.

As the nature and scope of their activities changed, funding requirements increased and nonsmokers' rights groups became more professionalized. Drafting legislation and engineering its passage demanded legal experience; organizing statewide initiative campaigns was expensive. Along with these changes came paid staff, greater bureaucratization, concerns about incorporation and tax exemption, and—perhaps inevitably—some nostalgia on the part of early campaigners for the enthusiasm of an earlier time.[19] This transformation is a classic process of organizational change, the price a social movement pays for public acceptance and success. Loss of innocence—together with internal dissension associated with setbacks in Congress and the Supreme Court—has led to recent public expressions of concern about the movement's future by some of its earliest leaders (Pertschuk et al. 1999; Pertschuk 2001; Blum, Solbery, and Wolinsky 2004). From a purely public health perspective, however, the movement's greatest limitation has been its essentially middle-class base, reflected in the marked social class disparity in current smoking prevalence. Not only the movement's elitism but also its moralism—the division of society into "good" nonsmokers and "evil" smokers—replicate classic features of reform movements in the United States (Morone 2003).

Constructions of Risk: Innocent Victims, Merchants of Death   The late twentieth century smoking–tobacco control movement transformed the cigarette and smoking from symbols of "modernity, power, and sexuality" to symbols of weakness, irrationality, and addiction (Brandt 1992, 70). From its inception in 1971 the mission of the nonsmokers' rights movement was twofold: first to "get nonsmokers to protect themselves" against the immediate, irritating effects of cigarette smoke, and second "to make smoking so unpopular that smokers would quit" (Gouin, interview, November 1995). In the first paragraph of the first issue of its newsletter *The Ventilator*, published in March 1971, GASP called on innocent nonsmokers, the "involuntary victims of tobacco smoke," to rise up and assert their "right to breathe clean air [that] is superior to the right of the smoker to enjoy a harmful habit" (1).

This construction of smoking—a danger externally imposed, outside the control of its innocent victims—was expanded and elaborated in the following years to encompass three seemingly distinct but in fact closely intertwined highly emotive threats: addiction, the seduction of innocent children, and a malign and duplicitous industry. Children and nicotine addicts were linked by their putative absence of choice:

> A comprehensive review of the evidence [shows] that cigarettes and other forms of tobacco are addicting and that nicotine is the drug in tobacco that causes addiction. These two factors refute the argument that smoking is a matter of free choice. Most smokers start smoking as teenagers and then become addicted. (Koop 1989, v)

In this construction cigarettes are "drug delivery devices" (HHS 1995), addiction "begins as a pediatric disease" (Kessler 2001), and tobacco manufacturers are, at best, pushers and, at worst, "merchants of death" (ACS official cited in Nathanson, 1999, 453). The tobacco industry had until the late 1980s been almost invisible as a target of the smoking–tobacco control movement. By 1996, the third link in the rhetorical chain between addiction, children, and the industry was fully formed, signaled by no less an authority than the American Cancer Society. "Protect Our Children from the Tobacco Companies" was its message, broadcast as a public service announcement on the Cable News Network (CNN).

During most of the period under discussion, the industry had continued to deny both that cigarettes caused disease and that they were addictive. This posture was powerfully undermined by the discovery of company documents dating back to the early 1950s in which these properties were clearly acknowledged (Glantz et al. 1996; Hilts 1996; Derthick 2005). This information was hardly new, but hard evidence of the industry's knowledge substantially increased its vulnerability not only in the courts of law and public opinion but in the halls of Congress. Smoking's decline in the United States, however, long predated evidence of industry deception (see, for example, Derthick 2005). This massive change in behavior can largely be attributed to the work of antismoking activists, for the most part outside of government.

France

The left-bank intellectual with a Gauloise drooping from the corner of his mouth has virtual iconic status as a symbol, if not to the French themselves at least to the tourist soaking up culture and smoke in equal parts at every café and on every street corner. This image is, nevertheless, of relatively recent date and, in some sense, misleading (Goodman 1993). Not until after World War II did cigarettes become the dominant form of tobacco consumption in France, and it is only recently that the prevalence of smoking among men has surpassed that in the United States. Even more counterintuitive, perhaps, is the fact that France in 1976 was among the first countries to pass tobacco-control legislation, including controls both on advertising and on smoking in public places.[20]

Policy from Above

In 1972, the French National Academy of Medicine passed a unanimous resolution calling attention to the nefarious consequences of smoking. Detailed knowledge of the reports of the British Royal College in 1962 and of the U.S. surgeon general in 1964 was, however, confined to the few specialists who read English.

The loi Veil   There was essentially no public or media attention to this issue until 1975 when Minister of Health Simone Veil became an enthusiastic disciple, converted to the cause against smoking by the distinguished oncologist Maurice Tubiana, who had observed Mme. Veil on television with a cigarette in her hand.[21] The eponymous loi Veil was passed with relatively little fanfare in June of 1976.[22] The gist of its provisions was to restrict tobacco advertising, impose (ambiguous and nearly illegible) package warnings, and place limitations on smoking in places "affectés à un usage collectif" (open to the public). Regulations implementing the Veil law, issued after a delay of two years, were cursory to the vanishing point.

As a piece of legislation the loi Veil was way ahead of its time, banning most outdoor advertising and restricting smoking in places of public accommodation years before anything comparable was passed elsewhere. In the event, however, it amounted to little more than an intellectual exercise, honored far more in the breach than the observance. The law was the work of one person, Simone Veil. Although the French president (Valéry Giscard d'Estaing) supported it, the powerful finance ministry—ever mindful of tobacco's contribution to the treasury and fearful of what any increase in tobacco prices might do to the cost of living index—was opposed.[23] French authorities took few or no steps to enforce the loi Veil, industry evasion of its provisions with respect to advertising was widespread, and the law's limitations on smoking in places open to the public were essentially ignored.

The loi Evin   The loi Veil was replaced in 1991 by the loi Evin, named for the health minister who shepherded its adoption, Claude Evin.[24] Credit belongs in large part to a group of five prominent and politically well-connected physicians—the cinq sages, as they came to be known—who came together out of common frustration with what they saw as government complicity to weaken or evade existing laws for the protection of public health.[25] The new law strengthened provisions against illegal advertising, prohibited smoking except in locations reserved for smokers, and took tobacco out of the government's cost of living index. This last provision made it possible for the government to raise the price of cigarettes independent of labor agreements tied to the index.

In contrast to the loi Veil experience, the loi Evin was extremely contentious, in part because it incorporated regulation of advertising for alcohol products as well as tobacco. (The drafters had calculated that Parliament would take so easily to the regulation of tobacco that it would not notice the threat to wine and cognac.) Debate continued for nine months in multiple sessions of the General Assembly and the Senate. Like the loi Veil, however, the loi Evin was a government bill, and when it ultimately passed in late 1990, it did so with the unanimous support of the Groupe socialiste (the party in power). Opposition (almost equally united) was from the unlikely combination of conservatives opposed to limits on the free market and communists opposed to legislation that ignored underlying social and economic problems.

Parliamentary debate (insofar as it concerned tobacco, not alcohol) focused almost entirely on the threat to French economic interests (the tobacco industry, media, automobile racing) posed by the bill's advertising restrictions. From the public's perspective, however, the law's principal innovation was not in its strengthened advertising bans, but in a single sentence, pithier even than comparable provisions of the loi Veil, that—for the first time—privileged the rights of nonsmokers over those of smokers: "Smoking is prohibited in places open to the public, including educational institutions, and in public transport, *except* in locations expressly designated for smokers" [emphasis added]. In comments in the course of parliamentary debate, Evin made his intentions explicit: "Our aim is the reversal of current logic. Smoking (now) is allowed everywhere except in places reserved for non-smokers. Henceforth it will be forbidden to smoke except in places reserved for smokers" (France 1990, 2902). The devil, of course, was in the details, and the décret spelling out the meaning of this provision, issued at the end of May 1992, was unclear both as to the locations covered and the accommodations to be made for separating smokers and nonsmokers.

There is consensus among French observers—including a government-appointed commission to evaluate the operation of the loi Evin—that the law's smoking bans are both unclear and poorly enforced.[26] Efforts to rectify the situation by legislative means were unsuccessful, and in the fall of 2006 the French prime minister, Dominique de Villepin, announced a smoking ban to be enacted by decree. Still, restaurants, bars, and cafes have until January 2008 to comply, and the terms of the ban in other respects—including provisions for enforcement—remain unclear (Crampton 2006).

Insofar as the loi Evin was intended to reduce smoking, its most important provision may have been taking tobacco out of the cost of living index and thus making it possible to raise the price of cigarettes. Under the French tobacco regime, both tobacco taxes and the total price of cigarettes to the consumer are controlled by the state. Taxes have consistently hovered around 75 percent of the total price, a percentage not atypical for Europe. The Finance Ministry's interest in holding down the price of cigarettes had been dictated by tobacco's inclusion in the cost of living index, which played a major role in employer-employee negotiations over wages and salaries. Between 1992 and 1998, cigarette prices were increased eleven times, by a total of 122 percent. The evaluation commission attributed declines in smoking primarily to these increases (more than doubling the price of a package of cigarettes between 1992 and 1998), arguing that advertising had been limited under the Veil law and smoking had hardly changed (Commissariat général du plan 2000). After several years of relatively flat taxes (1998 to 2001), a new wave of cigarette tax increases was launched in 2001. Cigarette sales again dropped, by close to 50 percent between April and October of 2003 alone. Sales have stabilized since then at a somewhat higher level.

On March 24, 2003, in front of more than 500 dignitaries assembled at the Elysée Palace, the French head of state, Jacques Chirac, declared war on tobacco (la guerre au tabac). Whether this declaration reflected a newfound serious commitment to tobacco control by the state, and what impact it would have on French smoking behavior are questions difficult to unravel without new research on the ground.[27] On the first point, the only legislation passed since Chirac's statement was a largely symbolic ban on cigarette sales to persons under sixteen. And, in a concession to the association that represents France's tobacco sellers, the government recently agreed to a four-year moratorium on tobacco tax increases. In a not unfamiliar pattern, Chirac—and the state he represents—were longer on rhetoric than on implementation. In the context of France's political culture, however, Chirac's highly public embrace of tobacco control was arguably an essential first step in persuading French citizens to take the antismoking movement seriously. With his proclamation in 2006, three and a half years later, of a ban on public smoking, Prime Minister Villepin took a critical second step.

Actors

Tobacco was introduced into France in the sixteenth century. Duties imposed on tobacco imports rapidly became an important source of revenue to the state, and finance ministers from Richelieu in the early seventeenth century to Necker just before the French Revolution took steps to ensure the size and continuity of those receipts.

Tobacco and the State   In 1674, Colbert declared the manufacture and sale of tobacco products a monopoly of the state. By the end of the eighteenth century, the French tobacco monopoly yielded seven percent of total state revenue, creating "both a state interest and private interests that could not readily be ignored when relevant policy questions came to be decided" (Price 1995, 167). This state of affairs remained relatively stable until about 1970. Since then, the interrelated pressures of market, consumer, and regulatory change have led to the monopoly's gradual privatization and, in 1999, to a merger between the tobacco industries of France and Spain. Tobacco continues, nevertheless, to be an important source of revenue to the French state (doubling between 1991 and 2000 in the wake of price increases), and the industry's directors are still fully enmeshed in "the network of links [among graduates of the grandes écoles] established across the boundaries between the state and private sectors" (Price, 296).

The Advertising Industry   The strongest opposition to the loi Evin was not from smokers or even directly from the tobacco industry itself but instead from advertising agencies and the media, which had historically depended on the industry for much of their revenue: "the most powerful lobby wasn't the alcohol lobby, it was the advertising one, and politicians needed money to be elected and needed the advertising world to be elected too" (Dubois, interview, May 1995). The consensus among antitobacco activists was that government inaction on the public health issues presented by tobacco and alcohol was attributable far more to the economic power of the advertising world than to the alcohol and tobacco lobbies.

Agents of Change   There are in France organizations that correspond to the American Cancer Society (la Ligue nationale contre le cancer) and the American Heart Association (la Fédération française de cardiologie). For most of their history, these groups have been even more conservative than their American counterparts, oriented almost exclusively toward raising funds for medical research. Within the last few years, the Ligue, under new leadership, has become much more active and visible in tobacco control and is now a dominant player. The vanguard of the French tobacco wars, however, were the cinq sages and a small group of militants, the Comité nationale contre le tabagisme (CNCT).

The Cinq Sages.   The difference between the loi Veil and the loi Evin was less in the content of these two laws than in the campaign on behalf of the loi Evin mounted by the small but determined band of medical specialists, the cinq sages. Their campaign was unique in France as reflected in the level of media and parliamentary attention it received.

The group formed on the basis of prior social and professional connections and drew its influence from the distinct but overlapping relations of its members with the French medical elite, government officials, and politicians. Chronologically, their story begins not with tobacco but with alcohol. In the mid-1980s, Claude Got and Gérard Dubois, two of the cinq sages, were members of a government-appointed commission on alcoholism.[28] When in 1987 the prime minister decided to authorize alcohol advertising on television, Got made a highly public resignation from the commission. He and Dubois then recruited the cream of the French medical establishment—Nobel prize winners, current and former presidents of the Academy of Medicine, medical school deans—in support of an intensive media campaign to get this decision overturned. Within three months, the authorization for television advertising was withdrawn: Got and Dubois had discovered the power of medical lobbying.

At much the same time, there was a revival of action on the tobacco front, largely moribund since the passage of the loi Veil. In 1986, Albert Hirsch, professor of medicine and specialist in lung diseases at a Paris hospital, was asked by the minister of health to do the first official evaluation of the loi Veil. Hirsch's report, *Lutter contre le tabagisme* [*To Fight against Tobacco Use*] published in 1987, was scathing in its denunciation of the French government's response to open and widespread violation of the Veil law's provisions with respect to tobacco advertising.[29]

> Ten years after the law's adoption, the inadequacies in its implementation are notorious. . . . The authorities have continuously held back, and the fight against tobacco (tabagisme) has not, up to now, been a serious object of public policy [l'objet d'une volonté politique fermement déclarée]. (Hirsch et al. 1987, 10)

Hirsch's report and its series of recommendations received substantial media attention (due in part to a carefully-timed article in *Le Monde*, "Le tabagisme, un véritable désastre sanitaire [Smoking, a True Health Disaster]" signed by medical heavyweights Maurice Tubiana and Jean Bernard). The report was, however, essentially ignored by a government then caught up in approaching elections. It was then that the advocates of alcohol and tobacco control determined to join forces, as described by Albert Hirsch:

> So, because nothing happened, I decided to join my efforts with a friend, Claude Got. I knew Claude Got very well, who was at that time involved with alcohol control. And because nothing happened in alcohol and nothing happened in tobacco Claude Got and I decided to join our efforts in order to lobby. This was completely new in France. We decided to increase the

number of the group to five. Claude Got introduced me to Gérard Dubois, because they were both involved in the alcohol program. And we decided to ask Maurice Tubiana because he is very representative of the medical establishment, [which is] very strong in France. And he was at that time the Chairman of the group of European experts from the program, Europe Against Cancer. (And, finally, Hirsch asked François Grémy, another friend, and, like Dubois, a professor of public health, to join the group.) (Interview, May 1995)

In addition to medical eminence and political connections, a third consideration in formation of the cinq sages was their diverse political affiliations (two right, one center, two Socialist): "It was important to present the issue not as a political problem [or rather] as a political problem, but not in the sense of belonging to the right or the left" (Hirsch, interview, May 1995).

From early 1988, just before the French presidential election of that year (which brought in the Socialist government of François Mitterrand) until after the passage of the Evin law in 1991, the cinq sages followed a strategy that alternated intense public pressure on the government through the media with insider lobbying of parliamentarians, civil servants, and politicians. In a classic ploy of public-interest lobbyists, their first step was to address a series of questions to the presidential candidates not simply in a letter but in a press conference that received wide coverage on television and in print. With the exception of Jacques Chirac, then the prime minister, all the candidates committed themselves to a complete ban on tobacco advertising. Following Mitterrand's election, the new minister of health, Claude Evin, asked the cinq sages for recommendations for the control of smoking (along with other "unhealthy" behaviors). Their report was completed in 1989. Much as had been the fate of Hirsch's earlier report, however, this one too was in danger of being buried. To rescue it,

[Claude Evin] asked us to lobby the government, that is his own administration. That's quite unusual, and we were quite uneasy with that. And, after some months, we realized that it doesn't work because you have to be silent, we were underground, official but underground, and that's not the right way. (Gérard Dubois, interview, May 1995)

So, again, the cinq sages went to the media with their (officially "confidential") report, publishing it in Le Monde, the French equivalent of The New York Times. This last démarche was, finally, successful. The five doctors were courted by influential members of parliament and of Mitterrand's administration. Within a year and a half, the Evin law—written in its essentials by the cinq sages—became law. The economic interests that had worked within the government to keep the issue under wraps were (at least partially) defeated. The prime minister at the time, Michel Rocard, was reported to have said to his colleagues responsible for budget and finance, "Écoutez, de toute manière, vous avez perdu; les médecins ont gagné. Nous n'avons plus le choix [Listen. You have lost. The doctors have won. We no longer have a choice]."

The relative success enjoyed by the cinq sages was by no means a foregone conclusion. France is not friendly to preventive medicine and public health. This difficult climate is attributable to public health's institutional weaknesses, to its generally low status relative to curative medicine and, more specifically in the case of tobacco, to what was perceived as the unscientific nature of advocacy for tobacco control. Within the government, Health is a relatively small entity located administratively within the much larger Ministry of Solidarity, Health, and Social Protection, which is responsible, among other things, for the state system of health insurance. Although individual health ministers have acted effectively—Simone Veil is a notable example—the office itself has few resources and little power.

There is considerable irony in the low status occupied by public health in the land of Louis Pasteur, an irony by no means lost on the various actors in this drama. The explanation offered for this low esteem is twofold. First is the powerful position held by what is called in French the "clinique"—the highly individualized assessment of each patient by his or her doctor—as the supreme medical act. Second is the well-developed suspicion of public health as, on the one hand, an infringement on the liberty of the individual and, on the other, a government penny-pinching scheme. The image of an authoritarian government trampling on the liberties of the people draws, of course, on deep roots in French history and culture. The continuing resonance of this image is reflected not only in the elite intellectual status of its proponents ("the philosophers are not with us," lamented one of my informants from the world of tobacco control) but in the frequency with which the image is mentioned and its applicability contested by advocates of action on behalf of public health (see, for example, Malet 1993). Suspicion of government penny-pinching (the state advocates disease prevention not out of any altruistic motives but solely to avoid paying for its cure) may have deep roots as well, but its immediate context was the French government's vocal concern with the rising cost of its state-supported system of medical care.

Finally, even in the mid-1990s, smoking and health was not a respectable topic for academic research (much less advocacy) in France.[30] There was no unit of INSERM (the French equivalent of NIH) devoted to smoking. Despite France's role as host for the 1994 International Conference on Smoking and Health, relatively few French scientists attended (only 10 percent of the delegates were French, and "we had to beat the bushes to find them," according to one of the organizers). Although INSERM provided some funding for the conference, strict limits were placed on how the funding could be used (that is, not for anything that smacked of advocacy). A dean of the French medical profession with whom I spoke (himself one of the cinq sages and a strong supporter of the smoking and health cause) analogized the status of smoking to that of sewers in the late nineteenth century: smoking is now—as sewers were then—beneath the dignity of physicians to address.

Given this context, the strategy of the cinq sages had four critical elements. First, of the five leaders in the cause of smoking and health in France, three were specialists in cancer and heart disease: the status associated with these latter specialties was a necessary condition for attention to be paid. Second was the group's resort to medical luminaries (Nobel prize winners and the like) as props to further reinforce the scientific authority and legitimacy of their case. Third was the discovery and highly strategic employment of outsider media-based lobbying. Last and, indeed, the coup de grâce for a Socialist government, according to Hirsch, was the social inequality of sickness and death, an inequality, the cinq sages maintained, created by diseases associated with tobacco and alcohol. For a "government of the left" this inequality was an argument impossible to ignore (Hirsch and Karsenty 1992).

Comité Nationale Contre Le Tabagisme.   It is a telling fact that in their otherwise detailed account of the struggle for tobacco regulation in France, Hirsch and Karsenty never mention CNCT, this despite the fact that Hirsch was its president from 1991 until 1993, when the position was assumed by Gérard Dubois. Activists in France are more likely to be regarded with suspicion than admiration, and lay advocacy on behalf of what is seen as properly a medical or scientific question is particularly suspect.[31] Nevertheless, as recognized in the evaluation report on the loi Evin, CNCT was almost solely responsible for what legal action was taken to enforce that law's provisions (Commissariat général du plan 2000). And so antitobacco militancy in France has proceeded over much of the past fifteen or twenty years along two tracks, intersecting at various points and mutually aware, but also mutually wary: a "respectable" track represented by the cinq sages and a less respectable track, that of CNCT.

CNCT long predated the emergence of the cinq sages. Indeed, it traced its origins to the nineteenth-century Association contre l'abus de tabac and celebrated its centenary in 1977. During most of the 1970s, CNCT was medically dominated and pursued a fairly conventional agenda of health education and smoking cessation programs. In the late 1970s, however, observing that the loi Veil was violated more often than it was observed and that the state prosecutorial system remained quiescent, CNCT launched its own campaign of legal action against violations of the law. That campaign was largely responsible for CNCT's visibility in France and for its status as the industry's enemy number one.

The loi Evin, though not the catalyst for CNCT's actions in court, considerably reinforced its standing to litigate against the tobacco industry. Close on the heels of this action, CNCT reinvented itself a second time, essentially throwing out the (relatively) moderate leadership in place since the mid-1970s and replacing it with a highly politicized set of activists. The latter included the more overtly militant of the cinq sages, Hirsch and later Dubois, as unpaid présidents and a salaried lay director with advocacy experience.

In its incarnation in the mid-1990s, CNCT presented a familiar picture to American eyes: a small group of young, highly dedicated activists working out of a renovated old house, surrounded by computers, a fax machine, telephones, file cabinets, and overflowing cardboard boxes. From the French perspective, however, it was an anomaly: a health association staffed by nonphysicians; an activist public gadfly supported at least in part by recoveries in court; an American-style lobby. CNCT's dues-paying membership was, in fact, very small (no more than a few hundred). It appeared indeed, apart from its partial public funding (about half of its revenue), to be a modern public-interest lobby, grafted uncomfortably onto French soil.

In the three and a half years between January 1, 1991 and June 10, 1994 alone, CNCT reported initiating 120 lawsuits against violators of the French statutes against tobacco advertising and recovering close to $1.5 million. Perhaps the most credible testimony to CNCT's impact was the hostility it generated from the tobacco industry. In a 1994 internal memo to its members describing the antitobacco lobby in France, CDIT gave CNCT equal billing with the cinq sages. Among the principal complaints of industry spokespersons was that CNCT was inappropriately "substituting itself for public officials in matters of public health" (Burton 1995, 3). CNCT was, indeed, acting in place of a judiciary that had proved extremely reluctant to act in its own name, either against violations of the earlier loi Veil or against the loi Evin. Clear evidence of CNCT's key role as a government surrogate was the latter's intervention to save the group when, in late 1997 and 1998, it confronted a legal and financial crisis. In the evaluation report cited earlier "the important role of associations [that is, CNCT] in implementation of the [Evin] law" was clearly recognized. The report suggested in its conclusion, however, that the state should take a more active prosecutorial role in the future.[32] There is no evidence that the state has followed this advice, and CNCT continues to be an active, and successful, litigator.

Passive Smoking: la Liberté versus la Santé Publique

The meanings of cigarettes and smoking in France are thrown into sharp relief by a comparison with the meanings of narcotic drugs. French horror of *illegal* addictive drugs is no less than that of Americans. The bases for the French aversion are, however, culturally specific: the danger of narcotic drugs lies in their association with the *rejection* of social ties. In sharp contrast, cigarettes and smoking are associated with the *creation* of social ties: "Tobacco makes a connection. . . . To offer a cigarette is to create a connection, a sociable (friendly, companionable) space."[33] The loi Evin attempted to redefine this space from friendly and companionable to dangerous. More recently, "official" constructions of smoking attempt to capitalize directly on the French aversion to narcotics: tobacco is defined as a drug within the purview of the national drug control agency; the tobacco unit within the Health Ministry is the Bureau of Addictive Practices. These actions aim to transform smoking from a basis of inclusion—making a connection—to one of exclusion.

In the immediate aftermath of the loi Evin, some French left-wing intellectuals and members of the press mounted a broad attack on public health as the entering wedge of the totalitarian state and on tobacco control as a new form of racism. The target of this attack was not the law's advertising bans, which were largely accepted, but the new privileging of nonsmokers. The American left is friendly to public health, identifying it as among the few government-financed and run programs that (among other things) directly serve the poorest and most vulnerable members of the population (poor mothers and children, drug users, persons with sexually transmitted infections, and so on). The French left, by contrast, sees public health and, in particular, the new public health focused on what are perceived to be lifestyle choices as unacceptable intervention by the "hygienic" state into individuals' most personal decisions: "medicine wants to direct our life, dictate our conduct, rule over us by 'the medical light' " (Bensaïd 1993, 53).[34] Invasion of privacy, health "fascism," discrimination, setting smokers and nonsmokers at one another's throats, and victim-blaming are among the major themes of this discourse.[35] In these polemics, the United States serves as an all-purpose bête noir, cited by the left as a horrible example of what is in store for France—not only a new Prohibition but also new forms of segregation reminiscent of Jim Crow—and even by public health advocates as an instructive example of the road not taken: in France, unlike the United States, the unreconstructed smoker will not be pushed outside the social pale.[36]

Not far beneath the surface of this debate are conceptions of the nonsmoker and of the relation between smokers and nonsmokers that are very different from those to which we are accustomed in the United States. Nonsmokers are portrayed by advocates friendly to their cause as victims (for example, children and pregnant women) especially in need of protection by the State: "legislation must above all protect non-smokers . . . the right of the most vulnerable to breathe clean air must be respected" (Tubiana 1997, 10). By the same token, to protest against another's smoke is to cast oneself in the unattractive role of victim and, moreover, of a busybody who is prepared to interfere with another's small pleasures for what are perceived to be specious reasons:

> The smoker—I know, I've been there—does not for a moment believe that the nonsmoker is truly bothered. No, he simply wants to annoy, to deprive the smoker of a little pleasure [Le fumeur—je sais, j'en suis parfois— ne pense par une seconde que le non-fumeur est vraiment gêné. Non, il veut simplement l'embêter, le priver d'un petit plaisir]. (*Tabac et santé*, October 1997, no. 137)[37]

This construction of smoking as "un petit plaisir" with which it is simply churlish to interfere accounts in large part for the fact that smoking restrictions are more readily respected in buses, trains, and airplanes than in cafés and restaurants. The latter are defined as zones of pleasure whereas the former are not.

The principle of solidarité dictates that smokers should, insofar as possible, not be segregated. Images of the smoker out in the cold, of "civil war between smokers and non-smokers" are invoked to argue against any overzealous enforcement of restrictions on when and where smoking will be allowed. Ideally, smokers and nonsmokers will resolve their disagreements through dialogue and negotiation and will arrive at a solution equally satisfying to all parties. This process is, however, likely to take a while, and there is no guarantee that it will be continuous.

> In the end, France will change like everyone else: the whole world is coming to know that the Marlboro cowboy died of smoker's cancer. But we have a long way still to go. [Enfin en France, on finira par évoluer comme partout: tout le monde commence à savoir que le cowboy Marlboro est mort du cancer du fumeur. Mais on est encore loin.] (*Tabac et santé*, October 1997, no. 137)

Britain

Late in 1998, within a year of coming into office, Britain's Labor government issued a white paper, *Smoking Kills,* laying out its policy objectives in the tobacco-control arena (UK Department of Health 1998). These included a nationwide campaign focused on "protecting children from the tobacco industry," including enforcement of existing under-age sales restrictions; legislation "soon" to end billboard and other tobacco advertising; smoking-cessation programs; and a range of numerical targets for smoking reduction. Although tobacco-control advocates were critical of what they saw as important omissions (for example, no legislative bans on smoking in public or in the workplace), the overall response was remarkably enthusiastic. The British Medical Association described the white paper as "an historical first step against the tobacco industry" (Boseley 1998, 4). *The Guardian* commented editorially, "the importance of this white paper cannot be overstated" ("Smoking to Death," December 11, 1998, 21).

Enthusiasm was premature. It took nearly five years—and considerable political maneuvering—before the promised legislation became law. As *The Guardian* described the situation on August 23, 2002,

> It took two sessions of parliament before an unnecessarily diluted bill was introduced, and then that was killed by the [dissolution of parliament for a general election]. There would have been no bill this session but for the intervention of the Liberal peer, Tim Clement-Jones, who introduced a private member's measure into the Lords that was identical with the earlier government bill. With much embarrassment, ministers have belatedly backed it. ("A Healthy Ban on Adverts," 19)

The Tobacco Advertising and Promotion Act, as the bill was known, passed the House of Commons in October 2002 and came into force on Valentine's Day of 2003. It banned the advertising and promotion of tobacco products except at point of sale; a ban on sponsorship of "transcontinental sports" (that is, Formula One auto racing) was deferred. Somewhat surprisingly, in 2006—a mere three years later—the government abandoned its longstanding position in favor of voluntary regulation of public smoking, and Parliament voted 453 to 125 in favor of a total ban on smoking inside "virtually every enclosed public place and workplace" throughout England, to take effect in 2007 (White 2006).

Doubtless these were landmark events. However, tobacco control had been on Britain's policy agenda in one form or another since the mid-1960s. Beginning in 1971, bills were regularly introduced by private members and debated in Parliament (seventeen bills were introduced by one member alone, and at least five lengthy debates on smoking took place between 1971 and 1995); two scientific committees were appointed and submitted reports; and at least twelve separate "voluntary agreements" on labeling, advertising, and sponsorship were negotiated between the government and the tobacco industry. The novelty of the 1998 white paper and the legislation that ultimately followed was less in the specific policies advanced than that for the first time those policies were advanced in the name of the government rather than in the form of private members' bills in Parliament (seldom successful) or as the outcome of closed-door negotiations with representatives of the tobacco industry sitting as (at least formally) equal partners. Referring to the white paper in a December 11, 1998, article, *The Guardian* described it as:

> the beginning of a process which should have started years ago but would never have been initiated by the Conservatives, whose mateyness with the industry, enthusiasm for cigarette revenue and determination to allow the

individual the freedom to smoke himself to death would not allow it. Labour must be given credit for making a real effort to tackle the biggest public health problem of all. ("Smoking to Death," 21)

The Guardian's comments were a bit unjust. Only within the previous two years had *any* British government, Labor or Conservative, shown the least enthusiasm for legislation (or any other form of coercive regulation) to tackle smoking as a public health problem. The government had acted, but it had done so for the most part indirectly: through the appointment of "expert" committees; through surrogates, either government-funded or acting with the knowledge and support of one or another minister; and through a long series of gentlemen's agreements with the tobacco industry.

Tobacco and the State

The role of tobacco in the British economy was established in the seventeenth century, when colonial tobacco planters agreed to pay twice the customary import duties to the Crown in return for a prohibition on tobacco cultivation in England (Goodman 1998). This and other agreements with tobacco merchants "resulted in a considerable flow of revenue into the Exchequer" (12). The flow of revenue continues to this day, and more than one observer has argued that it was the major factor "inhibiting governmental action to reduce tobacco consumption" (Friedman 1975, 112; Taylor 1984; HM Revenue and Customs 2005). However, though taxes currently account for 80 percent of the price of cigarettes, the relative importance of cigarette taxes as a revenue source has declined considerably in recent years (Townsend 1987b; Makay and Eriksen 2002).

The Tobacco Industry   Tobacco manufacturing in Britain is dominated by four large multinational corporations. Jobs in tobacco manufacturing (concentrated in a few parliamentary constituencies) as well as among the many small tobacconists and news agents who sell cigarettes featured as major issues in Parliamentary debate since the subject of tobacco control was first broached in the early 1970s. Historically, the relation between government and the tobacco industry has been close, exemplified by the movement of officials out of office and into industry positions or consultancies (see, for example, Gilmore and McKee 2004, 235).

Gentlemen's Agreements   The epidemiologic evidence against tobacco emerged, then, in the context of a more than 400-year relation between the British government and the tobacco industry. The relation was formalized in the early days of World War II with the creation of a Tobacco Advisory Committee (TAC) of manufacturers to advise the government on how to ensure cigarette supplies in wartime (Read 1992); it is at the core of what

Melvyn Read calls the "producer network," consisting of the tobacco industry and two key government departments, of the Exchequer and of Trade and Industry. The pattern of insider negotiation between ministers and the industry (the "mateyness" abjured by *The Guardian)* was established well before its incarnation in the form of the voluntary agreements so abhorred by British advocates of tobacco control. Indeed, these agreements fell within an entrenched policymaking tradition. The "gentlemen's agreement [is] deeply rooted in the British culture. And the feeling that laws should be used as little as possible. And the tradition of self-regulation . . . the voluntary agreements are in that tradition" (interview with a former civil servant responsible for tobacco policy within the Department of Health during the late 1980s, May 1995). In parliamentary debate on proposed tobacco legislation, among the arguments advanced by the legislation's opponents were that "confrontation" should be avoided in principle and that legislation was an evil: "legislation should be resorted to only if there is an overwhelming argument that we shall not make any worthwhile progress without it" (United Kingdom 1976, 866, 858; on the tradition of voluntary agreements, see also Friedman 1975, 132–36; Popham 1981; Calnan 1984).

The dangers of smoking had been well accepted within the British government by the late 1950s. Beginning in the mid-1960s, increasingly strong action against smoking and the tobacco industry was attempted by successive ministers of health, to be frustrated in each case by the "producer network" and its various allies (Taylor 1984; O'Conner 1995). The battles were fought almost entirely among government, industry and, to a lesser extent, scientific "insiders." Something of their flavor from the perspective of a powerful opponent of antitobacco action is reflected in the diaries of Richard Crossman, a cabinet minister in the Labour government from 1964 to 1970.

Among the first health ministers to take on cigarettes directly was Kenneth Robinson, minister of health when Crossman was leader of the House of Commons. Having succeeded through purely intragovernmental maneuvering (that is, without recourse to Parliament) in banning cigarette ads on television (in 1965), Robinson wanted to ban the tobacco industry's next "wildly successful" sales promotion scheme, redeemable gift coupons included with each cigarette pack (Taylor 1984, 82). Negotiations with the industry, Robinson's first recourse, were going nowhere, and Robinson publicly threatened legislation, much to Crossman's chagrin:

> We are in danger of becoming known as the Government which stops what
> the working classes really want. . . . Today they had another grouse about
> the Government–the announcement that we were going to stop coupons in
> cigarette cartons. When this proposal was urged by Kenneth Robinson at

Home Affairs Committee I had pleaded that we should hold it back for at least twelve months. . . . But no, the Minister of Health had to make his policy announcement and he chose to do so this morning (just before a crucial by-election), thereby battering the poor old Leicester Labour Party with another blow. (Crossman 1975, 532)

Despite considerable support within the government for action against the tobacco industry, Crossman was ultimately successful in blocking any and all legislation (1978, 147). In 1968, Crossman became secretary of state for the newly created Department of Health and Social Services, and Robinson was replaced by a less confrontational minister of health. No further action was taken by the government until 1971, when the newly elected Conservative government, galvanized by a biting second report from the Royal College of Physicians, resumed negotiation with the tobacco industry, leading to the first voluntary agreement.[38]

The pattern thus established, of threatened legislation, negotiation followed by voluntary agreement, and the departure or reshuffling to other posts of health ministers who were too aggressive in their approach to the industry, continued at least through the mid-1990s. The former civil servant described these agreements as the industry's "most brilliant strategy. . . . These agreements, which are largely useless in reducing tobacco promotion, are frequently cited by ministers when rejecting the need for legislation." Indeed, in parliamentary debate, the industry was lauded by its defenders for its willingness to cooperate with the government, with the suggestion that this harmonious relationship was threatened by legislation. A credible threat of legislation was, on the other hand, perceived by health ministers as essential to obtaining agreement. As David Owen, former minister of health, explained: "Voluntary agreements are not worth the paper they're written on, unless the industry knows the Minister of Health has the power to legislate" (cited in Taylor 1984, 87).[39]

Although antismoking activists' uniform discontent with the cozy relations between the British government and the tobacco industry was understandable, the pattern I have described closely follows Britain's national style of regulation: "There is a preferred type of machinery, reflecting normative values—which is to avoid electoral politics and public conflict in order to reach consensus or 'accommodation' in the labyrinth of consultative machinery which has developed" (Jordan and Richardson 1982, 81). Based on his study of environmental regulation (which has much in common with smoking–tobacco control), David Vogel identifies key elements of this regulatory style, comparing it with that of the United States:

British regulation is relatively informal and flexible while American regulation tends to be more formal and rule-oriented. Britain makes extensive

use of self-regulation and encourages close cooperation between government officials and representatives of industry. The United States does little
of the former and has generally been suspicious of the latter. (1986, 24)

And, again in sharp contrast to the United States, access to the regulatory
process is controlled by government officials, effectively "insulating many
of [Britain's] regulatory bodies from public scrutiny" (25).[40]

Although voluntary agreements were the principal bête-noir of antitobacco advocates, they were not, in fact, the centerpiece of the British
government's smoking/tobacco policy. Before passage of the Tobacco
Advertising and Promotion Act in 2003, that place was occupied by taxes,
or what government officials called "action on the price of tobacco products," a price almost wholly under central government control (UK Department of Health 1993). The government perceived high tobacco taxes as an
effective smoking deterrent and at least neutral in their revenue impact,
both conclusions supported by economic analyses (Townsend 1993).
They were popular among antismoking activists and conservative supporters of voluntary agreements and controversial among scholars and
politicians concerned with their differential impact on the poor (see, for
example, Marsh and McKay 1994; Berridge 2004).[41]

Professional Activism

The British movement against smoking was initiated by the Royal College of Physicians (RCP) in the late 1950s, sustaining the effort at first on
its own and later through its lobbying arm, Action on Smoking and
Health (ASH). In 1984, the British Medical Association entered the fray.
Voluntary organization either at the level of large health charities, comparable to the American Cancer Society, or at the grass roots played virtually no role in the British campaign against smoking. The evidence for
this vacuum is striking.

A civil servant interviewed by Virginia Berridge in 1995 remarked on
"how little voluntary pressure group activity there was for smoking by
comparison with other areas of social concern" (1998, 153). Voluntary
organizations did exist. Britain had two groups to promote cancer research,
the Peale Cancer Research Fund and the Cancer Research Campaign.
Both were dominated by medical scientists, saw their primary goal as
fund-raising for medical research, and evinced a corresponding distaste
for "politics" that might interfere with this goal. While these organizations have recently become more supportive of Britain's antismoking
campaign, during the first two decades of antismoking advocacy they
were conspicuous primarily for their absence. The National Society of
Non-Smokers (NNS) had been founded in 1926, and ASH had some local
branches. However, these groups were not only discounted by officials

and self-styled legitimate activists—as well as by such medical historians as Roy Porter and Virginia Berridge—but, in the case of NNS, positively disowned. Berridge described the NNS as ineffectual, "a non-medical body whose arguments were perceived [by government] as akin to those of the temperance lobby, carrying the taint of moralism with little reference to science" (1999, 1185). David Simpson, former director of ASH, went further. "[ASH] had the backing of other organizations (that is, NNS) that we didn't want—the zealots—and made strenuous efforts to drop them" (1998, 209). Simpson dismissed local ASH groups as doing "little things locally" and went on to state that they weren't worth bothering with because antitobacco activities were now "officially encouraged" and part of each local health department's agenda (Simpson, interview, May 1995). Absent elite patronage and the personal connections with ministers and key civil servants that this patronage allowed, ASH would have been relegated to the "nuisance" category along with the NNS.

The Royal College of Physicians   The genesis of RCP involvement in tobacco control was, to say the least, convoluted. The first approach to the RCP, in 1956, came from the physician in whose unit Richard Doll[42] worked at the Central Middlesex Hospital, and was summarily rejected by the RCP president at the time, Lord Brain—among the "gilded elite of the London teaching hospitals" (Booth 1998, 193). Lord Brain was shortly replaced by a "provincial doctor," Robert Platt, who not only broke "the London monopoly on one of the high offices in the world of medicine" but also proved far more receptive to antismoking overtures (195). These overtures were triggered in a fashion simultaneously circuitous and chummy that is highly characteristic of the policy process in Britain.

In 1958, George Godber, subsequently chief medical officer and Sir George, was a deputy chief medical officer in the Ministry of Health, frustrated by ministry inaction on smoking and health. In the course of a meeting on another matter, Charles Fletcher, a respiratory physician with impeccable elite credentials, asked one of Godber's ministry colleagues what the ministry planned to do about smoking. A few days later, Godber invited Fletcher to lunch at his club and between them they agreed that Fletcher would sound out Platt: Godber, a civil servant, could not make the approach directly. Fletcher made the call that same day, Platt was highly receptive, and the nucleus of the committee that wrote the RCP report *Smoking and Health* met in the college's offices a few days later. Critical in this delicate play of Tinker to Evers to Chance were the access to centers of power and shared knowledge of appropriate forms of action guaranteed by the players' social standing in and outside of the world of medicine and by their preexisting social ties.

Smoking and Health was launched in 1962 with considerable fanfare, a crowded press conference and television interviews with Platt and

Fletcher. But its immediate impact, Fletcher suggests, was considerably greater in the United States than in Britain:

> The American Cancer Society circulated the report to all their members. So J. F. Kennedy, then US President, came to hear of it. He asked Dr. Luther Terry, then his Surgeon-General, to produce a US report. Thus the superb series of Surgeon-General's reports on all aspects of smoking and health were started. (Fletcher 1998, 203)

Fletcher was unsparing in his contrast of the British with the American government's response: "in the absence of any effective government action, cigarette sales had continued to rise. . . . The [report] did publicize the risks of smoking but had little effect on smoking habits because the government ignored it" (204).[43] The RCP's response to perceived government inaction took two forms: a second report (published in 1971) that was scathing in its denunciation of the government and, in the same year, the initiation of the new antismoking organization ASH.

Action on Smoking and Health   ASH was launched in much the same fashion as the first RCP report, by a small meeting at the college. Its extremely close ties to the RCP are reflected in its first set of officers: the first president of ASH was the president of the RCP and its chairman was Charles Fletcher, the instigator of the RCP reports. ASH was not initially, and never became, a grassroots membership organization. It was founded as a small, staff-led pressure group with the goal of influencing government policy through media campaigns and through its close connections with ministers, civil servants, and members of Parliament. The primary end in view was to legislate a ban on all tobacco advertising and promotion. Given its small size and resources, ASH was constrained to work closely with other and larger bodies—the Health Education Authority funded through the National Health Service and the British Medical Association.[44] To all intents and purposes, ASH was paid to engage in its advocacy activities by the government it was designed to attack.

The bulk of ASH's funding—around 80 percent—was from the Ministry of Health. Commenting on this seemingly anomalous practice (not unique to ASH), a British political scientist said,

> [Ministry] officials may feel that their constitutional position debars them from taking on the overtly political and propagandistic role of ASH directly. If they did, sympathetic discussions with the industry's representatives, leading to voluntary agreements, might well be jeopardised. Ministers may also benefit to some extent if the resentment of firms is directed on to ASH. On the other hand, ASH may bite the hand that feeds it. (Popham 1981, 333–34)[45]

ASH's position was nothing if not a delicate one. David Simpson, the director of ASH from 1979 to 1991, described to me in some detail how he maneuvered within these constraints. In 1979, the newly elected Thatcher government appointed Sir George Young as junior minister with responsibility for smoking and health. Sir George was a "stalwart member" of ASH's all-party group of MPs (Taylor 1984, 129), and he and Simpson developed a strong working relationship.

> I kept very close to the minister . . . because he was such a good guy. And he knew how to use an agency like us to lobby. He'd sometimes tell me . . . that you're criticizing me for this because I want to be seen under pressure to do such and such, or can you get the medical charities to do such and such? So, we'd have private meetings where we'd agree on strategy like that. (Simpson, interview, May 1995)

From the perspective of tobacco manufacturers and their friends in Parliament, Sir George was in fact much too good a guy. After two years he was, as David Simpson described it, "sidelined into [a] 'safer' job by pressure from the [parliamentary] whips, I believe, though in reality from the tobacco industry" (1998, 210). At about the same time, questions were raised in Parliament about whether ASH's "lobbying" efforts were consistent with its tax-exempt status and government funding. Although these attempts to undermine both ASH's credibility and its funding were unsuccessful, they did lead ASH to exercise a certain amount of caution.[46]

The British Medical Association   Among the strategies ASH adopted following its failure in the early 1980s to achieve its legislative goals through ministerial access was to work through the British Medical Association. The BMA is a principal negotiating partner with the Department of Health on behalf of the profession "and expects to be consulted on any matters which affect its members" (Ham 1992, 125). It is also, however, highly autonomous, a point emphasized repeatedly in accounts of the BMA's role in the British antitobacco movement: "the BMA was uniquely placed to spearhead an anti-smoking campaign, because it was not inhibited by having to rely on the Government for its money either directly or indirectly" (British Medical Association 1986, 7). Furthermore, the BMA was, in contrast to ASH, an extremely large organization with substantial infrastructure and a 150-year history of participation in medical public policy.[47] Still, the BMA delayed becoming directly involved in the anti-smoking campaign until 1984.[48] When it did, former ASH director David Simpson explained, "it was like the Americans entering the Second World War" (cited in British Medical Association 1986, 7). Not only did the BMA greatly extend the reach and impact of ASH's antitobacco message but it was also able to attack the government in ways that ASH could not:

> If I wanted to do something particularly critical [of the government], I then went to the BMA. [I'd say to them] I'll give you all the information, I'll write

the press release. Will you do it? And they'd say, sure. It was often just done as a phone call straight to the BMA's press office. (Simpson 1995)

Nevertheless, despite the primary role of the RCP and the BMA in agenda setting and in the mobilization of antitobacco advocacy, their influence in shaping the government's tobacco policy appears to have been quite limited.[49] In 1981, all eight presidents of royal colleges signed a joint letter to the minister of sport requesting a ban on tobacco sponsorship of sporting events. The letter was ignored (Taylor 1984, 107). A similar joint letter in 2003, this time with eighteen signatures, called for "legislation to make public places smoke-free" (*The Times* [London], "Call for a Ban on Public Smoking," November 25). Government response to this letter, described in *The Lancet* as "an unprecedented attack by the medical establishment of the UK on government health policy," was tepid at best ("How Do You Sleep at Night, Mr. Blair?" December 6, 2003, 1865). Whitehall has its own government-appointed scientific committees and is generally unfriendly to experts it has not itself anointed (see, for example, Crossman 1975).[50]

Enter Passive Smoking

Legislation to make public places smoke-free did pass in 2006. What is striking to an American observer, however, is the almost complete absence of attention to this issue either by activists or by the government during the 1970s and early 1980s, when passive smoking became the central theme of antitobacco advocacy in the United States. Commenting on this difference, the former director of ASH observed that U.S. antitobacco campaigners "concentrated on passive smoking, really, well before that thing was even invented" (Simpson 1995). The British aversion to raising this issue is well illustrated by the fact that in 1985 at the annual meeting of the BMA a motion calling for a tobacco act to ban all advertising and sponsorship passed by "a massive majority," whereas a motion to ban smoking on National Health Service property failed by twenty votes out of 194 (British Medical Association 1986, 69). Not until 1988, when publication of the *Froggat Report* (the final publication of the government's Independent Scientific Committee on Smoking and Health), in which passive smoking was accorded the legitimacy of science, did the idea of nonsmokers as innocent victims gain credibility in Britain. Consistent with British dislike of legislative regulation, however, nonsmoking policies were for many years issued in the form of suggested guidelines (see, for example, British Medical Journal 1991). In the 1998 white paper, *Smoking Kills*, the government stated its view that "a universal ban on smoking in all public places is [not] justified while we can make fast and substantial progress in partnership with industry (i.e., employers)." Only in the wake of Ireland's 2004 workplace smoking ban, the first in Europe, did this position begin to change.

Framing Contests

From the late 1960s to the present, debate about tobacco control has centered on two ideological constructs with high symbolic resonance in Britain: the liberty of the individual versus the protection of public health and the pleasures, livelihood, and (more recently) health of the working class. As early as 1967, debate within the government on antitobacco legislation was not about whether smoking was harmful but about "the propriety of the state interfering with personal liberties" (Taylor 1984, 84). As late as 2006, "both sides in the dispute [over smoking bans] squabbled to the very end over the right line to draw between protecting public health and individual liberty" (White 2006, 13). Arguments against tobacco legislation are phrased in terms of smokers' freedom to choose (see, for example, Taylor 1984, 134); the government used almost identical language in opposing legislated smoking bans: "In public places we want to see real choice for the public as a whole—non-smokers and smokers" (UK Department of Health 1998, sec. 7.5). The resonance of this rhetoric is suggested by its reappearance in every parliamentary debate on tobacco-related legislation; it may account for the continuing, and to an American remarkable, respectability of Britain's industry-subsidized prosmoking association, FOREST (Freedom Organization for the Right to Enjoy Smoking Tobacco).

A second rhetorical constant in Britain's tobacco debates is the theme of smoking and class. In the context of ongoing political contest between the Labor and Conservative parties, this discourse has had pragmatic political as well as ideological significance. Early on in the tobacco wars (as noted earlier) Richard Crossman attributed the loss of a vital Labor constituency to working class anger over government interference with "what the working classes really want [that is, to smoke]" (Crossman 1975, 532). More recently, conservative MPs presented themselves as defenders of working-class jobs against the callous indifference of tobacco's foes: "If members do not think the potential loss of jobs is real, let them come with me to Northolt [the speaker's constituency] and meet people whose jobs will be threatened. They do not care" (Hansard 1995, 1262). By 2002, Labor had repositioned smoking from a vital element of working-class culture to a threat to working class health: "smoking is . . . one of the principal causes of health inequalities in our country" (United Kingdom 2002, 684). And in a final twist, the Trades Union Congress urged MPs to support the 2006 ban on smoking in public places (TUC 2006). Turning Crossman on his head, the TUC interpreted this legislation not as depriving the working class of its pleasures but as protecting workers from danger to their health. Framed in this way, the workplace smoking ban received nearly unanimous Labor support.

From its inception—and this is my last point—the principal target of the antitobacco movement in Britain has been the tobacco industry, not the individual smoker. Far earlier than in the United States, the industry was publicly denounced as a killer, a drug pusher, and a merchant of death. The following quotes from the 1976 parliamentary debate give a flavor of this rhetoric:

> They are, in effect, mass killers. They are committing genocide by their products. (United Kingdom 1976, 825)

> Tobacco manufacturers produce an addictive drug and do everything in their power to induce people to become addicted to it. . . . I suggest that tobacco manufacturers are more akin to drug pushers than to motor car manufacturers. (825)

The industry's victims were identified as children "clearly not in a position to exercise choice and discretion for themselves" and, later, as women, young or pregnant. In this litany, adult men and nonsmokers were equally notable for their absence.

Canada

A comparative study of tobacco-control policies published in the mid-1970s observed that the Canadian federal government "has responded more slowly to the [smoking and health] controversy than the United States or Great Britain" and suggested that perhaps Canada was waiting to learn the impact of these countries' policies before plunging into the fray itself (Friedman 1975). By 1990, Canada was being described not only as a world leader in antitobacco laws but as the world's pacesetter, pointing the road for other countries to follow (Mintz 1990). Although the government's tobacco policies were set back in the 1990s, as I shall describe, Canada reasserted its world leadership in 1997 with the passage of its second tobacco act in ten years. Canada's transition from laggard to leader was abrupt as such policy changes go: it took place over a period of about nine years between 1979 and 1988. About ten years later there was an equally rapid policy shift in the province of Quebec. My focus in this narrative is on the circumstances that surrounded these remarkable changes in public health policy.

Policy Evolution: From Laggard to Leader

My Canadian policy narrative begins with the major studies of smoking and mortality published between 1950 and 1954.

Phase One (1950 to 1980)   A resolution proposing the establishment of a special committee to consider the health and other consequences of smoking was introduced (and defeated) in Parliament as early as 1951. In 1954, the Canadian Medical Association (CMA) warned publicly of the hazards of smoking and the federal Department of Health and Welfare began its own study of smoking's health effects. The statements of medical and health authorities became increasingly forceful as evidence for the perils of smoking accumulated and in 1963 Canadian Health Minister Judy LaMarsh—taking her cue from the 1962 report of the British Royal College of Physicians—stated that smoking was a contributory cause of lung cancer. Not coincidentally, the Canadian Tobacco Manufacturers' Council was established in that same year, well before the emergence of an organized tobacco-control movement.

The first phase of tobacco control in Canada followed what was in retrospect a relatively conventional path. Beginning in the early 1960s, legislation to ban advertising and require warning labels on tobacco products was periodically introduced in Parliament and—for the next twenty-five years—failed with equal regularity. Extensive hearings on tobacco issues were initiated in 1968 by the House of Commons Standing Committee on Health, Welfare, and Social Affairs. The result was the Isabelle report, the Canadian equivalent of the U.S. Surgeon General and British Royal College reports but produced, interestingly enough, by politicians rather than medical men (although Isabelle himself was a physician). In its rejection of industry arguments (for example, the uncertainty of medical evidence that smoking was harmful) and in the forcefulness and wide-ranging nature of its recommendations (including a complete ban on tobacco advertising) the Isabelle report was far ahead of its time and, indeed, far ahead of Britain and the United States. Nevertheless, although legislation to implement the Isabelle committee's recommendations was introduced in Parliament in 1970 with the backing of the health minister, it died without debate. Midway through the hearings, the tobacco industry announced a voluntary code that included health warnings and a ban on radio and television ads. As in Britain, throughout the 1970s, successive voluntary agreements between government ministers and the industry were effective in blocking antitobacco legislation.[51]

Phase Two (1979 to 1988)   By the late 1970s, the relative quiet of Phase One was over, and a period of highly aggressive antitobacco politics had begun, aimed at placing tobacco control squarely on the national political agenda. The critical breakthrough for this movement came in 1986 when New Democratic Party MP Lynn McDonald's private bill—C-204, the Non-Smokers' Health Act—was chosen by lottery to receive parliamentary consideration.[52] McDonald's bill proposed to restrict smoking in federally regulated workplaces as well as on planes, trains and boats. Although luck got the bill to the House floor, once there "it played a critical role in pushing official government action forward. [By the time] it reached the floor of the House of Commons for debate, the 'Non-Smokers' Health Act' had become a lightning rod for anti-smoking activists" (Manfredi and Maioni 2004, 80). Under the pressure created by McDonald's bill, the government in the person of its health minister at the time, Jake Epp, quickly introduced its own bill—C-51, An Act to Prohibit the Advertising and Promotion, and Respecting the Labeling and Monitoring of Tobacco Products. From then on parliamentary debate on the two bills took place almost simultaneously.

The tobacco industry fought bill C-51 with all the forces at its command, and its passage was by no means ensured despite the government's large majority in the House of Commons. Against the industry was arrayed a coalition of health groups. I describe these groups' strategies in greater detail below. Suffice it to say that they more than matched in intensity those of the industry and were, in the event, successful. C-204 and C-51 were both passed in early 1988 and came into force in 1989. Manfredi and Maioni summarize the essential provisions of the Tobacco Products Control Act (TPCA), formerly C-51, as follows:

> [they] prohibited *all* forms of tobacco advertising in Canada; prohibited the free or discounted distribution of tobacco products; prohibited the use of tobacco trademarks on anything other than a tobacco product; permitted tobacco company sponsorship of cultural or sporting events as long as promotional material did not use specific brand names; and required that one of eight separate health warnings appear in an area covering at least 25 percent of cigarette packages. (2004, 81)

The Non-Smokers' Health Act (C-204) regulated smoking in workplaces under federal jurisdiction and on federally regulated transportation carriers (generally ships, aircraft, trains, and interprovincial buses). Taken together, this legislation went far beyond measures that existed in any other country at the time.

Phase Three (1988 forward)   The Canadian government's aggressive policies did not end with the TPCA and the Non-Smokers' Health Act. Since 1988 there have been two additional major pieces of legislation, the Tobacco Sales to Young Persons Act (1993) and the Tobacco Act (1997). The Tobacco Sales to Young Persons Act set eighteen as the minimum age for purchase of tobacco products and banned cigarette vending machines except in bars. The Tobacco Act was introduced to remedy portions of the TPCA struck down by the Canadian Supreme Court in 1995. It also gave

Health Canada new authority over packaging, with the result that Canada has among the most fearsome cigarette packages in the world. Signaling the current high level of collaboration among tobacco's opponents, in 1999 federal and provincial officials and national antitobacco advocacy groups signed the National Tobacco Control Strategy (a statement of intent) followed in 2001 by the Federal Tobacco Control Strategy, which allocated more than $480 million in federal funds to a range of tobacco-control measures. Other moves have included significant tax increases and litigation to defend the Tobacco Act and other aspects of the government's position.

The 1988 Non-Smokers Health Act was limited to federal workers and covered only about 10 percent of the population. However, the provinces eventually followed suit and "all provinces have [now] passed restrictions on smoking in public and private places under their jurisdiction (for example, schools, shopping malls, hospitals), and seven provinces have enacted legislation authorizing municipal authorities to pass smoking bylaws" (Manfredi and Maioni 2004, 74). Nevertheless, in contrast to its aggressive posture in other domains, "Canada has generally lagged behind the United States" in adopting restrictions on public smoking (Cunningham 1996, 113). This lag is particularly evident in the venues most visible to the casual visitor—restaurants and bars. Although more than 280 municipalities have by-laws restricting smoking in some fashion, only forty ban smoking in restaurants and twenty-five in bars.

Policy Detours   There were two major detours along the Canadian tobacco policy road: the Supreme Court's action just noted and, in the early 1990s, smuggling. The 1988 Tobacco Products Control Act was almost immediately challenged in court by the tobacco industry, and in the fall of 1995 the Supreme Court struck down two of its principal provisions: the total ban on tobacco advertising and promotion and the requirement for unattributed health warnings, that is, those not identified as to their source (RJR-MacDonald v. Canada 1995). This decision was, of course, perceived by Canadian antitobacco groups—many of whom had been parties to the suit as "interveners" (equivalent to amicus curiae) on the side of the government—as a major setback and, indeed, its immediate effect was to reinstate tobacco advertising, which had been banned while the litigation was in progress. Not surprisingly the industry attacked the 1997 Tobacco Act in court as well—the Supreme Court is expected to rule on that case early in 2007.

Rapid tax increases of the late 1980s and early 1990s led to a massive increase in smuggling across the U.S.-Canadian border. "By the beginning of 1994, tobacco smuggling had become a C$5 billion per year industry. Approximately one-third of all cigarettes consumed in Canada were obtained illegally, and more than 2 million Canadians purchased cigarettes smuggled to Canada from the United States" (Manfredi and Maioni 2004, 82). This surge of illegal activity presented the government with a major political problem (above and beyond the significant loss of tax revenue), and it responded with a tax rollback of close to 50 percent. Provinces with a smuggling problem, which included the two largest provinces, Ontario and Quebec, did likewise. Cigarette prices fell sharply and consumption increased.[53]

Actors

The 1997 Tobacco Act, which passed in the wake of these setbacks, was no cakewalk for the Canadian federal government. The act, wrote the *Montreal Gazette*, "was subject to a tumultuous public debate and one of the most intense lobbies ever waged by the health community on one side and by the tobacco companies on the other" (Wills 1997). Let me describe these two protagonists in greater detail.

The Tobacco Industry: Down But Not (Quite) Out   Tobacco is both grown and manufactured into cigarettes in Canada, and Canadians are highly partial to their local product: the country produces about 99 percent of the tobacco it consumes. Tobacco farming is concentrated in southern Ontario; manufacturing is in Quebec. The number of farms has declined dramatically since the early 1970s, from about 3,800 to about 1,500, due not only to reduced demand but also to the amalgamation of small farms into larger ones (Friedman 1975; Irvine and Sims 1997; Cunningham 1996). Tobacco farming continues to be profitable—decreases in per capita consumption have been largely offset by population growth—and by the late 1980s the number of farmers exiting from tobacco production, encouraged by a major federal crop-diversification initiative, had considerably slowed.[54]

Along with tobacco farming, cigarette manufacturing has also consolidated. Currently Canada has three major companies, down from four in the mid-1970s: Imperial, the largest with about two-thirds of the market, RJR-McDonald, and RBH (combining Rothman's and Benson and Hedges). Each of these companies is wholly or partially owned by British or American multinational firms (Irvine and Sims 1997). Manufacturing, like farming, is highly profitable—industry profits in 1995 "set an all-time record high" (Cunningham 1996, 18; see also Studlar 2002). Although the industry's present power to influence the politics of public health in Canadian parliaments is substantially diminished, the industry has taken full advantage of new political opportunities created by the Canadian Charter of Rights and Freedoms. The Charter gave "vast new power" to the lawyers and judges who would interpret it (see. for example, Morton 2000), presenting tobacco lawyers with a political venue where they hoped to find a friendlier reception than among elected bodies. Their success to date has been limited. In June 2006, more than a hundred Ontario health officials signed a letter urging the provincial premier to join other provinces in legal action against the industry to recover health care costs (action modeled explicitly on the U.S. example).

Crusaders Against Tobacco   The first phase of tobacco control in Canada was, as I observed, relatively conventional, led by traditional health interest groups and focused on education directed at the young. By the late 1970s this decorous climate had begun to shatter, to the point where in 1986 an industry trade journal, *Tobacco Reporter,* described Canada's "vociferous" antitobacco lobby as "one of the fiercest in the world" (Cunningham 1996, 201). Canada's path was superficially similar to that of the United States. First, the entrepreneurs of tobacco control in Canada were not physicians but lay zealots.[55] Second, the catalyst for an organized single-issue tobacco-control movement was the formation of "nonsmokers' rights" groups in the 1970s.[56] Third, by the mid-1980s, the relation between the Canadian Nonsmokers' Rights Association and the Canadian Cancer Society had evolved into the "bad cop, good cop" pattern that also characterized the relation of U.S. nonsmokers' rights groups with the American Cancer Society and other traditional health voluntaries. The Canadian movement rapidly distinguished itself from its American counterpart, however, by its organizational structure, its mode of operation, and its highly confrontational style.

The primary focus of the Non-Smokers' Rights Association (NSRA) was never on the rights of nonsmokers to be protected from tobacco smoke. From the first high-profile campaign (in 1979) to get the Toronto Transit Commission to refuse tobacco ads, the goal of NSRA was to use the regulatory and legislative powers of government against the tobacco industry. The Canadian federal government has exclusive power (not shared with the provinces) to enact criminal law. Ad bans and package warnings were (activists believed, and the Canadian Supreme Court later concurred) within the scope of federal criminal law powers, and the NSRA took the first good opportunity to move its campaign to Ottawa. A single-minded focus on federal legislation to regulate industry practices shaped both the organizational and rhetorical strategies of Canadian antitobacco activists. They eschewed grassroots organizing in favor of highly centralized—even authoritarian—organizational forms, cultivated close ties with government insiders and used the media to build fires under laggard politicians.

In the Canadian (as in the British and French) parliamentary system, power is concentrated in the government's executive branch:

> Most interest groups discovered long ago that parliamentary sovereignty was a myth. As a result, little time is spent lobbying backbenchers or oppo-

sition members. Instead, interest group activity typically focuses on cabinet ministers and the bureaucracy in the relevant government departments. (Landes 1995, 493)

Key to the legislative success of the NSRA and its allies in the mid-1980s was their relationship with a career civil servant within the health ministry (Neil Collishaw) and, through him, with the health minister, Jake Epp:

> He [Collishaw] couldn't be a lobbyist but he could produce things that would be valuable . . . research that you need to move the agenda ahead. We [NSRA and Collishaw] could work very well as a team. [Further] we could short circuit the system [that is, bypass the bureaucratic hierarchy, go directly to the minister]. A good bureaucrat would say, "look, you know, you gotta get something pretty quick done by Tuesday." And you say, "does it have anything to do with a cabinet meeting on Wednesday?" and he says, "yeah." (Interview with NSRA staff member, August 1995)

As these comments suggest, outside pressure not only was welcomed but actually was also promoted from within the government itself. Collishaw recalls that in the early 1980s citizens' antismoking groups were "weak and disorganized." Aware that he "needed citizens groups making noise" to advance the tobacco-control agenda at the federal level, Collishaw actively sought out these groups and found ways to direct funding and other resources (for example, insider information and access) to them. The symbiotic relationship between government and advocacy groups was explicitly recognized by Jake Epp in comments following passage of the 1980s tobacco-control legislation. He praised NSRA for its "leadership role . . . in mobilizing public support so that the government could more seriously address the tobacco-related chronic disease epidemic" (Mintz 1990, 36).

Strikingly absent from the Canadian insider scenario were the physicians who dominated these scenarios in Britain and France.[57] Tobacco-control advocates in all three parliamentary political structures used insider strategies, but the key actors were quite different: "zealots" in Canada; experts in Britain and France.[58] Canadian advocates made clear to me that physicians in their movement served primarily as window dressing:

> Having a few doctors that were proactive makes all the difference in the world because they were able to give credibility to all the other people. Having a few doctors was absolutely key, but they've got to be the right ones. (Interview with CCS staff member, August 1995)[59]

Physicians were perceived by these lay advocates as, by and large, overly conservative, committed to a "medical model" of disease causation, and unwilling to engage in the kind of "brass-knuckle hardball" tactics favored by NSRA. In Canada, unlike France, the work of British and American scientific authorities was sufficient to establish the dangers of smoking; no further recourse to medical authority was required, nor did physicians step forward to assume leadership of the tobacco-control movement, as they did in Britain and France.

Landes asserts that interest groups in Canada have traditionally operated in secrecy, "out of view of the ordinary citizen" (1995, 493). Not so the NSRA and its allies. On the contrary, they made highly aggressive use of the media, "simultaneously [working] the channels of mass communication and inside political gamesmanship" (Kagan and Vogel 1994, 29). Characteristic of these tactics was the notorious "Mulroney/Neville" ad linking the Prime Minister Brian Mulroney to William H. Neville, a "consummate well-connected political insider . . . personally close to the Prime Minister" who had just been appointed president of the Canadian Tobacco Manufacturers' Council (Cunningham 1996, 74). The full-page ad, headlined "How Many Canadians Will Die from Tobacco Industry Products May Largely Be in the Hands of These Two Men," appeared in Canada's leading newspaper, the *Toronto Globe and Mail*, only hours before the tobacco-control bill was to be marked up in the House of Commons. "The ad devastated Neville's influence by personalizing the tobacco lobby and making whatever success it might have politically damaging to Mulroney" (Mintz 1990, 31). The NSRA won by exposing to public view and demonizing the insider strategy traditionally used by Canadian business lobbyists—a strategy the health lobby itself did not hesitate to use, as I noted.

Quebec: History Repeats Itself

Although Canada's federal government has played the primary role in tobacco control, many provinces have enacted their own parallel or complementary legislation: "the federal laws and regulations act as a kind of minimum standard, with provinces having the ability to 'ratchet up' the regulatory framework" (Manfredi and Maioni 2004, 74).[62] Among the provinces most aggressive in taking advantage of this opportunity was Quebec.

Tensions between Quebec's linguistically and culturally distinctive society and that of the rest of Canada, and between Canadian nationalism and Quebec separatism, thread throughout Canadian history. Quebec has been particularly aggressive in its stance toward the organization of medical care, within the context of Canada's national health-care system, asserting the province's right to establish a unique system somewhat less friendly to professional stakeholders than the other provinces (see, for example, Gray 1991; Maioni 2002). In tobacco control, however, Quebec was a notorious laggard. Smoking prevalence in Quebec remained the highest among the ten provinces until the year 2000. Cigarette manufacturing is concentrated in Quebec; the largest of the three Canadian companies (Imasco) has its headquarters in Montreal. Writing in 1995, a French-Canadian journalist described Quebec as "la terre des fumeurs et le havre des fabricants [the land of smokers and the haven of manufacturers]" (Nadeau 1995, 30). Quebec was the despair of tobacco-control advocates. That year, a representative of the Canadian Cancer Society commented to me,

> One of the problems in Canada, smoking rates are much higher among French speaking Canadians, and you have a different mentality in the province of Québec. [Smoking] is one of the little pleasures of life. There is a real difference between French Canadians and the rest of Canada. (Interview, August 1995)

This mentality—one in which questions of cultural identity and economic viability became intertwined with those of tobacco control—was prominent in debate over the 1997 Tobacco Act. In a provincial referendum two years earlier, sovereignty for Quebec had barely been defeated.

> In a country worried stiff about national unity and job losses, [the tobacco lobby] made survival of the tobacco industry a national-unity issue by pointing out that most of Canada's cigarettes are made in Québec. If the government squeezed the industry, said the lobbyists, it would kill jobs in the already-depressed Montréal economy. This would simply give the [separatist] Québec government another stick with which to beat Ottawa. (Gray 1997, 239)

Among the provisions of the act was an end to tobacco industry sponsorship for cultural and sporting events, many of which (the Montreal Jazz Festival, the du Maurier Tennis Tournament, Formula-One auto racing) take place in Quebec. In parliamentary debate, members of the Bloc québecois (the Quebec separatist party) framed this provision as a deliberate attack on the provincial economy. In the event, the Tobacco Act passed by a wide margin. However, in a bow to the potential for political fallout in Quebec, it was almost immediately amended to delay the full effect of the sponsorship phase-out until October 2003.

Somewhat surprisingly—given this history—the provincial legislature in 1998 passed the Quebec Tobacco Act, establishing "a comprehensive regulatory regime that complements and covers the same range of subjects as the federal statutes" (Manfredi and Maioni 2004, 74). The Quebec legislation mirrors federal legislation in respect of controls on advertising but goes substantially beyond it in the restrictions imposed on smoking in the workplace. This action is counterintuitive on its face. It can be explained, however, by a unique concatenation of political opportunities and by the rapid mobilization of a heretofore essentially dormant anti-smoking movement.

In the winter of 2002, a long-time tobacco-control advocate commented to me that, "never in my wildest dreams would I have believed that we [in Quebec] would have arrived at the point where we are today." Following a path ten years behind but otherwise strikingly parallel to that of English Canada, French Canada moved from tobacco-control laggard to leader in the remarkably short period of seven years. The turning point for tobacco control in Quebec came in 1994. Open and widespread smuggling and black market purchase of cigarettes had the dual consequences of forcing the provincial government to confront tobacco as a political problem and of forcing tobacco-control activists to confront their own organizational weaknesses, as reflected in their inability to prevent a major provincial (in addition to federal) tax rollback.

Tobacco control in Quebec before 1994 was largely in the hands of health voluntaries, such as the Heart and Stroke Foundation, and was limited to programs for education and cessation directed at youth and smokers. Provincial health authorities did not define smoking as a public health problem and neither staff nor funds were dedicated to tobacco control. The economic and political hand of the tobacco industry lay heavily on Quebec in the form of jobs and of close industry ties with politicians, unions, and the media. The latter were markedly hostile to tobacco control: activists were pilloried in print as the ayatollahs of tobacco. Two sets of circumstances combined to open a window of opportunity for change. First, public and political furor over cigarette smuggling across the U.S. border with Quebec triggered a chain of events that included the tax rollback and a widely reported rise in cigarette consumption. Second, provincial elections in the fall of 1994 replaced the Quebec Liberals with the Parti québecois and brought in a new health minister—Jean Rochon—who had prior knowledge of and interest in tobacco control and a strong commitment to tobacco legislation.[61] Rochon could accomplish very little, however—as he recognized—without powerful pressure from outside the government, and it was essential that this pressure be articulated in French.[62] Hardball antitobacco advocacy had, heretofore, been almost entirely in English.

Antitobacco mobilization in Quebec was galvanized by the events of 1994. Mobilization did not come out of nowhere. A tiny nucleus of individuals worked on tobacco within the provincial health department and the local health voluntaries and were profoundly dissatisfied with the tepid approach taken by these entities. With the newfound financial and political support and encouragement of the provincial health ministry, and with some support from the NSRA in Toronto (an NSRA office was opened in Montreal in 1995), the Coalition québecois pour le contrôle du tabac was launched in 1996. The coalition was modeled directly, and deliberately, on an earlier successful Quebec coalition for gun control.[63] It was funded by monies subscribed by each of the seventeen Quebec regional health directorates from their tobacco control budgets.

Coalition staff describe their mode of operation as nonconfrontational by comparison with that of the national NSRA.[64] There are similarities nonetheless. Although it was formally a coalition, the Quebec movement was in fact the creation of two energetic individuals who demanded a sign-off of decision-making authority from each potential coalition partner before it could join. Further, to pass the Quebec Tobacco Act, the coalition, like the NSRA, successfully combined insider and outsider strategies. In addition to working closely with Rochon's political staff, the coalition seized every opportunity to get its message to the local media. Here, again, circumstances were in their favor. Coincident with the tax rollback and the accession of Rochon as provincial health minister in 1994 was the discovery in the United States of the notorious tobacco-industry documents, dating back to the 1950s, in which the harmful properties of tobacco were clearly acknowledged (Glantz et al. 1996; Hilts 1996). The discoveries were widely publicized in Canada and Quebec, where American television is universally available, and were capitalized on by the coalition and its ally the NSRA to undermine the industry's credibility with the local media (and, mutatis mutandis, with politicians and the public).

Arguably, the coalition benefited from the favorable social and political climate in the country at large (though from the perspective of many Québecois the enthusiasm of anglophone Canada for tobacco control was a good reason to reject it). Its success was made possible, however, by a succession of favorable events including—of perhaps the greatest importance—elite political support from within the separatist party itself, the Parti Québecois.

Health versus Greed: The Framing of Tobacco Control

As the goals of collective action evolve, so does the rhetoric of its leaders. When in the early 1980s Canada's tobacco-control activists moved away from health education and the mobilization of nonsmokers to mobilizing political elites or their constituents to accomplish specific legislative goals, their framing of the tobacco "problem" shifted as well. The central components of this latter frame are the construction of smoking as, above all, a question of health (not rights), the attribution of responsibility for the health problem to the tobacco industry rather than to the industry's "victims" (and to the government insofar as it fails to address the problem), and the assignment of responsibility for solving the problem to the government (not to individual smokers).

The health of Canadians as an overriding value was invoked in support of tobacco-control legislation in 1969 by then Health Minister John Munroe. In his testimony before the Isabelle committee, Munroe asserted that "over and above these economic questions remains the human factor. We can never lose sight of the fact that the issue is the health and happiness, and indeed the lives of countless Canadians" (Friedman 1975, 88). When and why this construction was revived is suggested by Rob Cunningham:

> In the 1970s, the discourse was oriented more toward rights, as symbolized by the name of the Non-Smokers' Rights Association. The emphasis today is on addressing the tobacco epidemic, on reducing disease, and on saving lives. If this issue positioning is done successfully, as it often has been, the health lobby has an advantage over the industry, which seeks to frame the debate in terms having nothing to do with health, such as freedom, jobs, or law and order. (1996, 200)

That this "advantage" was fully recognized by the industry is reflected in the comment of the head of the Canadian Tobacco Manufacturers Council following passage of the Tobacco Products Control Act in 1988: "Clearly one of the aims—and to give them their due one of the successes— of the anti-tobacco lobby was to make this appear to be a health issue. And when that happens that's a difficult area for the industry" (cited in Cunningham 1996, 201).

Just why the health frame is so awkward for the industry requires some explanation; it is less self-evident than it may appear. First, and most important, is that Canadian citizens expect their government to act as a guardian of the people's health. Antonia Maioni comments on the ideological underpinnings of Canada's health care system:

> Three specific ideas were embedded [in these health plans]. The first idea is that health care is a public good and should be subject to extensive regulation. The second idea is that the state must ensure universal coverage and equitable access. The third idea is that the federal [central] government belongs in the health policy arena as a guardian of the "right" to health care. (2002, 90)

These ideas are readily interpreted as a broad government "mandate to protect the health of Canadians" (Non-Smokers Rights Association 1986, 10). Health brings in the government as a major player in a way that rights do not. Indeed, rights work in favor of the tobacco industry, as reflected in the 1995 Canadian Supreme Court's decision striking down a number of provisions of the Tobacco Products Control Act as trammeling on the industry's right of free expression (RJR-MacDonald v. Canada 1995).

Second, as I noted earlier, under Canada's legal framework the federal Parliament is empowered to safeguard the public's health by means of criminal legislation: "The scope of the federal power to create criminal legislation with respect to health matters is broad, and is circumscribed only by the requirements that the legislation must contain a prohibition accompanied by a penal sanction and must be directed at a legitimate public health evil" (RJR-MacDonald v. Canada 1995, 32). The Canadian Supreme Court agreed that the Tobacco Products Control Act was just such a piece of criminal legislation; its provisions were overturned on other grounds. Therefore, threats to the health of Canadians are at one and the same time an appeal to shared communitarian values and a strategy for bringing the full power of government down on the tobacco industry. No wonder the industry found this construction "difficult."

Causal responsibility for the "public health evil" of tobacco was laid, in a 1986 *Washington Post* article, directly at the door of the tobacco industry: "We don't talk about smoking killing 'poor old Uncle Ed.' We talk about the tobacco industry killing poor old Uncle Ed" (Gar Mahood, cited in "Smoking Bans Grow in Canada," Herbert Denton, September 19, p. F1). In a report titled, *A Catalogue of Deception: The Use and Abuse of Voluntary Regulation of Tobacco Advertising in Canada,* released by the NSRA in the same year, the industry's duplicity over the years was chronicled in elaborate detail. This report was identified as "for submission to the Honourable Jake Epp, Minister of Health, Health and Welfare Canada" and played an important role in convincing Epp of the need to replace the voluntary code with legislation.[65] When health is pitted against greed— "the profit motive" as more elegantly put by Canada's Supreme Court— health often wins.

There was no doubt in the minds of those who wrote the *Catalogue of Deception* (as well as more recent documents of similar intent) as to the location of responsibility for addressing the tobacco evil. The report was addressed to the health minister. A more recent document of comparable authorship (NSRA plus several other tobacco-control advocacy groups) addressed the prime minister directly: "Prime Minister, Integrity means honouring your commitment to tobacco legislation. Prime Minister, where is the tobacco legislation?" Both reports made clear their view that a government that does not act shares "direct responsibility for the continuing epidemic of tobacco-related illness and death."[66]

Finally, protection of nonsmokers has been a common theme in Canadian (as in American) rhetoric, albeit more muted and with a very different notion of where the boundaries between smokers and nonsmokers should be drawn. From the Canadian perspective involuntary smoking is smoking in the workplace and in public transport, not (or not primarily) in bars and restaurants. Among the most frequently cited victims of workplace smoking were pregnant women, effectively merging child welfare and involuntary exposure into a single package:

When we cannot even come down to the decision in this Legislature, after debate, that an unborn foetus has protection from secondhand smoke, in the face of all the evidence, then where are we? . . . [Tobacco is the number one killer of our population] yet we have a minister who is frightened to put upon the employers the obligation to provide a pregnant woman with a smoke-free workplace. (Grossman and Price 1992, 3–54)[67]

Although pregnant women are a relatively small proportion of the workplace population exposed to secondhand smoke, they and their unborn children hold a privileged status as innocent victims. In this reading of the passive smoking debate, pregnant women workers and workers generally can stay away from bars and restaurants but are required to attend their place of employment. So it is around the latter spaces that boundaries must be carefully drawn.

As the tide of smoking bans rose around the world, beginning with Ireland in 2004, Canada's cautious approach began to give way. By June 2006, legislation with 100 percent smoking bans inside restaurants and bars had been enacted by seven provinces, including Ontario and Quebec, and two territories.

Chapter 6

HIV/AIDS in
Injection Drug Users

THE FIRST five cases of what later came to be known as Acquired Immune Deficiency Syndrome (AIDS) were reported in the *Morbidity and Mortality Weekly Report* (*MMWR*) on June 5, 1981, under the enigmatic title, "Pneumocystis pneumonia—Los Angeles." On June 12, 1981, the "afternoon mail brought from the United States [to Dr. Willy Rozenbaum, Paris physician and infectious disease specialist] the *MMWR* describing the pneumonia outbreak in Los Angeles" (Shilts 1987, 72). Earlier that same day, Rozenbaum had diagnosed Pneumocystis in a gay man and, as Shilts describes, based on his interviews with Rozenbaum, immediately made the connection with the *MMWR* report. Communication within the international medical community about this new and strange syndrome was virtually instantaneous.[1] The lay press was quick to follow with its accounts.[2] The United States, Great Britain, Canada, and France were each confronted at essentially the same time with the same clinical data: an apparently new, frightening, possibly infectious disease among young homosexual men. What each country made of this new information was, in large part, a product of old social and political patterns, well-established in response to earlier critical periods in public health.

Stories of AIDS have been told and will continue to be told many times, from many perspectives. Early histories as well as political and cultural analyses were dominated by the experience of gay men (for example, Shilts 1987; Fee and Fox 1988). Not only were gay men publicly identified with AIDS from its inception, they were also articulate in speaking on their behalf and in positions to make themselves heard. The international scandal of France's delayed response to the danger of AIDS-tainted blood, the construction of transfusees as innocent AIDS victims, and an organized movement of hemophiliacs have ensured that the contentious cultural politics of AIDS and blood received substantial attention as well (Morelle 1996; Setbon 1993; Steffen 1996; Kirp 1997, 1999; Feldman and Bayer 1999).

Once a blood test for the causal agent (HIV) became available in 1985, each country confronted questions about who should be tested, when, under what circumstances, and with what consequences. There is a very large literature on the difficulties that these questions presented (and still present) and on the differences in countries' responses (see, for example, country reports in Kirp and Bayer 1992; Feldman and Bayer 1999 as well as a recent analysis by Baldwin 2005a). The stories least often told, however, and the ones that I will tell, are about AIDS and injection-drug users.[3] These stories are inseparable not only from the larger history of the AIDS epidemic, but also from the much longer history of the West's war on drugs.

AIDS made its public debut in the summer of 1981, reported almost simultaneously from New York and California in the form of two relatively rare conditions, Kaposi's sarcoma (a type of skin tumor) and Pneumocystis carinii pneumonia (CDC 1981a; 1981b). Nearly all of the reported cases were among homosexual men.[4] Before the year was over, three cases had been reported from Europe, again in homosexual men, of whom two had visited gay venues in the United States within the past year. By December 10, 1981, when the *New England Journal of Medicine* published three papers accompanied by an editorial on this "unexpected outbreak," more than 160 cases had been reported, reports were coming in at the rate of five or six a week, and the outbreak had become firmly identified with young male homosexuals practicing what these sober medical reports described as "liberated" or "promiscuous" lifestyles.[5]

The magnitude of the AIDS epidemic as it has evolved over time is measurable in several ways, none of them wholly satisfactory.[6] However, AIDS case reporting is reasonably complete in industrialized countries (Low-Beer et al. 1998). I use the number of reported cases per 100,000 total population per year for a broad comparison across the four countries included in this study. Figure 6.1 shows reported cases per 100,000 for the United States, the UK, France, and Canada from the beginning of the epidemic in 1981 through 2004.[7] The drop in incidence in the mid-1990s is attributable to the influence of new drug therapies in delaying progression from HIV infection to AIDS (CDC 1998, "Commentary").[8] The apparent surge in cases in the United States in 1992 and 1993 was due to an expanded definition of AIDS adopted in this country but not by Canada, France, or the UK. The point of this figure is to show, first, the relatively high rate of reported AIDS cases in the United States and, second, the relative ranking of the other three countries. For much of the 1990s, France's rates were considerably above those of Canada and the UK.

The HIV/AIDS epidemic is a moving target for many reasons, even in these four industrialized countries, where overall rates are low compared with many parts of the developing world. Not only has the advent of antiretroviral medications meant HIV infection is less likely to progress to AIDS, meaning that AIDS cases are an increasingly less accurate

Figure 6.1   Estimated AIDS Cases, 1981 to 2004

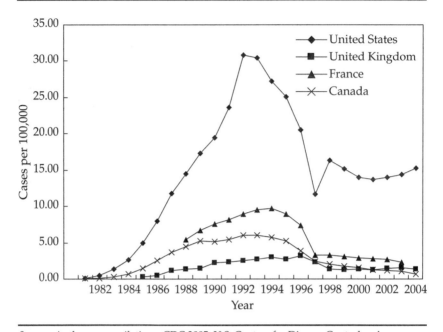

Sources: Authors comp ilations; CDC 2005; U.S. Centers for Disease Control and
Prevention (2005); Institut de veille sanitaire (2005); Avert.org (2005); Health Canada
(2004); U.S. Bureau of the Census (2005).

reflection of the epidemic's progress, but there have also been shifts over
time in demographic characteristics and exposure patterns of newly
reported cases. As the shape of the epidemic changes, the salient issues
for public health policy change as well. My research for the narratives that
follow was concentrated in the mid- to late 1990s, and my brief account
of AIDS epidemiology reflects the patterns as they existed at that time.

Much like tuberculosis in the nineteenth century, AIDS in the 1990s
was a disease of young adults, in industrialized countries predominantly
of young adult men.[9] Variations among the four countries in the age and
sex of reported cases were relatively minor. Their median age lay between
thirty and thirty-nine; the percentage of cases among females (as noted)
ranged between 7 and 22 percent. The major differences were, first, in the
sheer number of cases relative to total population, as suggested by the
case data reported, and, second, in the distribution of cases by transmission (or exposure) category. Among the most unique aspects of AIDS
reporting is the conventional breakdown by presumptive mode of virus
transmission: sex between men (formerly "homosexual-bisexual" now

"men who have sex with men [MSM]"), intravenous drug use (IDU), heterosexual sex, blood, and mother to child (perinatal). Although sex between men remained the principal mode of transmission during the 1990s, its relative magnitude declined over time in all four countries. Second, injection drug use was an important mode of transmission from the beginning of the AIDS epidemic, and its importance increased steadily through the mid-1990s, particularly in the United States and France. In 1995, close to a quarter of AIDS cases in each of these two countries were attributed to injection drug use, compared with 12 percent in Canada and only 9 percent in the UK.[10]

Drug addicts with Pneumocystis first came to the attention of CDC in the summer of 1981, within a month of the initial *MMWR* report (Shilts 1987, 83). According to Shilts's account, "at the CDC, there was a reluctance to believe that intravenous drug users might be wrapped into this epidemic, and the New York physicians [who saw these cases] seemed obsessed with the gay angle . . . drug addicts were not taken very seriously back in Atlanta" (83). This obsession is clearly reflected in the titles of the first set of scientific publications on the epidemic: in all but four of the thirteen that appeared in 1981, the subject matter was identified as a syndrome exhibited by homosexual men. From the beginning, injection drug users have been the most stigmatized and, concomitantly, the least publicly visible victims of AIDS. Before turning to each country's story, I briefly review the clinical dimensions of HIV/AIDS among injection drug users.

The human immunodeficiency virus (HIV) is carried in the blood of infected persons. The primary means of transmission among injection drug users is

> *direct needle sharing,* which involves the reuse of needles and syringes that have been contaminated through prior use by an infected individual. Penetration of the needle through the skin is sufficient for contamination and subsequent transmission of HIV infection . . . *indirect needle sharing,* involves common use of other drug preparation or injection equipment that can become contaminated. (Normand et al. 1995, 24, 26, emphasis in original)

Both the frequency of injection and specific practices associated with injection increase the probability of HIV infection among injection drug users as compared to, say, health-care workers who have experienced a needle-stick (Normand et al. 1995, 25). Recommended strategies for prevention of HIV infection among injection drug users have included abstinence from drug use, substitution of a noninjectable narcotic drug (for example methadone) for drug injection, needle sterilization before each use (for example, with bleach), and arrangements to provide injection drug users with sterile equipment. "For injection drug users who cannot or will not stop injecting drugs, the once-only use of sterile needles and syringes remains the safest, most effective approach for limiting HIV transmission" (2). In industrialized countries, the two principal means advocated by public health authorities for preventing HIV infection among injection drug users are substitution and the use of sterile injection equipment.[11]

United States

Of the four countries, only the United States has failed to produce any coherent national policy response to the threat of HIV/AIDS in injection drug users. Underlying this failure are fundamental disagreements about whether the AIDS–drugs link should be defined as a drug problem or as a health problem and, consequently, about who "owns" the problem—authorities in drug control and law enforcement or in public health—and about the location of responsibility for solving the problem. These disagreements exist not only between public health experts and politicians; they are present at all levels of government and among the leaders of civil society, and they account in large part for the patchwork nature of action in this country to address the AIDS–drugs threat.

Federal Policy Stalemate

On April 20, 1998, following considerable media build-up, the Clinton administration announced that a "meticulous scientific review has now proven that needle exchange programs can reduce the transmission of HIV and save lives without losing ground in the battle against illegal drugs."[12] It also announced that a ban on federal funds for these programs, first imposed in 1988, would remain in place. On April 21, the Presidential Advisory Council on HIV/AIDS described the administration's position as "morally indefensible." "It is akin to refusing to throw a life preserver to [a] drowning person" (Huettner 1998). The administration's hydra-headed statement was a precise reflection of the conflict between HIV prevention and drug-war politics that has shadowed the federal government's AIDS policy from the earliest stages of the epidemic.

The combatants fall into two very broad categories. On one side is the national medical–scientific–public health establishment: the National Academy of Sciences and (in the 1980s and early 1990s) the National AIDS Commission[13] together with the federal health and scientific bureaucracy (Department of Health and Human Services, National Institutes of Health, Centers for Disease Control and Prevention). On the other side is the antidrug bureaucracy (Office of National Drug Control Policy, Drug Enforcement Administration, and other related federal agencies), Congress, and the president. Neither of these categories is monolithic in the positions adopted by its members, and these positions shift with changes in the larger political climate, the heads of federal agencies being, of course, political appointees. Beginning in the mid-1980s, the split between these two groups has gradually widened. As the medical-scientific-public health establishment became increasingly alarmed by the concentration of new HIV infections in injection drug users, Congress and the president became increasingly committed, rhetorically and in practice, to a highly punitive war on drugs (Meier 1994; Gordon 1994; Bertram et al. 1996). The two groups talked past each other, each barely recognizing the other's existence.

My account begins in 1986, when an elite committee of the National Academy of Sciences, in its first report on the AIDS epidemic, urged the expansion of drug treatment and "experimenting with removing legal barriers to the sale and possession of sterile, disposable needles and syringes" (IOM 1986, 112). That year, President Reagan declared a "national crusade against drugs" and Congress passed the Federal Mail Order Drug Paraphernalia Control Act (Mail Order Act) as part of the Anti-Drug Abuse Act of 1986. The Mail Order Act prohibited the shipment of drug paraphernalia in interstate commerce. "Despite the foreseeable health effects of restricting access to injection equipment during this epidemic, public health and HIV prevention were not discussed at congressional hearings" (Gostin et al. 1997, 55). In 1988, the Academy excoriated the "gross inadequacy of federal efforts to reduce HIV transmission among IV drug abusers" and repeated its earlier recommendations. Congress in the same year inserted what was to become a ritual prohibition against the use of federal funds "to carry out any programs of distributing sterile needles for the hypodermic injection of illegal drugs or distributing bleach for the purpose of cleaning needles for such hypodermic injection" into two pieces of health programs legislation; and passed an antidrugs bill even more punitive than in 1986 (Bertram et al. 1996, 140ff.). In 1991, the presidentially appointed National AIDS Commission, which had limited its first (1988) report to relatively noncontroversial recommendations for expanded drug treatment, attacked the federal government, singling out in particular the president's Office of National Drug Control Policy (ONDCP), for its neglect of the HIV epidemic among injection drug users. It stressed "the absolute necessity of [drug] treatment on demand" and recommended that "legal barriers to the purchase and possession of injection equipment" be removed (U.S. National Commission on AIDS 1991). In 1992, then director of the ONDCP wrote:

[Distributing clean needles] undercuts the credibility of society's message that drug use is illegal and morally wrong. . . . We must not lose sight of the fact that illegal drugs . . . still pose a serious threat to our nation. *Nor can we allow our concern for AIDS to undermine our determination to win the war on drugs.* (cited in Gordon 1994, 171, emphasis added)

In 1998, following the Clinton administration's determination that needle-exchange programs were scientifically sound if not federally fundable, legislation was passed by the House of Representatives to make the funding ban permanent. Although this legislation failed, a ban on federal funding of needle-exchange programs has been incorporated in every subsequent appropriations bill for the Department of Health and Human Services. Further, since 1999, the House has used its authority over District of Columbia appropriations to prohibit the District from funding a needle exchange program (amfAR 2002). More recently, as reported in a *New York Times* editorial, it has threatened to withhold funding from international AIDS programs that include needle exchange ("Ideology and AIDS," February 26, 2005).

Expansion of drug treatment programs has fared little better than programs to provide clean injection equipment. According to one estimate, the treatment system as presently constituted can accommodate about 20 percent of narcotic drug users (Fiellin et al. 2001). In 1989, the Food and Drug Administration (FDA) and the National Institute on Drug Abuse (NIDA), in direct response to the "HIV epidemic in the intravenous drug-abusing population," proposed regulations that would have speeded access to methadone maintenance programs (U.S. Department of Health and Human Services, FDA 1989, 8973). The changes were vehemently opposed by the drug treatment community, by representatives of the African American community, and by a number of African American physicians (HHS 1990), leading NIDA to withdraw its proposal. In 1997, an NIH Consensus Development Statement on the "Effective Medical Treatment of Opiate Addiction" recommended that restrictive federal methadone regulations in place since 1972 should be eliminated entirely. Addiction should be treated as a disease, and "many more physicians and pharmacies" should be allowed to prescribe and dispense methadone (National Consensus Development Panel 1998, 1941). In apparent response to these recommendations new federal regulations were issued in 2001 transferring oversight of methadone maintenance programs from the FDA to the Substance Abuse and Mental Health Services Administration (SAMHSA 2001). How meaningful this bureaucratic change will be in increasing access to treatment is an open question. Although federal funds for drug treatment have increased since 1986, they form a declining percentage of the total drug-control budget (Bertram et al. 1996, 264; Drucker 1999; U.S. Office of National Drug Control Policy 2004, table 3), and the gap between the need for treatment and its availability continues.

As I have said, federal funds cannot be used for syringe exchange programs (SEPs), and even research to evaluate these programs is politically controversial (Vlahov et al. 2001; Burris, Strathdee, and Vernick 2003).[14] There is, nevertheless, striking inconsistency among federal agencies in whether and how access to sterile syringes for HIV prevention is officially presented. The Centers for Disease Control and Prevention regularly publishes updates on the status of SEPs in the United States (see, for example, CDC 2005b). Information emphasizing the importance of syringe access is readily available on its website, including the statement, "For injection drug users who cannot or will not stop injecting drugs, the once-only use of sterile needles and syringes remains the safest, most effective approach for limiting HIV transmission" (CDC 2005c). By contrast, in their most recent relevant policy statements, neither the National Institute of Drug Abuse nor the HIV/AIDS Bureau of the Health Resources and Services Administration (which administers the federal Ryan White program for care and treatment of persons with AIDS) makes any reference to SEPs or sterile syringes. Indeed, needle sharing is discounted as a cause of HIV transmission in favor of "dangerous risk behaviors" due to impaired judgment (U.S. National Institute on Drug Abuse 2006).

Action on the Ground and in the States

In the United States, methadone maintenance and comparable drug treatment are heavily regulated by federal, state, and sometimes local law, are limited to federally licensed narcotic treatment programs, and are subject to detailed requirements for patient supervision. Syringe access is governed by a complex network of state laws—"syringe prescription laws and regulations," "other pharmacy regulations or miscellaneous statutes imposing a variety of restrictions on the sale of syringes by pharmacists or others," "drug paraphernalia laws prohibiting the sale or possession of items intended to be used to consume illegal drugs," and laws on drug possession (Burris, Strathdee, and Vernick 2003, 814). Adding a further layer of complexity, several states have modified their laws in recent years in response to the threat of AIDS. Summarizing current evidence, Burris and colleagues conclude that though syringe access laws "do not prevent IDUs from getting some sort of syringe and injecting drugs," they do "interfere with access to and use of new sterile syringes" (855). It is in the context of this convoluted and shifting legal climate that syringe exchange programs were created and continue to operate in the United States.

The first "exchange system for syringes and needles" to prevent the spread of HIV among injection drug users was initiated in Amsterdam in 1984 jointly by the local health authorities and a drug users' association (Buning, Coutinho, and van Brussel 1986). In the United States, the first syringe exchange program was started by a local AIDS activist in Tacoma, Washington, in 1988, establishing a pattern common to most of the programs that followed.[15]

> Nearly everywhere that a needle exchange is operating, a single activist or a handful of individuals has served as the catalyst. In this initial phase, charisma matters. . . . Usually, an act of civil disobedience—the willingness to court arrest for distributing clean needles illegally—has been necessary to attract the attention of public health officials, the press, and particularly politicians and police, all of whom must eventually acquiesce if needle exchange is to be sustained. (Kirp and Bayer 1993, 82)

David Kirp's and Ronald Bayer's observations on the critical role of activist intervention were confirmed in a recent analysis evaluating the relative importance of several variables—resource availability, institutional opposition, need "as measured by the extent of AIDS among IDUs or the proportion of the metropolitan population who inject drugs" and the presence of a chapter of ACT UP (a relatively militant AIDS advocacy group)—in predicting the presence of a SEP (Tempalski 2005). This analysis, made across ninety-six of the largest metropolitan statistical areas in the United States, demonstrated that "metropolitan areas with ACT UP chapters, higher proportions of MSMs [men who have sex with men] and higher percentages of areas with college educated populations are more likely to have syringe exchange programs" (68). "The establishment of SEPs in the United States," Tempalski concludes, "results from political pressure or direct action from AIDS advocacy groups, grassroots organizations, and individual local activists" (20). There was no statistical relation between the need for a program and its presence. "The overall public response to the HIV epidemic [among injection drug users]," Ricky Bluthenthal observed based on his study of harm reduction in Oakland, "has emerged not from the rational and sensible application of the most promising and effective prevention strategies as understood by public health experts, but through the mobilization of elements of impacted communities and their allies" (1998, 1151).

The number of SEPs in the United States has grown slowly over time, not quite doubling between 1996 (101) and 2004 (184) (CDC 2005b).[16] Close to half of existing programs are in the western United States, very few in the South, where nearly half of all AIDS cases are located (Des Jarlais et al. 2002). Of the 127 programs surveyed by Des Jarlais and colleagues in 2000, 55 percent were state and or locally funded: large programs in large metropolitan areas were the most likely to receive public funds. Despite some progress, these programs continue to be highly controversial in many parts of the country as evidenced by the frequency with which they experience closures, police harassment, attacks by local politicians and the like (see, for example, Des Jarlais et al. 2002; Burris et al. 2004; Tempalski 2005; New York Times 2005; Chen 2006).

Public Health Success: An Illustrative Case   "In New York City, SEPs have been associated with a dramatic decline in the incidence of HIV infection, indicating an HIV epidemic among IDUs that has essentially been reversed" (Burris, Strathdee, and Vernick 2003, 840–54). The full story behind this reversal has not been told (and will not be told in this brief narrative). It would not have been predicted from the program's inauspicious beginning.

In 1985, New York City Health Commissioner David Sencer proposed the distribution of clean needles to the city's drug users. Public response was swift and negative, the arguments a preview of what was to come:

> the recommendation provoked vehement opposition. Law enforcement officials argued that addicts were not responsible enough to use clean needles to safeguard their own health: making needles freely available would only encourage young people to try drugs. The government would appear to officially sanction intravenous (IV) drug use. "How can cities ravaged by heroin," asked a *New York Times* editorial writer, "condone its use?" (Anderson 1991, 1507)

A pilot program initiated by the City Health Department in 1988 was discontinued by a new mayor in 1990. Legalization of SEPs through the state legislature was politically impossible, so in 1992 the health commissioner of New York State declared a public health emergency (now routinely reissued every year) providing a legal basis for the establishment of needle exchange programs in New York City, seven years after they were first proposed.

The city's ultimate acquiescence to needle exchange was the result of social and political pressure from two directions. First, local AIDS activists—ACT-UP backed by a locally based AIDS policy research organization with some depth in resources and expertise—had initiated illegal but well-publicized exchanges, essentially forcing the city's hand. Second, the appearance of African American unanimity in opposition to needle exchange was breached by statements and actions of the black mayors of Baltimore and New Haven: "The fact that New Haven's black mayor . . . an opponent of needle exchange when he was a state legislator, had supported the [needle exchange trial in New Haven] and boldly announced its success, put great pressure" on David Dinkins, the black mayor of New York City (Kirp and Bayer 1993, 88).

After 1992 needle exchange programs in New York City expanded rapidly: the estimated number of syringes exchanged "increased from approximately 250,000 in 1991 . . . to 3,000,000 in 2000 and 2002" (Des Jarlais et al. 2005, 1439). HIV incidence among IDUs declined concurrently, in linear relation to the number of syringes exchanged. Commenting on this phenomenon, Don Des Jarlais and his colleagues observed that the "legalization, expansion, and public [New York State] funding of syringe exchange programs in New York City was the result of a collaborative effort among public health officials, community-based organizations (which operated the exchanges), political leaders, researchers, and a private foundation (the American Foundation for AIDS Research) among others" (1443). This collaborative effort is likely to have played a key role in New York City's success.[17]

AIDS-drugs and the Minority Community   Mobilization for AIDS prevention and treatment in the United States, much like mobilization against secondhand smoke, has depended heavily on the organizational resources and capacities of the affected groups. Response to the AIDS-drugs nexus departed from this pattern in important—and instructive—respects. Injection drug users with HIV/AIDS in the United States are overwhelmingly African American or Hispanic. In New York City, close to 90 percent of persons living with AIDS in 2004 who had been exposed through injection drug use were black or Hispanic (New York City Department of Health and Mental Hygiene 2005b). The comparable figure in 1988, when the city's pilot program was initiated, was 85 percent (HHS 2005). Indeed, in 1988, African Americans and Hispanics were 66 percent of the total reported AIDS cases in New York City (HHS 2005).

New York City's white gay men had come together almost immediately after the first reports of the epidemic, using their ample financial and social resources to create a grassroots organizational response that combined services to the gay community with advocacy on its behalf (see, for example, Shilts 1987, Bayer and Kirp 1992; Epstein 1996).[18] The response of minority communities was quite different. Among the most vocal opponents of the city's pilot SEP had been leaders of the African American and Hispanic communities: "The distribution of clean needles and syringes seemed to them a cynical, cheap solution to a drug problem that had brought not only AIDS but also crime, social breakdown, and other illnesses—such as tuberculosis—to the city's Black and Hispanic neighborhoods" (Anderson 1991, 1512). Although the minority community was not monolithic in its opposition to needle-exchange (Latino communities have been far more supportive than African Americans), the opponents included some highly visible and vocal individuals, in particular New York City's black congressman Charles Rangel. Rangel played important roles both in the prohibition of federal funds for needle exchange (Kirp and Bayer 1993, 80) and in NIDA's withdrawal of its proposed interim methadone maintenance regulations, described earlier.

Early scholarly commentary on official neglect of HIV/AIDS in New York City's minority communities called attention to the absence of organizational response comparable to that of gay men. For example, "intravenous drug users in New York City were too unorganized and socially stigmatized to force government action, or to enter into negotiations over the appropriate policy response" (Anderson 1991, 1515). Absence of organization was due (and is still due) at least as much to the reluctance of minority elites and institutions to confront HIV/AIDS in their communities as it is to disorganization and stigma among the persons affected.

> most indigenous black institutions . . . provided a mixed, limited, and often reluctant response to (the AIDS) epidemic. The AIDS programs initiated by these organizations were designed not only to provide needed services to segments of black communities, but also to fit within a constrained moral and political framework, where anything from a lack of expertise on this issue or the word of God were offered [the former by the NAACP, the latter by black clergy] as reasons for doing less. (Cohen 1997, 256)

Cathy Cohen suggests three reasons for the black establishment's uneven response to AIDS. First, the absence of mainstream white institutional and media attention to AIDS among African Americans "supported the denial of black community leaders, who viewed AIDS as a disease they did not have to own" (182). The "marginalized status of poor people and injection drug users," she observes, "rendered them invisible to the [Centers for Disease Control and Prevention]. If these individuals were invisible to the CDC, then the cause of their death was also invisible to the communities of color, like the African-American and Latino communities, to which many belonged" (130). Second, injection drug use and (even more) homosexuality are highly stigmatized identities in black communities: community leaders and politicians moved quickly to distance themselves from any implication that these behaviors were inherent among blacks (Perrow and Guillén 1990). Finally, Cohen speculates that "traditional [black] leaders, incorporated into dominant institutions to fulfill, in part, managerial roles" may have viewed the demands of AIDS activists for an indigenous response to the disease "as working against their specific interests and mobility" (291).

Into the gap in mainstream (white and black) organization and leadership in behalf of injection drug users moved ACT-UP, militant white middle-class activists committed to policy change and willing to do civil disobedience if that was necessary to obtain it. "ACT-UP members who became involved in needle exchange understood that we *could* do things that other communities couldn't and were willing to use the privileges that come with being white and middle-class in order to absorb some necessary risks" (Naomi Brain, personal communication). Once having accomplished its goal of getting SEPs legalized in New York State (in 1992), the majority of ACT-UP's members moved on, leaving others to deal with the routine of grants and budgets.

Drugs and Drug Users

The American response to HIV/AIDS in injection drug users has been powerfully shaped by this country's long history of demonizing narcotic drugs and the individuals who used them. Drug wars have been an integral part of United States foreign and domestic politics since the late nineteenth century, accompanied by a powerful and unremitting identification of the drug threat with so-called dangerous classes: aliens, youth, political dissidents and, invariably, blacks (Gordon 1994). The history of the Harrison Act of 1914—the first federal legislation restricting and criminalizing the prescription and sale of narcotic drugs—is particularly instructive in this regard. American narcotics policies in the early twentieth century were driven by a complex combination of economic, moral, and political interests, originating with the conquest of the Philippines and the opening of trade with China (Musto 1973). The act was promoted by the State Department with a view to bringing domestic narcotics policy in line with the restrictive policies the United States was urging on other countries. A major argument for narcotics legislation—intended to attract the support of southern Democrats sensitive to the bill's potential encroachment on state's rights—was the alleged threat posed by cocaine use among blacks. In a report to Congress, the legislation's major promoter wrote of "cocaine's 'encouragement . . . among the humbler ranks of the Negro population in the South,' "concluding that, " 'it has been authoritatively stated that cocaine is often the direct incentive to the crime of rape by the Negroes of the South and other sections of the country' " (cited in Musto 1973, 43–44). The Harrison Act passed virtually without discussion. Summarizing the state of public opinion in 1914, David Musto writes

> prominent newspapers, physicians, pharmacists, and congressmen believed opiates and cocaine predisposed habitués toward insanity and crime. They were widely seen as substances associated with foreigners and alien subgroups. Cocaine raised the spectre of the wild Negro, opium the devious Chinese, morphine the tramps in the slums; it was feared that use of all these drugs was spreading into the "higher classes." (1973, 65)

Both the association of drugs and drug users with marginalized groups and the portrayal of these groups and their destructive behaviors as an imminent danger to mainstream society are as much a part of American culture today as they were in 1914 (see, for example, Gordon 1994; Meier 1994). Contemporary rhetoric is less likely to personify mainstream society as the better classes, however, than as "innocent" children. The mantra of virtually every attack on distribution of clean needles to injection drug users is that to do so will send "the wrong message" to children. At the same time, a central argument for clean needle distribution, repeated in every Institute of Medicine and AIDS Commission document, is not that it will protect the health of drug users, but that it will protect their babies and the mothers of their children. Drug users are loathed and feared by affluent whites, by many in the black communities most affected by drugs, and even by some members of the drug-treatment bureaucracy (Gordon 1994; Meier 1994; HHS 1990). Among the consequences of fear and demonization are (at best) apathy and (at worst) hostility toward the portrayal of narcotic drug use as a public health problem. For many in American society, black and white, the criminal justice system is all that stands between "us" and "them."

France

By 1985, epidemiologists in France were fully aware of the connection between AIDS and injection drug use (Coppel 1996, 84). It took ten years for a combination of expert-activists outside of government and public health authorities within government to overcome the political and ideological obstacles in the way of a coherent national response. The government did change its policies, however, and the incidence of HIV infection in injection drug users has declined significantly.

Policy Collision

In 1987 the French minister of health, Michelle Barzach, authorized over-the-counter sale (vente libre) by pharmacists of needles and syringes as a step toward the protection of drug injectors against HIV transmission. Much like Simone Veil's 1976 initiative on smoking, Barzach's action was an isolated event, neither preceded by public discussion or demand nor followed by related policy initiatives. Indeed, Barzach, a physician, acted on her own in the face of the combined opposition of drug-treatment experts and the minister of justice. It was, in the words of a civil servant on the scene, "a power struggle between two ministers," finally resolved by the prime minister, Jacques Chirac, who came down on the side of Barzach.

The power struggle was intense but with few repercussions, confined as it was within the walls of the ministries immediately concerned. The first official public document on the AIDS epidemic in France was written and made public in the short space of three months in the fall of 1988 by Claude Got, perhaps the most respected voice of public health in France (1989). The report's introduction makes it clear that the spread of HIV among injection drug users was well known to Claude Evin, the health minister who commissioned the report. In the report's 133 pages, however, barely three are devoted to the issue of injection drug use, and Got's recommendations are nothing if not conservative, focused primarily on access to treatment for already infected drug users. He left little doubt as to his reasons: "la politisation de tout ce qui touche à la drogue n'est pas un élément favorable pour traiter le dossier avec sérénité [the politicization of everything connected with drugs is unfavorable to dispassionate discussion]" (90). A government report on France's drug war, issued one year later, devoted all of two self-congratulatory pages to AIDS in injection drug users; in government drug-war plans issued in 1990 and 1993 AIDS is barely mentioned (Coppel 1996).

It took until 1992, five years after the Barzach démarche, before a multifaceted power struggle pitting the threat of AIDS against the threat of drugs finally erupted onto the French public stage. The terms of this conflict—which continued at full throttle from 1992 through 1994—were chronicled in some detail by Le Monde. Late in 1992, in an appearance before the National Assembly, the minister of health, Dr. Bernard Kouchner, stated that AIDS was a greater threat than drugs and announced plans to develop methadone maintenance programs; the possibility of needle exchange programs had been floated earlier. Within a month, Kouchner's approach was publicly disavowed by the interior minister, Paul Quiles, together with the Paris police commissioner and head of the country's antidrug war, Robert Broussard. A few days later, the prime minister, Pierre Beregovoy, denied any conflict between his two ministers, insisting that the public health and criminal justice approaches were complementary and should not get in each other's way. Clearly outgunned, Kouchner denied any problems between him and the interior minister.

Interministerial conflict was only one dimension of the controversy. Earlier in the fall of 1992, Le Monde had published an article by a group of Paris doctors proposing that general practitioners be given the freedom to prescribe methadone and other "medicaments de substitution" as part of a broader arsenal of risk reduction policies to combat AIDS. This proposal had no sooner appeared than it was publicly attacked by specialists in the treatment of drug addiction, for whom methadone prescription was equivalent to legal drug dealing ("dealers en blouse blanche" was a favorite epithet), a confession of failure, and an "abandonment" of drug users to their fate. A physician member of Kouchner's staff recalled his struggle "lost in advance" against a coalition of physicians, members of the government, and the police for whom "anything that might contribute to encouraging drug addiction was unacceptable, even at the price of AIDS" ("Le societé française face au sida," October 21, 1993). The logjam created by this combination of professional contention and political impasse remained unbroken until the publication of the Henrion report in February 1995.

In 1994, the minister of state for social, health, and urban affairs, Simone Veil, had appointed a seventeen-member commission, headed by the obstetrician-gynecologist Robert Henrion, to examine and reflect on narcotic drugs policies and, specifically, to consider whether distribution of clean needles and substitution should be considered in light of the ravages of AIDS and hepatitis among injection drug users (toxicomanes) in France.[19] The commission's report minced no words: "The drug war policy, based on the premise that nothing must be done to facilitate the lives of drug users, has caused health and social catastrophe" (Henrion 1995, 35).

The commission recommended that needle exchange and substitution be actively pursued, that mobile facilities as well as fixed sites where drug users could attend to their immediate physical needs be supported, and that liaison with drug user associations be encouraged. Within one month, distribution of syringes and needles by nonprofit groups or individuals engaged in "AIDS prevention or risk reduction among drug users" was made legal by ministerial decree, and methadone was transformed from a prohibited narcotic drug with "no medical value" to a "medication." By October methadone had been authorized for prescription by general practitioners to "stabilized" patients. These policies—previously blocked by political contention—had long been in the works, accounting for the government's ability to take rapid action once the Henrion Commission had spoken. A report by the Conseil national du sida (National Council on AIDS) published in 2004 states that the government's policy change—despite uneven implementation due in large part to the many remaining ambiguities of government narcotic drugs policy—has been effective in decreasing the risk of HIV transmission among injection drug users (Conseil national du sida 2004). This estimate is supported by the fact that only 2 percent of new HIV infections in 2004 were attributed to injection drug use (Institut de veille sanitaire 2005).

The Price of Ideological Politics

Ten years had passed from the point when epidemiologists first became aware that France had a significant problem of HIV/AIDS among injection drug users to the publication of the Henrion report and the government actions that almost immediately followed. In the meantime France recorded the largest number of AIDS cases in Europe and the highest case rate of any European country except Switzerland. (France's case rate did not approach that of the United States, but was far higher than either Great Britain's or Canada's.) In 1993, the percentage of injection drug users among total AIDS cases in France was over 25 percent, close to that in the United States. France's marked delay in responding to the problem of HIV/AIDS in injection drug users was comparable to, but far less internationally notorious than, its delayed response to the dangers confronted by hemophiliacs and blood transfusees (see, for example, Steffen 1999). The reasons were complex. They arose from ideological and substantive conflict over the meaning and treatment of narcotic drugs and narcotic drug use and from politicization of the AIDS/drugs nexus in the wake of electoral gains, in fact and in prospect, by the ultraconservative National Front. One—but only one—key to this conflict is what from the perspective of many French commentators is an inherent contradiction in the 1970 law governing narcotic drugs, a contradiction that was not resolved by the members of the Henrion commission.

The 1970 law (Loi n° 70-1320 du 31 décembre 1970) was passed unanimously by the French parliament in an atmosphere of intense concern about youth out of control, in which the criminal, the dealer, and the young revolutionary melded into a single threat symbolized by the use of narcotic drugs (Ehrenberg 1995, 74). The essential provisions of this law, distinguishing it from earlier French statutes and most European drug laws, were the criminalization of drug use, with no distinction between hard and soft drugs, and what was called the therapeutic injunction. Under the latter provision, an individual could avoid prosecution by submitting to treatment to "cure" his or her addiction. The 1970 law thus created at the same time a new class of criminals and a new category of patients. In practice, the law has been a dead letter, its provisions largely ignored; its irrelevance to the realities of narcotic drug use and drug use policy is widely acknowledged. Its reason for being—a reason reaffirmed by each of three national commissions on drug use, including the Henrion commission, is its perceived importance as an assertion by the State of the norm to which French citizens are expected to adhere. In 2004, the government again affirmed its support of the 1970 law, turning down continued appeals for reform (Bienvault 2004).

In France, drug addiction is defined as a psychiatric problem, drug treatment specialists are psychiatrists, and the treatment of choice is psychoanalysis. The professional ideology to which these psychiatrists subscribed demanded that treatment for drug addiction be "voluntary, anonymous, and free."[20] The patient must "want" to be cured. The treatment community, though subscribing to the symbolic significance of the 1970 law, thus rejected its coercive implications along with the role in implementation of the law to which treatment specialists were assigned. (At any rate, the number of slots for psychiatric treatment remained far below the potential demand.) Hostility to the therapeutic injunction was equaled if not surpassed by hostility to "medicalization": the construction of drug addiction as a chronic disease requiring ongoing medical treatment—that is, substitution. From this perspective—a perspective that is perhaps the most difficult for an outsider to understand—defining drug addiction as an organic illness had two destructive consequences. First, it was equivalent to giving up on the therapeutic goal of abstinence and thus abandoning drug addicts to their addiction. Second, treatment in the form of substitution—insofar as the patient was both dependent on the physician and subjected to continuous monitoring for compliance with the treatment regimen—was, like the therapeutic injunction, simply another form of social control. Operating within this framework, French drug treatment specialists had a particular horror of what they saw as American-style methadone maintenance programs, requiring daily visits for medication and monitoring of patients' urine to ensure compliance. These specialists found it far easier to accept syringe exchange—which they saw as an autonomous act by the drug user—than methadone maintenance that in their eyes implicated the physician in the user's actions.

The authorities on drug treatment in France—the authorities routinely consulted by government officials, politicians and journalists—were thus firmly committed to treatment of the drug user's soul and firmly against treatment of the user's body. These specialists controlled the drug treatment bureaucracy to which narcotic drug users were routinely referred, an existing bureaucracy that was completely separate from the new agencies the French government created to cope with AIDS.

Compounding the resistance of the drug treatment community and contributing to the extreme reluctance of French elites to publicly confront the AIDS-drugs connection, and other dimensions of AIDS, were both deep-seated cultural values and narrow political calculations. The conspiracy of silence was driven in part by the French ideal of social solidarity along with its obverse, rejection of stigmatization. The concept of risk groups, taken for granted in American-style epidemiology, flies in the face of these normative commitments. Early warnings of the AIDS-drugs connection were widely denounced as sensationalist exploitation for political purposes (Coppel 1996, 80). The apparent threat was twofold. On the one hand was the danger that AIDS victims would be further stigmatized by too close an association with drug users. On the other was the contention that services specific to drug users (for example, over-the-counter sale of syringes, syringe exchange programs) were a form of social exclusion amounting to "ghettoization." Adding fuel to this fire was the mid-1980s rise of an ultraright political party, the National Front, led by Jean-Marie Le Pen. Le Pen advocated the criminalization of homosexuality and the quarantine of AIDS victims. Health professionals and mainstream politicians were united in their fear that to call attention to the AIDS-drugs connection was to play into the hands of Le Pen.

A further serious obstacle to confrontation of the AIDS-drugs nexus applies equally to the tobacco control problem; it was described in that connection but deserves reemphasis here: Public health in France is both ideologically suspect and institutionally weak. The identification of public health with social control is firmly embedded in the political culture of the French left. It was frequently called to my attention that two figures who played a major role in shifting France's drugs policies in response to HIV/AIDS, Michelle Barzach and Simone Veil, were both on the right. State regulation in the interest of disease and accident prevention (such as smoking restrictions, mandated seat-belt use, even methadone maintenance to prevent HIV infection) is characterized by intellectuals of this persuasion as deprivation by an overprotective (even quasi-totalitarian) state of individuals' right to enjoy dangerous pleasures.[21] From this perspective, only the enemies of liberty sound the public health alarm. At the same time, public health is institutionally weak both with respect to other government ministries and with respect to other sources of expertise on questions of health and illness (Steffen 1992; Morelle 1996). The importance of these obstacles to the development of public health in France goes well beyond their significance for the French response to HIV/AIDS in injection drug users.

Street-Level Mobilization

In the summer of 1992, a diverse group of fifteen or so French physicians and specialists in drug treatment attended the eighth international AIDS conference in Amsterdam. Included in the delegation was Anne Coppel, a sociologist who has devoted her professional career to writing about drug use and drug users in France and to activism in their behalf and who went on to play a central role in bringing about the government's ultimate policy revolution in response to AIDS and drugs. As she describes it, the Amsterdam meeting was critical in alerting the French in attendance that other countries' narcotic drug policies were changing in response to AIDS.

> Every time we ran into people from England, they would ask, "What's going on in France?" And we would say, "What do you mean, what's going on in France?" We didn't know what they were talking about. And they would say, "How come you haven't done anything about AIDS?" And suddenly we realized that something could be done, that it was possible to do it, and that it would produce results. And I began to read feverishly[22]. . . . It was necessary to make a revolution. Otherwise nothing would change. So we made a revolution. (Coppel, interview, January 1998)

Within a year, the loose group of French professionals and activists brought together in Amsterdam created an association, Limiter la casse (literally, limit the breakage; figuratively, reduce the risks), and broke the public silence surrounding the AIDS-drugs connection. In June of 1993 Limiter la casse organized an "états généraux toxicomanie-sida," an assembly representing the full range of participants in the AIDS-drugs debate.[23] Seven hundred people came, including the minister of health, Simone Veil. At the end of November 1993, a full-page ad titled "Limiter la casse" appeared in the country's major newspapers. It was signed by many prominent individuals and organizations, including three former ministers of health (Barzach, Evin, and Kouchner), Daniel Defert, the founder of the principal French organization against AIDS (AIDES), Médecins du Monde, and so on. The ad was hard-hitting. Drug users were dying; their deaths were avoidable; they could be prevented by access to clean needles, by substitution, and by recognition of drug users' own role in prevention. In Europe, France was the exception: prevention was discouraged, drug addicts were harassed, the sick were imprisoned, and finally, the authorities were responsible, just as they were in the case of the tainted blood (that is, the threat of a virus-contaminated blood supply to hemophiliacs and transfusees, referred to earlier). Three months after these ads appeared, Simone Veil appointed the Henrion commission. Amsterdam was a major catalyst for change. But it was not, in fact, the beginning. Efforts at prevention on a small scale had begun as early as 1985, mounted by AIDES and Médecins du Monde, by local medical practitioners and street-level drug treatment specialists, and by drug users.[24] Needle-exchange in Paris was initiated by Médecins du Monde in 1989 and quickly incorporated as one of three experimental needle-exchange programs sponsored by the Department of Health. In the face of intense user demand, local practitioners began to prescribe narcotics for purposes of maintenance rather than withdrawal, and organized around REPSUD (Réseau des professionnels pour les soins aux usagers de drogues). Both initiatives were, by the letter of the law, illegal. In 1992, a drug users' association, ASUD (Auto Support des Usagers de Drogues) was formed and a newsletter was published. These activities were highly localized and largely independent of one another. Looking back, Coppel reflects that "we all, in our own way, [had] tried to do what we could to help drug users; no one had the idea it was necessary to change." From this perspective, Amsterdam was a classic consciousness-raising experience. It brought together the disparate actors "on the street" and convinced them that France's narcotic drug policies did indeed need to be fundamentally changed.

Commenting on the recent past, the person at AIDES in charge of activities in connection with injection drug use remarked that drug policies had made more progress in the preceding two years, 1995 to 1997, than they had in the previous twenty: "C'est le sida qui a tout déclenché [it's AIDS that got everything unlocked]" (Interview with AIDES staff member, January 1998). Offering a more nuanced analysis, a long-time civil servant believed that the rapid change following the Henrion report was a direct consequence of the French scandale du sang contaminé [contaminated-blood scandal] that erupted in the early 1990s (Interview with civil servant, January 1998; see, for example, Steffen 1999). This devastating experience put the fear of God into public officials, causing them to become "very afraid of not taking extremely seriously this question of drugs" (Interview with civil servant, January 1998). Whether France's policy shift in the mid-1990s is attributed to the mobilization of street-level workers represented by Limiter la casse, to the blood scandal, or to a combination of the two, there is ample evidence that absent external pressure the French government would have done little in response to the AIDS epidemic in injection drug users.

Needles, Drugs, and Drug Users

Officially, France has accepted a policy of risk reduction and greatly expanded programs for the distribution of clean needles and for substitution with methadone or comparable products. On the ground, however, the circumstances for both the providers of these services and their recipients are highly unstable. Depending on the locality, arrangements for needle distribution or the location of automatic needle dispensers can become a bureaucratic or political nightmare. With the law on their side local police can, if they so choose, act arbitrarily to harass providers or their clients.[25] This instability stems from the ideological and political conflicts I described earlier, from the Byzantine bureaucratic and legal conditions of drug-use treatment that stem from these conflicts, and from the marginalized status of drug users in French society.

Comparing France with Britain, Holland, and the United States, Alain Ehrenberg asserted that "French society is particularly intolerant of narcotic drugs and very tolerant of alcohol and psychotropic drugs. The press in general paints a one-dimensional picture: the consumer is an addict; drugs are a social menace [fléau] to be eradicated" (1995, 96). Drugs and drug users are no less demonized in the United States, but there are clear differences between the two countries in how the menace is construed. Indeed, from the French perspective, the threat lies far less in users' danger to society than in their withdrawal from society. Society is endangered when its members—particularly its younger members— are seen to reject the social and normative ties that bind them to the larger community in favor of the private world of drugs.

> Youth that escapes from guardianship, a private life without social or political connection are the sources of French anxiety about drugs: this anxiety has much more to do with the supposed absence of the drug addict from others and from the world, in other words with the question of citizenship, than it does with dangers of drug use to the addict's health. (Ehrenberg 1995, 80)

In the documents I have cited and in my interviews with actors in the AIDS-drugs drama, the question of citizenship—citoyenneté—was raised over and over again. Is the drug user to be viewed as criminal, as diseased, or as a citizen? Underlying these labels is an ongoing struggle between and among physicians, officials, politicians, and activists over the norms that define drug users' relation to society and to the state. The French legal system offers only the first two alternatives, the criminal and the sick. The latter, as I have noted, has been a dead letter. In adopting the framework of harm reduction, the health authorities have committed themselves to a strategy of medicalization: the drug user is or may become physically ill and, as such, is primarily a public health rather than a criminal justice (or a psychiatric) problem. Writing in 1997, Le Monde's medical reporter Laurence Follea asserted that though this strategy has had some success, it is still controversial, as much among some physicians as among representatives of the criminal justice system ("Le bilan encourageant de la politique de réduction des risques," March 29, 1997, n.p.). Portrayal of the drug user as citizen goes farther, carrying with it connotations of responsibility to act and, conversely, to be accepted as a member of the social body (Duchesne 1997). The essence of citoyenneté, Duchesne argues, is the relation of individuals not to the state but to one another. "Citoyenneté is constituted by the willing assumption of the bonds that unite citizens to one another" (310). Narcotic drug users have been defined as rejecting those bonds, a rejection that strikes horror into the minds of the French. It is striking that in some national polls drugs were rated second only to unemployment as the most important problem confronting French society (cited in Serfaty 1996, 67).

In arguing for the citizenship label, advocates, including the recently formed users' groups, cite evidence for the active engagement (responsibilisation) of users in the work of HIV/AIDS prevention (reduction in needle sharing, enrollment in programs of substitution). Implicit in the notion of citoyenneté is opposition to the idea that drug users are either criminal or sick: they are, simply, citizens.

Britain

Among the sixteen narratives that provide the data for this book, there is no more striking example of rapid and successful action in the face of a public health crisis than the British government's response to the threat of HIV/AIDS in injection drug users. Critical in shaping this response were particularities of Britain's political system, the history of its narcotic drug policies, and the presence on the ground of political and policy entrepreneurs ready to seize the opportunity for change in those policies created by the AIDS–drugs nexus.

Policy Pragmatism

The first British government report on HIV infection in injection drug users, the McClelland Report, was issued by the Scottish Home and Health Department in September 1986. The first sentence of the report's first recommendation reads as follows: "Injecting drug misusers who cannot or will not abstain from misuse must be educated in *safer drug taking practices*" (Scottish Home and Health Department 1986, 12, emphasis added). Even more revolutionary was the premise on which this recommendation was based: "Infection with HIV poses a much greater threat to the life of the individual than the misuse of drugs" (4). Two years later, an advisory committee to the central government—the Advisory Committee on the Misuse of Drugs (ACMD)—reached the same conclusion: "HIV is a greater threat to public and individual health than drug misuse" (UK Department of Health and Social Security 1988, 1). The committee's recommendations called for "access to sterile needles and syringes" for those who would not stop injecting and for "prescribing" (that is, the medical prescription of narcotic drugs) as a means of "attracting drug misusers to services and helping them move away from HIV risk behaviour" (2). As we have seen, similar recommendations were made at about the same time by equally elite committees in the United States. The difference is that in Britain the government accepted its committee's premises and acted on its recommendations.

Fifteen pilot syringe-exchange schemes were initiated in 1987. The pilot label was intended to take the heat off arguments against syringe exchange. "We knew they really weren't," comments a civil servant intimately involved with this activity at the time. By 1997, the number had grown to 500, government-funded and embedded in a variety of community-based drug services agencies: "Syringe-exchange rapidly became the hub of HIV prevention" (Stimson 1995, 704). James Parsons and colleagues estimate that by 2002, "27 million syringes were distributed annually from over 2000 outlets in the United Kingdom" (2002, 845). Injecting drug users have other sources of equipment as well, that is, in addition to SEPs. There are no legal barriers to over-the-counter sales in Britain: "it has been estimated that pharmacy sales are the source of half of all needles used by drug injectors" (UK Department of Health and Social Security 1993, 34). Nor are there legal barriers to the prescription of oral or injectable methadone: "the amount of methadone distributed by manufacturers and wholesalers to pharmacies increased nearly fourfold from 93,166g in 1988 to 338,458g in 1992" (Stimson 1995, 704). Finally, concrete evidence of the British government's commitment to HIV prevention among injection drug users was the fourteen-fold increase in targeted funding for this purpose between 1987 and 1994.

These policy initiatives emerged in a public and political opinion climate not all that different from the United States. In the early 1980s, serious alarm about drug "misuse" (the British term of art) in general and about heroin addiction in particular surfaced in political speeches and the popular press (MacGregor 1989). "The election of the Thatcher government [in 1979] had seen the reawakening of political interest in the drugs issue and the institution, at the political level, of a US style 'war on drugs' " (Berridge 1996, 94). An all-party parliamentary committee on drug misuse was formed in 1984, chaired by Sir Bernard Braine, a Conservative MP who described heroin addiction as a "grave illness and a terrifying social evil" and who was vehemently opposed to needle-exchange. Braine's views "powerfully expressed the opinion of influential members of the drug 'policy community' " (Berridge 1996, 120). In 1985, the Standing Conference on Drug Abuse (SCODA), the coordinating agency for the voluntary sector, expelled an advocate of needle exchange. Finally, between 1985 and 1986, the government adopted two new pieces of legislation intended to control drug trafficking, including an increase in the maximum penalty for trafficking from fourteen years to life, and mounted a mass-media antiheroin campaign focused on eradication of drug use.

The government's actions were in harmony with public sentiment. MacGregor cites the comments from a debate in the House of Lords: "to be honest, the ordinary members of the public would rather give some money to Oxfam, blind babies or lifeboats . . . than they would to running a centre for drug addicts, perhaps next door to themselves" (MacGregor 1989, 9). In 1987, intense community opposition forced a local council in Scotland to abandon plans for a home for AIDS patients: "One argument used in the campaign was that children might contract AIDS by pricking themselves on disused syringes dumped by visiting drug addicts" (MacGregor 1989, 9). Indeed, the 1986 McClelland report was received with exceeding ill-grace by the Scottish cabinet minister who requested it, John Mackay. In an interview published in the *Scotsman* shortly before the report was published, he was quoted as saying that drug addiction [is] morally wrong and that in no way could it be condoned by issuing needles and syringes (Berridge 1996, 96).

Mackay's remarks caused embarrassment in Whitehall and were denounced in Parliament; Mackay lost his ministerial post in a cabinet reshuffle; and within two years "issuing needles and syringes" had become official government policy. Behind what appears on the surface as a remarkable transformation in public health policy are two stories: the more immediate story of "delicate manoeuvering, parliamentary persuasion and political stealth" that led to the ACMD report legitimizing needle exchange as the keystone of Britain's response to HIV/AIDS in injection drug users; and the larger history of British narcotic drugs policies.[26]

"In-House" Policy Making and Needle Exchange

In terms that recall my account of hydra-headed U.S. policy, Virginia Berridge describes 1980s British policy pre-AIDS as having a "dual face— a 'political' penal policy with a high public and mass media profile; and an 'in-house' health policy based on a rhetoric of demedicalisation and the development of community services and harm-minimisation" (Berridge 1993, 142). A major difference, of course, is that in Britain the "political penal policy" lost out in the face of AIDS. To comprehend how this happened requires some background: first, on the political system from which health policies emerged; and, second, on the state-of-play in narcotic drugs policies during the early 1980s.

Writing in the context of British HIV/AIDS policy making, John Street and Albert Weale describe the British political system as "hermetically sealed."

Although the country is formally a parliamentary democracy, real power lies with the executive [who are] elected politicians sustained by party discipline. . . . The executive is largely untouched by arguments it is not disposed to hear. Its privileged position is reinforced by an administrative system [i.e., the civil service] that is secretive and uncoordinated. Each department competes with all the others for resources; each chooses the advice it receives and structures it within a close-knit advisory system whose primary goal is corporate consensus. In such a system, change comes from within; external factors serve to expedite, rather than to cause, change. (1992, 188)

The government's response to HIV/AIDS in injection drug users emerged, then, out of "an essentially private world where policy was made by accommodation between experts and civil servants" (Stimson and Lart 1994, 336). Public opinion played virtually no role, at least none acknowledged either in the many published accounts of the events I will describe or in my interviews with key players. The voices of voluntary organizations and advocacy groups, insofar as they were heard at all, were channeled through advisory groups such as the ACMD.[27]

Responsibility for drug policy is shared between the Home Office (the government's law enforcement arm) and the Department of Health. Although there was a long history of tension between the two bodies over control of drug policy, during the 1980s,

the Department of Health was much more active [and] very well supported by the Chief Inspector of Drugs [a Home Office official]. We were fortunate in Home Office Secretaries; we didn't get active opposition to what we were doing. Main emphasis was on the health side. (Dorothy Black, interview, May 1998)[28]

The key players in the AIDS-drugs policy arena were Dr. Black (see note 27); Dr. Donald Acheson, a distinguished epidemiologist who was appointed chief medical officer (CMO) in 1983; Norman Fowler, who became secretary of state for health and social security in 1981 and remained in that position until 1987; David Mellor, who succeeded Fowler in 1988; and the ACMD working group on AIDS and drugs misuse, set up in May of 1987. The ACMD was described by one of its members as the "kind of committee of the great and the good . . . who sit unpaid . . . and give advice to government" (Interview with ACMD member, May 1997). Civil servants who supported harm minimization played a critical role in the ACMD working group both in their influence on appointments to the committee and in its deliberations: "There was a great deal of interchange between civil servants and members [of the ACMD working group]" (Interview with ACMD member, May 1997).

The ACMD's policy recommendations grew out of new approaches to the treatment of drug addiction initiated by the Department of Health in the early 1980s in response to perceived changes in the pattern of drug use and dissatisfaction with what had become a treatment model dominated by London-based psychiatrists. Well before HIV/AIDS was recognized, the Department of Health had committed itself to community-based treatment services decentralized out of London, provided by voluntary organizations with substantial nonmedical participation (for example, from social workers, counselors, psychiatric nurses and the like), and focused as much on prevention and treatment of the problems associated with drug use as on abstinence. The driving force behind these policy shifts was known as the Central Funding Initiative (CFI). Through the CFI, the Department of Health made substantial grant funds available directly to locally based groups (mostly local health authorities) for the development of drug treatment services on a national basis, displacing the old "hospital-based London-focused specialist treatment system" (Berridge 1993, 141). Thus, when HIV/AIDS came along, the basic approach that would be taken by the Department of Health, and that it was ultimately successful in selling to those in power, was already in place:

> one clear benefit of the CFI promotion of new services was that it provided a base from which AIDS work could be developed and allowed a smoother and more rapid response to be made to this major public health issue than might otherwise have been the case. If these projects had not been in existence in the late eighties, service development to meet the AIDS problem would have been very different in England. (MacGregor et al. 1990, 174)

From the Department of Health perspective, the "whole idea of community-based needle-exchange was very [much] in keeping with what we had been trying to develop, at grass roots, not stuffed in hospital. [We] already had in place drug projects, out in the community, [that] were accepted" (Dorothy Black, interview, May 1998).

Ministerial support and the support of the chief medical officer, Dr. Acheson, were critical, both to the CFI and to the eventual adoption of harm minimization as government policy. Norman Fowler was interested in and knowledgeable about narcotic drugs and in favor of an eclectic approach to drug treatment. David Mellor, who became minister of health at a crucial point in 1988, had become knowledgeable through his earlier chairmanship of an interministerial group on drugs. However, it was Dr. Acheson, the epidemiologist, who "realized the significance of HIV" and brought that significance home to the Department of Health.[29] As Dr. Black describes it,

> Donald Acheson was very important. . . . He had no previous interest in the drug scene, but saw it as a public health problem. He was not worried about

drug users—they could all pop off as far as he was concerned—he was concerned about other people [i.e., drug users as a threat to the wider community]. Once [he was] able to grasp that, it brought drug users into the area of his passion. He worked night and day. [He was] the right person in the post at the time. (Dorothy Black, interview, May 1998)

There was, nevertheless, a gap of over two years between the McClelland Report, which had first brought the question of HIV/AIDS in injection drug users to government attention, and officially legitimizing harm minimization as the policy response, as well as government funding for services targeted specifically to HIV/AIDS in drug users. Whether this was a remarkably rapid response or a rather slow one depends on one's perspective. Berridge argues that "of all the 'liberal' policy responses to AIDS, harm minimization for drug policy and the establishment of needle exchanges was to have the most difficult and rocky policy ride" (1996, 93). Participants in the policy ride took a more sanguine view: "it all happened pretty smoothly" said one member of the ACMD working group (interview with ACMD working group member, May 1997), and a heavily involved physician remarked that the Department of Health was better on needles than on sexual transmission: "they moved fast on that, and they were prepared to take the political flack" (Interview with STD physician, May 1997).

Syringe exchange was, in fact, controversial in Britain for much the same reasons as in the United States. The stage for its adoption was set not only by in-house consensus among influential elites but also by the framing of HIV/AIDS among drug users as a threat to the "general heterosexual population." In his memoir, *Ministers Decide*, Norman Fowler wrote,

Some opposed any special arrangement for addicts unless they were being weaned off drugs. They were not prepared to see addicts helped to maintain their habit. Their argument was that drug taking was illegal and the drug taker was committing a criminal offence. My view was that AIDS presented a new dimension. *Dirty needles spread the virus and infected mothers and babies.* (1991, 262, emphasis added)

The universality of the AIDS threat was a major theme of the McClelland report and of the first parliamentary debates on AIDS in 1986 and 1987: "It cannot be overemphasised that spread of HIV is not restricted to those groups originally recognised as being at risk, and that it represents a serious threat to the general population" (Scottish Home and Health Department 1986, 4). At the time those words were written, no Scottish cases of AIDS either in drug users or heterosexual contacts had been reported. However, more than half of injection drug users visiting outpatient clinics had been found to be HIV positive. Authorities in Britain were very concerned to avoid an epidemic of the proportions they saw in the United States.

In parliamentary debate, the theme of universal threat was closely associated with emphasis on the need for a communitarian response: AIDS is a problem for the entire nation—"it is of concern to all of us"; it is a "nonpolitical" problem demanding a bipartisan approach; there must be no stigmatization of AIDS sufferers: "It is only as a united country that we can tackle this dreadful disease" (UK 1987a, 1190).[30] The purposes of this very deliberate rhetoric (by government ministers as well as some back-benchers) were to construct AIDS as a public health problem and to counter the publicly popular alternative framing of AIDS as a disease self-inflicted by moral degenerates (Interview with STD physician, May 1997).

Finally, in sharp contrast to the United States, the authority of science—embodied in evaluation of the pilot projects by a highly respected research team—was effective in providing a cover of legitimacy for needle exchange as a technical solution to a public health problem.

> Responsibility for controversial decision making was deflected on to the "objective" process of research. [The strength of the research results] mattered less than the legitimation the research provided for politicians nervous about a policy change urged by the drug "policy community" . . . the important issue was less the detailed results of the research and more the policy change it appeared to support . . . the redefinition and refocusing of controversial policy change into a scientific and technical issue . . . secured the relatively painless passage of a policy objective into practice. (Berridge 1993,150–51)

Drug Policy and Drug Users in Britain: The "Longue Durée"

Berridge quotes a senior civil servant in the Department of Health as calling AIDS "a blessing in disguise," and another who saw AIDS as "the trigger that brings care for drug users into the mainstream . . . a golden opportunity to get it right for the first time" (1996, 222). There is no question that AIDS gained not only legitimacy and acceptability but also substantially increased funding for the harm-minimization approach to narcotic drug use. Far from representing a sharp break with past policies, however, the British response to the drugs–AIDS nexus demonstrated striking continuity with the past, both in process and in substance.[31]

The history of contemporary British narcotic drugs policies dates from the 1926 Rolleston Committee report. The committee, composed of eminent physicians and named for its chairman, was appointed to advise the government on what was "legitimate" medical prescription of narcotic drugs in light of a 1920 law limiting doctors to dispensing such drugs only "so far as may be necessary for the exercise of [their] profession" (Trebach 1982, 87). The essence of the committee's advice was that addiction was a disease, that prescribing may be necessary in some circumstances, and that the decision whether and how much to prescribe was up to the physician. This advice was incorporated in a memorandum (without force of law) to the profession from the Home Office and the Ministry of Health. No further action was taken until the late 1960s, when prescription of heroin and cocaine to addicts was restricted to physicians (primarily psychiatrists) licensed by the Home Office in new treatment centers. No new restrictions were placed on other narcotic drugs, including methadone.

From the appointment of the Rolleston Committee in 1924 to the present day, narcotic drugs policy has been the province of an alliance between bureaucrats and so-called experts, with the experts sometimes within the government in the capacity of medical civil servants and sometimes without, as advisory committees of the great and the good. Advisory committees were, until the mid-1980s, dominated by physicians and had among their major concerns the preservation of physician autonomy in medical treatment, including the treatment of drug addiction: "In the tussle between the State's desire to do something about the drug problem, and the medical profession's desire to retain its power, clinical freedom emerged unscathed" (Stimson and Lart 1994, 334). With increased emphasis on multidisciplinary approaches to drug use, medical dominance may have diminished in recent years (see, for example, MacGregor 1995). Berridge argues, however, that even this new system could not have moved forward without the endorsement of doctors and doctor civil servants (1993, 143).

A second element of continuity is the emphasis on what is now referred to as harm reduction. Although the Rolleston Committee did not use this phrase, the words of its report point strongly to a concern for protection of the drug user: failing all efforts to wean the user from the drug, it may "become justifiable in certain cases to order regularly the minimum dose which has been found necessary, either in order to avoid serious withdrawal symptoms, or to keep the patient in a condition in which he can lead a useful life" (cited in Trebach 1982, 94). This concern must, however, be placed in context.

> The approach outlined by Rolleston was class based. It was designed for the respectable and deserving addict. It was geared to the therapeutic addict— the iatrogenic victim—whose addiction was an accidental side-effect of medical treatment, and to the "professional" addict, which was official euphemism for doctors, nurses, and veterinary surgeons who had become addicted after habitually raiding their drugs cabinet or writing false prescriptions. (Stimson and Lart 1994, 332)

A shift toward more restrictive policies in the late 1960s was driven in large part by changed perceptions of the typical addict:

The descendants of the Rolleston committee could tolerate the idea of a general practitioner providing regular supplies of narcotics to somebody's old gentle mother, who had become used to her morphine when in the hospital twenty years ago for a cancer operation, but they positively gagged at applying the Rolleston rules to that mother's mod son, with his long hair and hippie clothes, who lived on the state, never worked a day in his life and did not intend to, and now wanted his heroin free from the National Health Service. (Trebach 1982, 174)

However, by the late 1980s, harm minimization had again reasserted itself, pushed this time not by changes in the user population but by the threat of AIDS. In the context of AIDS, drug use was defined as a public health problem—alternative moral and even criminal definitions were explicitly rejected—and drug users were reconstructed as responsible consumers. This new image, of the "*health conscious drug user*, responsive to public health and educational information, and engaging in rational planning, management and behavior" could hardly have been in sharper contrast to the earlier (and still prevalent) cultural image of the drug user as an irresponsible, manipulative hedonist (Stimson and Lart 1991, 1266, emphasis in original).

In the course of the first parliamentary debate on AIDS in the fall of 1986, an MP characterized the country as "at war with a new virus." He went on to say, "We must get ourselves on to a war footing to tackle the great problem" (United Kingdom 1986, 828). Berridge has argued that "war" was an appropriate metaphor for the government's mobilization against AIDS from 1986 through 1988: the nation was called upon by its leaders to work together in response to a common threat. More recently, the threat has receded, the scenario of AIDS as a danger to the general population is no longer widely accepted, and the availability of life-prolonging treatment has reconstructed AIDS from an infectious to a chronic disease. Among the apparent consequences is a shift in the emphasis of government discourse around narcotic drugs. The significance of harm minimization changed to mean minimization of harm to the community—that is, from crime and other negative consequences of drug use—as much as to the individual user, and recent documents pay substantially more attention to reduction of drug use (MacGregor 1995; Stimson 2000). Nevertheless—regardless of whether its drug policies have become more conservative in recent years—the government of the 1980s was successful in averting an HIV epidemic in Britain's injection drug users.

Canada

Canada's story is in many ways the most complex of the four countries, encompassing three levels of government, competing jurisdictions within and among levels, and actions on the ground that may conflict with or indeed be entirely unrelated to official policy at any of the three levels.

Further contributing to this Byzantine policy environment is Canada's proximity to the United States: "We have a sleeping elephant to the south who stirs every time we try to [change narcotic drug laws]" (Interview with drugs policy consultant, January 2002). Canadian public health authorities became aware of high HIV rates in injection drug users in the late 1980s. Local health officials in major cities moved rapidly but quietly to initiate needle-exchange. They had behind the scenes support from federal civil servants and some federal funding. Officially and publicly, however, the left hand—the federal government—has preferred to say as little as possible about what the right hand—in the cities on the ground—was doing.

Federal Policy: The Left Hand

The struggle of federal health authorities to formulate and advance a national response to a localized problem largely outside their formal jurisdiction (I remind the reader that health is a provincial responsibility) is reflected in two series of reports, corresponding to two perceived HIV/AIDS crises, that appeared between 1990 and 2001. Each report was funded by Health Canada, though only two reflect its views. The others are the work of consultants drawn for the most part from Canada's health establishment: physicians and public health workers professionally concerned with drug use and its health consequences. In a kind of bureaucratic ping-pong, consultants propose and the government disposes, either ignoring its consultants' recommendations or attending to them with considerable selectivity.

Phase I. 1988 to 1996   In 1988, Canada's National Advisory Committee on AIDS (NAC-AIDS), responding to the evidence of high HIV infection rates among injection drug users in Montreal, established a Working Group on HIV and Injection Drug Use (Hankins 1998). The group's report, transmitted to the minister of health in August of 1990, was modeled on the 1988 report of the British Advisory Council on the Misuse of Drugs. (Indeed, much of the language in the two reports was identical.) The Canadian report stated that "the spread of HIV is a greater danger to individuals and public health than injection drug use itself" and recommended that "all injection drug users should have ready access to sterile injecting equipment," that "methadone treatments should be more readily available across the country," and that "all legal and administrative obstacles to obtaining needles and syringes for the purpose of self-administration of drugs should be removed" (Canada NAC-AIDS 1994, 91–94). The NAC-AIDS report was never officially acknowledged and for four years its text was withheld from publication (Hankins 1998).

The same year that NAC-AIDS completed its report, 1990, the government issued its own AIDS strategy document (Canada Health and

Welfare 1990). Insofar as this strategy pertained to AIDS-drugs, the fact was well concealed. Buried on page 11 are three paragraphs under the heading "AIDS Prevention Program for Injection Drug Users and their Sexual Partners" (1990). What were, in fact, large-scale needle-exchange programs in Montreal, Toronto, and Vancouver were characterized as "pilot [research] projects."[32] Needle-exchange was never mentioned.

Phase II. 1997 to 2001   By 1996, events on the ground created new opportunities for public health experts to demand federal intervention on behalf of injection drug users. Data from Vancouver and Montreal had indicated unanticipated and anomalous increases in HIV infection rates among users as compared with non-users of needle-exchange programs (Strathdee et al. 1997; Patrick et al. 1997; Bruneau et al. 1997). At the request of the Canadian Public Health Association and the Toronto Center on Substance Abuse, the Task Force on HIV/AIDS and Injection Drug Use was created. The task force report, published in 1997, described Canada as "in the midst of a public health crisis concerning HIV and AIDS, and injection drug use" (Canada. Task Force on HIV/AIDS and Injection Drug Use 1997, 2). It argued that the illegal status of drugs was itself a major contributor to the spread of HIV/AIDS among injection drug users, called for drug-law reform, and demanded federal leadership: "The Task Force strongly reconfirms the responsibility of the federal Minister of Health to show leadership on this issue, in partnership with key ministries (Justice, Solicitor General, Corrections) through initiating action, monitoring implementation, and evaluating outcomes" (3). Other reports quickly followed with essentially the same recommendations (for example, Canadian HIV/AIDS Legal Network 1999).

In 2001, the Canadian government released two documents responding explicitly to these reports (Canada. F/P/T Advisory Committee on Population Health 2001; Health Canada 2001). Although their tone was circumspect—they largely skirted the question of drug-law reform and in characteristic Canadian fashion placed heavy emphasis on the need for ongoing consultation and collaboration among stakeholders, both documents were forthright in their identification of injection drug use as "a health issue, as opposed to a law and order issue" and in their embrace of a harm reduction approach to prevention and treatment (Health Canada 2001, 2). For example, though disclaiming direct responsibility for delivery of needle exchange and methadone maintenance treatment services as "a provincial/territorial responsibility," the Health Ministry document went on to describe a range of efforts in support of these programs (11). Further, both documents expressed tentative support for "pilot research trials" of heroin prescription, specifically, the North American Opiate Medication Initiative, and, in the FPT document, for "a feasibility study of establishing a scientific, medical research project regarding a supervised injection site in

Canada" (Canada. F/P/T Advisory Committee report 2001, no pagination). These statements, however carefully worded, went far beyond anything senior government officials in the United States said publicly.

It is reasonable to ask whether this piling up of reports represented action or a strategy to avoid action. How they are evaluated depends on where the observer sits. Those most militant on behalf of drug users were—not surprisingly—the most dismissive:

> "There are six or eight [government] reports that all make very sound do-able cost saving recommendations and none of them have been implemented, so to create the political will, we need to get political." (member of the Vancouver Harm Reduction Action Society, quoted in Michelle Cook, The Vancouver Sun, July 12, 2000)

> [Another activist] expressed her frustration by burning several recent government reports: "We've had so many years of talk, and now we're into trendy consultations." (The Vancouver Sun, July 12, 2000)

The MP who represents the area of Vancouver where drug users congregate shared this perspective: "There's not a shadow of a doubt in my mind that if it had been left to the people who are on these . . . committees and working groups and whatnot, or the minister . . . nothing would have happened" (Interview, February 2002). A local public health official who has sat on many of these committees took a considerably more sanguine view, focusing on the function of government-commissioned reports by "outside" experts: these reports can be "used to push ministers, politicians. . . . They create space [for] change. [For example,] as an activist I can go to [provincial health authorities] and say we need to do supervised injection facilities [citing the FPT reports]" (Interview with public health official, January 2002).

Negotiating the "Interjurisdictional Thicket"   Commenting on the many levels of government in Canada with responsibilities for health, David Rayside and Evert Lindquist observed that "the issues posed by AIDS have led policy makers and activists into an interjurisdictional thicket" (1992, 50). Calls for partnership and cross-governmental and multistakeholder consultation—repeated almost to the point of obsession in the documents reviewed—reflect a central fact of Canadian political life: the federal government—however much it may wish to involve itself in a particular health issue—"can't just parachute in" (Interview with city public health official, December 2002). HIV/AIDS prevention in whatever form—needle-exchange programs, methadone maintenance, heroin prescription, safe injection sites—is, by definition, health care, and health care delivery is a provincial responsibility: "If the provinces didn't buy in, [needle-exchange] would die. Feds need partners [that is, the provinces]" (Interview with physician head of university HIV/AIDS program, December 2002). In fact, civil servants in Health Canada played an essential role in the original push for needle exchange, directing federal funds for pilot projects to local community groups. This strategy allowed the federal government to—at least temporarily—bypass the provinces, in the expectation, of course, that the provinces would ulti-mately take over. The "feds like to work with community groups," said one provincial health official, "because it's a way around the provinces" (Interview with physician head of university HIV/AIDS program, Decem-ber 2002).

The partnership imperative was both increased and made more com-plicated in the case of AIDS/drugs policy by the illegal status of narcotic drugs: "The first thing politicians ask [about policy initiatives in this domain] is what do the police think" (Interview with provincial health officer, December 2002). The police, however, were hardly monolithic: what the Royal Canadian Mounted Police (RCMP)—governed by federal policy—think may or may not filter down to the beat cop in Toronto, Mon-treal, or Vancouver. Asked to identify his biggest problems, a local public health worker responded without hesitation, "partnerships." He explained: "Many determinants of public health are out of our control/jurisdiction. . . . Harm reduction, safe injection sites, heroin prescription [all] require nego-tiating with people [that is, the police] whose goal is not public health. Their goal is not to prevent disease. Their goal is public order. Requires each partner to compromise." Partnership and consultation are not only rhetorically appealing but also pragmatic strategies for advancing national policy in a highly decentralized federal system.

Action on the Ground: The Right Hand

HIV/AIDS in injection drug users was thrust onto Canada's public stage in the late 1980s when local public health officers in Canada's largest cities were confronted with the disease in their own backyards.

Activism by Experts   In the fall of 1988, Catherine Hankins, a physician-epidemiologist with the Montreal Regional Health Department, discov-ered "horrendous HIV-positive rates" among women prisoners who injected drugs. Hankins was a member of NAC/AIDS and made use of her position to bring the question of HIV/AIDS in injection drug users to national political attention. On a television program describing her results, Hankins was asked what needed to be done. Her reply was, "political will, political leadership." As she recounts it, the newly appointed health minister, Perrin Beatty, saw the program, came to the next meet-ing of NAC/AIDS, and said he had the political will.[33] Negotiation with federal and provincial health officials led to Montreal's needle-exchange program, launched in 1989 as a pilot project with federal funds.

Public health officials in Vancouver, alerted by New York's experience to the HIV risk posed by injection drug use, also swung into action in 1988 as soon as individuals with injection drug use as their only risk factor began to show up HIV-positive in British Columbia's HIV test results (Blatherwick 1989). John Blatherwick, medical health officer for the City of Vancouver, described hearing reports "from England and European centres . . . on the success of needle exchange programs" at the 1988 International AIDS Conference in Stockholm. "It was apparent that bold action would be necessary if Canada was to avoid the problems that New York now faces" (S26). The groundwork for Vancouver's needle-exchange program was carefully laid: Blatherwick met and corresponded with local elites (police, physicians, politicians) and informed the public through media appearances, interviews, and the like (S26–27). The program opened officially in 1989, funded by the Vancouver City Council.

By the late 1980s in Toronto, as in Montreal and Vancouver, HIV/AIDS in injection drug users had been identified by local public health officials as an emerging disease problem.[34] Proposals to respond with a needle-exchange program came from local community agencies serving street youth, and also from the Toronto-based Addiction Research Foundation. Initially there was competition between the Toronto Health Department and the more radical street youth agencies as to who should run the program. The Health Department prevailed. This was no surprise. Since the mid-1970s, the Toronto Board of Health had become recognized as a highly progressive force in the community; public health had credibility that the street groups lacked (MacDougall 1990).

The details of needle-exchange initiation differed in each of these cities, depending on how individual actors, local and provincial public health and political authorities, along with the judiciary and the police, defined and negotiated their respective roles. My informants—key players in these negotiations—identified as critical factors, first, the level of support by local political officials (for example, big-city mayors) for preventive services to injection drug users, and second, insider connections between health actors at the local level (public health officials, university-based experts) and key bureaucrats and politicians at all three levels of government: local, provincial, and federal.

Until very recently, the Canadian response to HIV/AIDS in injection drug users relied almost wholly on needle-syringe exchange. Methadone played little role. Indeed in 1995, "Canada featured one of the lowest per capita rates of methadone treatment availability in international comparison, significantly lower even than the United States" (Fischer 1999, 200). Methadone treatment for drug addiction had been introduced in Canada in the 1960s. Methadone was, nevertheless, subject to the same federal regulatory regime as other narcotic drugs, and "the concerted resistance of law enforcement, parts of the medical profession, and the federal health bureaucracy used the emerging accounts of methadone-related problems to impose a comprehensively restrictive regulatory framework" (204).

In the mid-1990s, responding to its expert consultants' advice and to the new evidence of epidemic HIV among injection drug users, the federal government devolved responsibility for regulation of methadone treatment to the provinces (Oscapella and Elliott 1999, A59). By all accounts, provincial response has been highly variable (Canada. F/P/T Advisory Committee on Population Health 2001). The availability of methadone maintenance treatment is still very limited and depends heavily on local circumstances and local professional and political leadership.

Mobilization from Below   In a book on AIDS politics published in 1992, authors of the chapter on Canada celebrated the emergence of AIDS activism and its powerful impact on that country's health-care system:

> Whatever public health measures are adopted [in response to AIDS], the top-down regulatory model run by experts will not go unchallenged. While the toll of AIDS has been heavy, many people with AIDS have resisted acting like victims; they have joined with other AIDS activists in questioning the received wisdom about how best to deal with the disease. In doing so, they have permanently altered the Canadian health care system for the better. (Rayside and Lindquist 1992, 94)

In the course of this fifty-page chapter, injection drug users—perhaps not surprisingly given this emphasis on community activism—were barely mentioned. The activists in question were gays and lesbians, not drug users. Their focus was on the prevention and treatment needs of gay men; they were unable—and often unwilling—to advocate on behalf of injection drug users:

> Originally the Canadian AIDS Society [CAS] was *the* AIDS organization in the country, and they haven't taken on drug use issues at all. [CAS was] a typical organization that was founded in the 80s, mainly by gay men concerned about gay men, and [they] had a very difficult time adjusting to the new [face of the epidemic]. And they really failed in a fairly spectacular way to do anything useful about drug issues, including when they did it doing it really badly because they didn't have anyone who understands the issues, to the extent that I just hope they will stay out of it. (Interview with AIDS-drugs activist, February 2002)

These comments were echoed in one form or another by every person with whom I spoke about the AIDS-drugs policy nexus in Canada. Although gay men were well organized on their own behalf, they played little or no role as catalysts for government action to address the problem of HIV/AIDS in injection-drug users.

A central theme in the rhetoric of advocates for injection-drug users was one of inclusion: users themselves should be "empowered" and programs "should actively involve the people they are designed to serve" (Canada NAC/AIDS 1994). However, narcotics users are highly stigmatized in Canada, as elsewhere; they were often unwilling to take the risk of advocacy when that meant going public as drug injectors (Canadian HIV/AIDS Legal Network 1999, 15). When health officials in Vancouver and Toronto contracted with local groups to offer needle exchange, those groups were identified as youth service organizations, although at least one, and perhaps both, were led by highly charismatic former users, and neither claimed to represent drug users. Despite the rhetoric of inclusion, user-organized and -run groups did not emerge until the late 1990s.

The most prominent of these groups, the Vancouver Area Network of Drug Users (VANDU) was founded in 1995 by a self-described nonuser, white, female, revolutionary health activist resident of the Downtown Eastside area of Vancouver, where drug users were concentrated. Convinced that nothing was being done by the government, she put up signs for a meeting, and VANDU took off from there. In 2002, it claimed 1,400 members. VANDU is remarkably well organized and has been highly effective politically, combining insider connections with City Hall and media-targeted protests to lobby for increased services from the municipality (for example, housing, toilets, places to wash and do laundry). VANDU gained legitimacy from the strong support of local health officials: "Early in the AIDS epidemic, we were able to talk to gay men. There was nothing for injection drug users. We need to talk to them. They told us what they wanted. They are the real grassroots" (Interview with health department official, December 2002). Moral support translated into funding. At the time of my field visit in 2002, VANDU received at least some funds for its activities from all three levels of government. Perhaps the strongest testimony to VANDU's success came from the leader of a local business group that had strongly, and unsuccessfully, opposed enhanced services on the ground that they would further concentrate drug users in the Downtown Eastside: "VANDU has been amazingly effective at organizing themselves and being heard." VANDU's position was further validated by the results of the city's 2002 mayoral election. Drug use in Vancouver was a central issue, and a strong advocate for harm reduction defeated his more timid rival.

Vancouver's circumstances may be unique. User mobilization was facilitated by the concentration of drug users in a single area of the city and there was a long history of local political and expert support for treating drug use as a health problem and for measures to reduce the harm from drug injection. I found little evidence of comparable mobilization outside of Vancouver, although the desirability of user organization was widely embraced by actors in the field.

HIV and Canada's Drug Policies:
In the Shadow of the Elephant

In the spring of 2001, the Canadian House of Commons debated a motion to create a committee on the nonmedical use of drugs. In the course of that debate, the parliamentary secretary to the leader of the government in the House of Commons, speaking for the government, commented as follows on Canada's ability to change its drug policies:

> Our neighbor to the south, the U.S.A., is a constraint, believe it or not. The way the U.S.A. treats this issue is the same way it has treated it for 75 or 100 years. It is based on enforcement and interdiction. That is not working. It is not working there and it is not working here. It is imported across our border just about the same way that a lot of other things are imported across our border. I am not talking about drugs. I am talking about the policy, the method of enforcement. . . . *It is difficult for us here to do things in a way that is radically different from the way policing and medical counterparts deal with it across the border,* but we have to find a way to do it. (Canada. House of Commons 2001, 1550, emphasis added)

A New Democratic Party (NDP) back-bencher was more blunt: "I wonder, given that we are going in a slightly different path than the United States, how much flexibility *Canada will be allowed* (1140, emphasis added). From the parliamentary representatives of a sovereign country, these are astonishing statements. They reflect a nearly hundred-year-long history of unbalanced interdependence between U.S. and Canadian drug policies. The two countries have moved in regulatory lock-step—from opium to marijuana to heroin and cocaine—facilitated by the "close working relationship between H. J. Anslinger, head of the U.S. Bureau of Narcotics for thirty-two years, and his Canadian counterpart, Colonel C. H. L. Sharman, chief of the Division of Narcotic Control from 1927–1946" (Mitchell 1991, 9).

In the 1960s, Canada, the United States, Britain, France, and other western European countries experienced a rise in drug use—marijuana in particular—among middle-class adolescents. The Trudeau government responded by appointing a royal commission, known as the Le Dain Commission after its chair, to examine illicit drug use in Canada and to make recommendations for change. Its recommendations, which included expansion of methadone treatment, reduction of criminal penalties for drug use, and decriminalization of marijuana, were ignored by Trudeau. In a 1998 interview, Le Dain commented, "It was a hot potato for all the parties and they didn't want to run any risk. The position adopted by the politicians was to do nothing" [cited by Mr. Dick Proctor, MP-Paliser-NDP, in the course of debate on Canada's drug policy] (Canada. House of Commons 2001, 1150). A Canadian authority on substance-use policies wrote somewhat less charitably that, "the Le Dain Commission served the role of most Royal Commissions: it delayed action on a controversial issue long enough for the public demand for action to subside" (Riley 1998, not paginated).

Canada's drug laws were most recently revised—and strengthened—in 1997 on the grounds that changes were necessary to bring Canada into compliance with its international treaty obligations and to counter U.S. Drug Enforcement Agency accusations of laxity on the part of Canadian authorities. Among other things, the new law—the Controlled Drugs and Substances Act (CDSA)—prohibits the "unauthorized possession, manufacture, cultivation, transportation, trafficking . . . export and import" of a large array of substances listed as "controlled" (Oscapella and Elliott 1999, A5). This provision was greeted with outrage by public health and drug policy activists: "There is no express exemption or protection in the statute (or regulations) for needle-syringe exchange programs or their personnel, who will often knowingly be in possession of used [drug-contaminated] equipment returned by users" (A5). Passage of the CDSA—an event its opponents regarded as an underhanded ploy ("passed the day of the Quebec [sovereignty referendum] when everyone was otherwise occupied")—played a major role in subsequent demands for drug law reform.

Among the more interesting arguments put forward by government representatives in favor of the CDSA was that it would not be strictly enforced: "We have not yet heard of any case of a person being charged by the police while exchanging a contaminated syringe for a sterile one . . . in some Canadian cities, a conscious policy decision has been made not to enforce the legislation" (Canada. Senate 1996). And indeed, HIV-drug policy professionals in Vancouver asserted that the CDSA language had not, in fact, led to arrests for syringe possession: "It didn't happen. [Lawyers thought it would.] It didn't." The distinction between law and practice was made even more explicit in remarks (in this case with respect to sentencing after conviction) to the Canadian Senate by an official of the Justice Department:

> It would appear, to someone who is not familiar with our legal regime, that our statutes are somewhat severe in that maximum imprisonment of life is provided for in respect of a number of substances. But the actual sentencing practices are considerably different. We allow our judges considerable discretion in applying the sentence. In most instances, sentences imposed are at the lower end of the spectrum rather than at the high end. (1995)

Navigating around the "elephant," Canada introduced needle exchange on the QT and passed harsh drug laws but enforced them selectively and inconsistently (see, for example, Riley 1998; Wood et al. 2003).

Science, Ideology, and Politics:
The Badger and the Elephant Compared

I referred earlier to studies conducted in Vancouver and Montreal that showed higher rates of HIV infection among individuals who attended needle-exchange programs as compared to those who did not. These studies were published in 1997, both in journals readily available in the United States. I do not describe them in detail except to say that their designs were unsuited to inferring a causal connection between program attendance and subsequent conversion from HIV negative to HIV positive. The methodological issues raised had been carefully reviewed in a report from the National Academy of Sciences issued before the articles were published (Normand, Vlahov, and Moses 1995, 291). The policy and political fallout from these publications was substantial and highly revealing of the difference between American and Canadian response to HIV/AIDS in injection drug users.

The original intent of these investigators had been to call attention to the need to expand needle exchange programs (for example, to increase the number of needles available for exchange) and to broaden the range of services available to drug users (for example, to include methadone maintenance) (Normand, Vlahov, and Moses 1995; Schecter et al. 1999). Canadian health authorities were highly responsive to this message:

> Not only has a decision been made *not* to cut funds for needle exchange funding, but a commitment has been made on behalf of federal, provincial and municipal governments to redouble our efforts and to expand services within and around needle exchange. In March 1997, the British Columbia Ministry of Health dedicated $3 million dollars to develop a more comprehensive harm reduction program. A Canadian national task force on HIV infection among drug users [cited earlier as Canada. F/P/T Advisory Committee on Population Health] recommended that needle exchange be maintained as a cornerstone of HIV prevention. (Strathdee 1998)

In Vancouver, the mayor, the district MP, the local health board, and the principal daily newspaper strongly supported efforts to expand existing services and to experiment with new approaches (for example, Steffenhagen 1997; Bula 2000, 2001; Vancouver Sun 1998). There was no absence of controversy: at least one local community group strongly opposed expansion of services to drug users, local police were not invariably supportive, and VANDU and its allies protested perceived political inaction and bureaucratic delays. The dominant message, however, was clearly in favor of more and better services, and additional services were indeed forthcoming, funded by all three levels of government, municipal, provincial, and federal.[35]

In the United States, the same data that led to expansion of services in Canada were seized upon by politicians and others opposed to needle exchange as ammunition to bolster their cause. Bob Goodlatte, a member of Congress from Virginia, asked his colleagues to co-sponsor legislation that would permanently "prohibit federal funds from being used to develop and support needle exchange programs," arguing that though "some are promoting the theory that needle exchange programs are effective ways to fight HIV . . . recent evidence clearly refutes that argument. . . . Not only do needle exchange programs not work, they are harmful to our communities and undermine our nation's drug control efforts" (1999, n.p.). On a local level in the United States, the Canadian data were repeatedly cited in opposition to NEPs (see for example, Ahmed 1999; San Diego Union-Tribune 2000). In an interview with Steffanie Strathdee, the lead author on the Vancouver paper, she described being caught between NEP opponents and U.S. NEP program staff: "when the Vancouver data about the outbreak hit, there were a lot of very angry American activists . . . and we were the most surprised people in the world, because we said, 'well it's your government that's got it wrong . . . don't yell at us' " (Strathdee, interview, December 2002).[36] Recounting a visit to his office by U.S. drug czar Barry McCaffrey's "boys," a university-based Canadian authority on HIV-drug policy said he told them they were misinterpreting the data. Their reaction was to shrug and say, "that's politics."

Central to Canadian advocates' discourse on behalf of injection drug users was the construction of narcotic drug use as a health problem. The health frame was in this case pitted against the law and order frame; in the parallel case of tobacco control, health was pitted against tobacco industry greed. As I noted in connection with tobacco, appeals to health in the Canadian context were more than just rhetorical statements. Much like appeals to partnership, appeals to health are intended to evoke shared communitarian values: health and health care are fundamental to Canadian ideas of citizenship. At the same time, these appeals constitute assertions of turf rights, statements about where in the Canadian political system's interjurisdictional thicket the problem of HIV/AIDS in injection drug users belongs.

PART IV

STRUCTURES, MOVEMENTS, AND IDEOLOGIES IN THE MAKING OF PUBLIC HEALTH POLICY

Chapter 7

Engines of Policy Change: The State and Civil Society

INOW TURN from data—the sixteen stories of public health I have recounted—to analysis and interpretation organized around the three broad determinants of public health action proposed in chapter 1: states, collective actions, and constructions of risk. The goals of this analysis are to arrive at an understanding of the social and political processes that drive policy making in public health, and to explain why countries otherwise comparable in so many respects reacted differently to essentially the same threats. My strategy is to move back and forth across the narratives in an effort to discover and account for both common and contrasting patterns. Although this entails an inevitable loss of contextual detail and chronological sequence, the compensating gain—if my intention is realized—comes in understanding how structure, opportunity, and human agency interact to create, or inhibit, the possibility of change.

Strong States, Weak States, and Public Health

In the dramas of public health, nation-states play multiple roles. They are dominant policy actors with the power, if they choose, to make or break public health initiatives. At the same time, states shape the social and cultural context for nonstate actors—members of civil society including (but not limited to) social movement and other forms of collective organization—that seek to advance their own public health agendas. As I explained earlier, I employ the notion of strong and weak states as developed by John Peter Nettl, Herbert Kitschelt, Theda Skocpol, and others as a heuristic device both to illuminate and to raise questions about the behaviors of the actual states whose actions I studied. Although these scholars' ideas had suggested the initial hypothesis that state strength would be associated with more aggressive and effective public health policy making (see, for example, Nathanson 1996), it became apparent early in my research that this hypothesis was magnificently—but instructively—wrong.

The first step in my analysis is to order the four countries according to their relative state strength. France is the ideal-typical strong state.

It is possible to regard the contemporary state in France as a close approximation to the model of the strong state. From the time of the absolute monarchy to Gaullism—and even to recent socialist policy—appeal to the state has seemed to be a natural course for all those in positions of political power. The state is the seat of legitimacy upon which aspiring future elites set their sights; its educational socialization operates more or less satisfactorily, and its control over society is extensive. Such a state renders the introduction of mechanisms of participatory democracy almost impossible. (Haas 1992, 63–64)

The French state is and has long been strong institutionally: centralized geographically and politically and guided by a corps of officials impervious (ideally, if not in fact) to outside pressure. Inseparable from these institutions is a political culture that identifies the state as the sole repository of legitimate power, specifically the power to initiate and implement public policy, and that delegitimizes other voices, making it difficult for those voices to be heard. Among the four countries included in this project, France anchors the strong-state end of the strong state–weak state continuum. Yet France's capacity to act in the domain of public health has been, as the narratives have shown, surprisingly limited. I will return to the questions raised by this paradox once the remaining three countries have been located on the strong state–weak state continuum.[1]

Just as France has been the exemplary strong state, the United States is the quintessentially "weak state." "The absence of a sense of the state . . . has been the great hallmark of American political culture," Stephen Skowronek has observed, though he located that sense of absence in the early twentieth century, suggesting that much has changed since then (1982, 3). Other scholars emphasize enduring structural characteristics—geographical and political fragmentation and the near absence of a cohesive and politically independent officialdom—to argue that the American state acts to minimize capacity for policy innovation and implementation and to maximize the access of non-state actors to policy gatekeepers (Kitschelt 1986; Walker 1991). A state's capacity in the abstract may be less important, however, than the disposition to exploit that capacity for policy making purposes: "governments [have] routinely expanded capacities when their policy prescriptions called for it" (Dobbin 1994, 229). Aversion to the use of federal government power to intervene in the country's social and economic life is a central and long-standing aspect of American political culture, routinely expressed in both denunciations of big government and appeals to states' rights. Although this rhetoric waxes and wanes (it is more muted in times of national crisis) it is ever-present in the discursive toolkit of American politicians and public officials (see, for example, Quadagno and Street 2005). Again, however, there are paradoxes. In the domain of public health, the United States has been somewhat less of a laggard than its putative weakness might have predicted.

Although France and the United States are almost stereotypically strong and weak states as these constructs are conventionally defined, Great Britain and Canada lend themselves considerably less well to categorization in the same terms. Nettl characterized Britain as "the stateless society *par excellence*" (Nettl 1968, 562), and early students of comparative politics tended to lump Great Britain with the United States: "In neither country is the state 'instantly recognizable as an area of autonomous action,' and in both, the law, rather than being an emanation of the state, has a great deal of autonomy" (Katznelson 1985, 271). Despite its unitary structure and the strong executive ensured by a parliamentary system that subordinates the legislature to the party in power, Britain was seen as an essentially liberal state highly reluctant to intervene in the country's social and economic life.

Scholars may have been deceived by "the Englishman's habitual stance of lackadaisical irreverence towards the majesty of the state" (Harris 1990, 102). Examination of the historical longue durée considerably complicates this weak state scenario. Whether the British state was strong or weak depended a great deal on when and where you looked. Pat Thane argues that "by the mid-eighteenth century . . . England had developed an apparatus of central government comparable with most European states" (1990, 5). Its methods, however, were less visible. In the nineteenth century, the era of Edwin Chadwick and John Simon, social intervention expanded in particular arenas, more especially in public health. Intervention was politically and ideologically contentious—it went against the liberal grain—and it was accompanied by ongoing struggles for power between central-state authorities and local governments. State intervention in local affairs occurred nonetheless. To describe the British state in the late nineteenth and early twentieth centuries as a " 'minimal,' 'nightwatchman,' or 'weak' state is seriously to misunderstand it. It was characterized by a small, but strong and flexible, core firmly directing the key activities of state and supervising the delegation of functions defined as less essential to local authorities and voluntary organizations" (Thane 1993, 343).

Little has changed. Structurally the British state, like the French, has ample capacity to act and is well able to exercise control over who is and who is not included in the policy process. Exercise of these "strong state" capacities, however, has been powerfully shaped by a political culture very different from that of France. On the one hand is an aversion to accomplishing policy ends with coercive measures and a corresponding commitment to policy making by consensus, that is, voluntary agreements among those directly affected (Vogel 1986). On the other is a belief that state power can legitimately be exercised to preserve social stability by responding to the needs of the poor, the disenfranchised, and the potentially militant (Thane 1990, 58) How these contradictory elements have played out in the arena of public health has been highly dependent on period and circumstances.

Of these four nation-states, Canada is the most complex in political structure and has experienced the most change in political culture in recent years. As I observed in an earlier chapter, Canada is a young country, established by the British North America Act in 1867. In sharp contrast with the United States, "the Canadian system was predicated upon a strong faith in government, a top-down approach to the development of policy, and an historical acceptance of government intervention" (Radin and Boase 2000, 69). Political power in Canada is highly concentrated: "The point of departure for an understanding of the Canadian system is an appreciation of the almost unchecked power . . . of a united cabinet that commands a majority in the legislature" (69) Power is also decentralized. In an arrangement unique to Canadian federalism, executive branch dominance at the federal level is mirrored in each of the ten provinces. Indeed, provincial power within the areas of provincial jurisdiction—including education, health policy, and social welfare—substantially exceeds that of the individual states in the United States: "Provincial governments have greater power in national debates than state governments, or any other actors on the political scene in either country" (Leman 1980, 142).

Among the consequences of this unique arrangement has been a long-standing pattern of jurisdictional power struggles. Histories of infant mortality and tuberculosis in the early twentieth century are remarkable for their descriptions of buck-passing, actors at each level of government insisting that responsibility for action, and for failure to act, lay at any level other than their own. A second outcome has been the development over time of elaborate, increasingly institutionalized structures to facilitate negotiation and compromise: "Policy development is very much a federal-provincial dialogue. . . . The federal government . . . cannot issue mandates in the areas of provincial jurisdiction; it must negotiate, compromise, and exploit its superior spending power to convince the provincial governments to pass legislation" (Radin and Boase 2000, 69). Canada is, in other words, governed by parallel strong states that compete for authority and power.[2] How public health policies are made depends largely on where in this jurisdictional thicket any given problem falls—or can be interpreted to fall. I argue that these circumstances create structural incentives for central government involvement in public health that are unique to Canada.

To complicate matters further, the past twenty years have seen a marked increase in opportunities for social movements and other interest-group actors to penetrate the Canadian political system. Political scientists writing about Canada before the mid-1980s emphasized the limited access of these groups to a policy process dominated by cabinet government oper-

Table 7.1   State Structures Compared

State Structure	France	Britain	Canada	United States
Centralization of power	high	high	low	low
Concentration of power	high	high	high	low
Civil service independence	high	high	high	medium
Political opportunities for nonstate actors	low	low	high	very high

Source: Author's analysis.

ating largely out of the public view (for example, Leman 1980). The adoption in 1982 of a Charter of Rights and Freedoms (similar to the U.S. Bill of Rights) has been associated with a major increase in interest-group activity (including litigation) (Meyer and Staggenborg 1998).[3] Indeed, one observer concluded on the basis of recent data that "Canadians, far from being deferential to authority, are among the most likely [to participate in politics through collective action], ranking slightly ahead of Americans in their propensity for protest" (cited in Meyer and Staggenborg 1998, 216).[4]

The cross-national differences in political structure that I have described are summarized in table 7.1. France anchors the strong-state end of the continuum, followed by Britain, Canada, and the United States.[5] Many qualifications are of course in order, only two of which I mention now. First, insofar as this table conveys an illusion of stability, it is false. Some elements of some countries' political structure are reasonably stable—surely centralization and concentration of power are longstanding characteristics of the French polity. In other countries, however, notably Canada, political structures have shifted considerably over time. Second, political culture is left out altogether, resulting in, among other things, a distorted impression of Great Britain that omits the real reluctance of that country's officials to fully exploit the considerable powers at their command.

If state strength predicted state intervention to promote public health, France should be highly aggressive, responding rapidly and effectively to public health threats, and the United States should respond slowly and ineffectually, if at all. The reality is quite different. Each state has acted effectively in a few (very few) instances and ineffectively in others, and neither has acted consistently as their respective strength or weakness, as measured by the criteria presented in table 7.1, would predict. Given these observations, the next step is to identify the social and political circumstances under which governments do marshal the capacity and the political will to take effective public health action.

The Weaknesses of a Strong State: France   In his classic book, *The Bureaucratic Phenomenon*, Michel Crozier described France as "a centralized power that

Table 7.2   Dates Selected Preventive Measures Adopted

Preventive Measures	United States	Britain	Canada	France
Mandatory TB notification	NYC:1897 59 cities by 1904 84 cities by 1908 No national mandate	Brighton: 1899 (voluntary) Sheffield: 1904 (compulsory) 1913: Mandatory	Ontario: 1912. "Large cities and towns" by 1910. No national mandate	1963
Pasteurization	Chicago: 1908 NYC: 1912 1921: 90% of cities over 100,000	1948	1914: Toronto 1938: Ontario 1914: Montreal West end only 1935: 94% in Montreal	1939: ~1% pasteurized.

Source: Author's analysis.

has become paralyzed because of its omnipotence and its concomitant iso-lation" (1964, 234). Nowhere has this paralysis been more evident than in the domain of public health, a judgment the more startling when we recall that France was the birthplace of Louis Pasteur. Even when a health threat was recognized and embraced by the state, as in the case of infant mortal-ity, there was a wide gap between state action and actual implementation.[6] Absent that embrace—which was limited to infant mortality among the four issues I investigated—state action was delayed and ineffective. Table 7.2 compares the dates of adoption of two relatively standard public health measures—mandatory notification of tuberculosis and pasteuriza-tion of cow's milk—across the four countries (for an updated review of empirical support for the public health importance of these measures, see Fairchild and Oppenheimer 1998). Both were widely adopted in the United States before World War I. France was the last of these countries to adopt tuberculosis notification, and did not institute pasteurization on any scale until after the second World War.[7] The French pattern of delayed or ineffective public health action was repeated in the late twentieth cen-tury. Although France was early to pass tobacco-control legislation (in 1976), this legislation had little support outside the health ministry and was never enforced. Its effects, if any, were largely symbolic. Policies to prevent HIV/AIDS in injection drug users were initiated early as well, in 1987, but again had little significant impact in the absence of political support from government officials outside the Ministry of Health.

In broad terms, France's weakness in the public health arena can be accounted for by five closely interrelated factors: first, the popular and political assumption of state omnipotence; second, the perception of the state as the sole legitimate policy actor; third, the corresponding underdevelopment of activism by ordinary people; fourth, the power of France's medical practitioners to shape health-related public policies to suit their professional interests; and last a powerful, persistent, and perhaps surprising strain of antistatism. I elaborate on each of these factors.[8]

Recounting the obstacles to an effective harm-reduction program for injection drug users in Paris, the physician-manager of one such program explained, "C'est l'état qui décide [It's the state that decides]" (Interview, January 1998). My efforts to identify more specifically the person or persons to whom he was referring were unavailing and, indeed, appeared to mystify my informant. His mystification reflected an understanding of the state that is firmly embedded in French political culture. The state is an abstraction largely independent of the individuals holding power within it—a père de famille, mostly benevolent, sometimes despotic, its pronouncements to be met with the wry skepticism of loving but wayward children (see for example, Nettl 1968, 575). Laws to benefit the public's, or some segment of the public's health, by preventing, as opposed to curing, disease have more often than not been passed less in anticipation of pragmatic results than as symbolic statements, either of good fatherly intentions or of normative expectations with which French citizens as obedient children were expected to comply. The persistent gap between public health action in the form of legislation and the implementation of these laws reflects on the one hand the laws' largely symbolic meaning, in the minds not only of lawmakers but also of the citizens to whose behavior the laws are directed, and on the other hand the institutional weakness of French public health and its low priority within the French political system.

Second, the state is identified as the deciding power—the sine qua non of public health policy—and as solely responsible if things go wrong (if public health problems go unrecognized or are mismanaged). The French state is at the same time the owner of public health problems with the authority to create and influence the [problem's] public definition and the bearer of political responsibility for solving the problem (Gusfield 1981). The state may also be accused of causing the problem by its neglect (in the cases of TB and AIDS, for example). Each of the four French narratives offers evidence for these interpretations but the contrasting stories of infant mortality and tuberculosis in the late nineteenth century are particularly telling. Infant mortality was created by physician-politicians as "a crisis of national proportions where previously none had been perceived" (Cole 1996, 433) for reasons of state: France's declining birthrate viewed in the context of national geopolitical concerns. Absent reasons of state—and given the hostility of physicians to any preventive measures that identified the patient—tuberculosis was ignored. Blame for this inaction was placed squarely on the state, both by contemporaries and by French historians of the period writing today and, ushering in my third factor, was linked by at least one contemporary to an excess of volunteerism.

The third element running through these narratives is the relative weakness of civil society. As reflected in the comment just cited, there are no structurally or culturally legitimate alternatives to action by the state. Denigration of volunteerism needs to be understood in the context of a distinction central to French political culture between intérêts publics (the collective good) and intérêts particuliers (private interests). Determination of intérêts publics and representation of these interests are quintessential functions of the French state. Nonstate groups seeking to advance their ideas of the collective good are perceived as representing intérêts particuliers and may be regarded not only as self-serving but also as an impediment to state action.[9] Among the most striking contrasts between France and the United States (and in the late twentieth-century Canada), is in the density of collective action on behalf of public health goals by lay—that is, nonphysician—actors: sparse in France but high in the United States and (recently) in Canada. Where the state occupies the entire public space, groups outside the state have little room to breathe and their potential for promoting an independent public health agenda is diminished or lost. Should the state itself also fail to act (as, for example, in the case of tuberculosis) the likely result is policy paralysis.

The exceptions I have described—the roles in galvanizing state action played by the cinq sages (tobacco) and limiter la casse (AIDS-drugs)—prove the rule. The state's prestigious economic ministries, staffed by the strongest graduates of the grandes écoles, exemplify the strong state scenario, generating innovation from within and ignoring the voices of intérêts particulier (see, for example, Prasad 2005). Opportunities for (highly selected) nonstate actors in the public health arena reflect the relative weakness of public health administrators both within the state's bureaucratic hierarchy and in the personnel they are able to attract. Among the long-standing beneficiaries of this weakness have been French medical practitioners. The capacity of the corps médical to obstruct public health initiatives it deems contrary—or simply irrelevant—to practitioners' or their patients' welfare has contributed to the paralysis of the French state in this domain. Individual medical care in France is state funded. Curative medicine (the clinique in French parlance) symbolized by the personal relation between doctor and patient is culturally privileged. The status of public health is correspondingly low. Along with cultural weakness come institutional and political weakness and, except in extraordinary circumstances, policy impasse and inaction.

Finally, it must be emphasized that French citizens' relation to the state is complex and contradictory. Reliance on the state as the sole legitimate public health actor is complemented by intense suspicion of the state and of its motives.[10] How these suspicions are formulated—in the language of market individualism (state intrusion into the medical marketplace) or antifascism (state intrusion into personal lives) depends on time, place, and occasion. They are, nevertheless—along with the other factors I have mentioned—a constant thorn in the side of public health.[11]

Confronted by extraordinary circumstances, that is, crises with the real or imagined potential for political damage to the state, the French government has been quite capable of rapid action.[12] In the late nineteenth century, infant mortality was identified as such a crisis. Legislation to address it—the loi Roussel—was passed by the French parliament unanimously and without debate. One hundred years later—within a month of the Henrion report describing French drug-war policy as the cause of health and social catastrophe among injection drug users—clean-needle distribution and methadone were legalized by ministerial decree, due in large part to fears of a second blood scandal.[13] In other words, Infant mortality and (with some delay) HIV/AIDS in injection drug users became targets of state action only when they were identified as potential political crises. Their status as health crises was secondary.

The Strengths of a Weak State: The United States   The American "weak" state—insofar as it is embodied by the federal government in Washington, D.C.—has been no more inclined to take bold action in behalf of public health than the muscle-bound strongman in Paris. Early twentieth-century reformers argued for a federal department that would "unite all health related agencies of the national government in the public health field" (Waserman 1975, 355). Despite seemingly propitious timing—Progressive-era elites were unusually supportive of government intervention on behalf of health and welfare—and the adherence of nationally recognized luminaries, a bill to accomplish that failed, defeated in large part by congressional aversion to centralized power.[14] For much of the Progressive era—the period covered by my narratives of infant mortality and tuberculosis—there was no public health beyond the level of individual cities and states. The singular exception to this pattern of inaction at the federal level was the creation in 1912 of the Children's Bureau. This exception is remarkable not only because it appears to conflict with this country's conventional characterization as a weak state but also because there were no strong state counterparts: the Children's Bureau was as unique cross-nationally as it was on the American scene.

With that exception, the United States in the Progressive era possessed neither the bureaucratic and administrative structures nor the political will to carry out interventionist public health policies at the national level. City governments, by contrast, were often remarkably aggressive, even draconian, in their approach to public health. By the end of the twentieth century the size and complexity of the federal government—including components concerned with health and medical care—had grown enormously. However, the political will to apply that vastly expanded federal bureaucracy in behalf of public health has increased very little, as reflected in my narratives of smoking and of HIV/AIDS in injection drug users. Federal regulation of the tobacco industry has run afoul of Congress and the Supreme Court due to extremely close financial, social, and political ties between tobacco manufacturers and politicians at the federal level and also to philosophical and constitutional limits on central government intervention in the free market. America stands out among the four countries not in the depth of industry-political ties, which are hardly unique to it, but in the extreme reluctance of its political leaders to intervene in economic life for the collective good. On the other hand, consistent with Frank Dobbins's observation that states act on their capacities when their policy prescriptions call for it, the government has applied its full power to block initiatives at the federal level for the prevention of HIV/AIDS in injection drug users.

The critical difference between the France and the United States is less in administrative capacity than in the fact that this country has many more strings to its bow, strings that do not depend on the action or inaction of the central state—more actors eager to swing their weight in public health arenas and more arenas where that weight can make a difference. The strength of the American weak state lies in its citizens' capacity for collective action.

Openings for energetic entrepreneurs of public health were particularly abundant in the early twentieth century. There was little in the way of a health bureaucracy at the federal level, leaving space for other actors. Organized medicine—the major competitor to public health in the United States as in France—had not nearly the political clout it later acquired. As I observed in the U.S. infant mortality narrative, this set of circumstances created political opportunities both for ambitious medical professionals at a local level (Hermann Biggs was a prime example, but there were others as well) and for white middle-class women who were already well organized through women's clubs and associations. Complementing this condition of institutional fluidity was the transient emergence of a political culture, Progressivism, that extolled the benefits of intervention by a benevolent state (and of equally transient executive support for intervention, as I will explain). In this structural and cultural context, questions of public health—infant mortality and tuberculosis among them—became vehicles for professional and political mobilization and advancement and also battlegrounds on which elite physicians and activist women fought (sometimes separately, sometimes together) for credibility, legitimacy, and power in the arena of public health. These actors proposed and successfully implemented a range of what were for the time highly innovative public health policies: the federal Children's Bureau and, at the local level, pasteurization and tuberculosis notification.

Comparing AIDS policy activism in the United States with that in Canada and Britain, David Rayside observed that "the American system creates more openings for social movements to intervene in the policy process than any other liberal democratic political system, and more incentives for even the most skeptical of activists to participate in the mainstream" (1998, 13). Dramatic changes in U.S. tobacco-control policy have come over the past fifty years due in large part to a pattern of grassroots collective action parallel to the one that in the early twentieth century contributed to the creation of the Children's Bureau. Blocked at the federal level, tobacco-control advocates were able to take advantage of the many alternative venues offered by the fragmented American state. Comparable opportunities are much less available to advocates for injection drug users, and policy change in this arena has been correspondingly less.

The strong state–weak state construct is useful in directing attention to state-based variation in the nature of political opportunities and in the forms political activism is likely to take: for example, limited access to the state affects both the pattern and frequency of grassroots activism. It is less useful, however, in predicting the circumstances under which governments—strong or weak—are more or less likely to exhibit the combination of political will and executive-administrative capacity necessary for autonomous public health action. Why did the weak U.S. government invent the Children's Bureau? Why did the British government respond promptly and effectively to the problem of HIV/AIDS in injection drug users and the French government delay? What enabled the Canadian government to pass four major pieces of antitobacco legislation between 1988 and 1997, when in the United States strong federal legislation was repeatedly blocked?

Explaining the Active State

Regardless of whether the impetus for action originated inside or outside the government, among medical experts or among lay enthusiasts, the common ingredients in cases of active state intervention in public health have been, first, the presence of politically savvy public health entrepreneurs positioned to seize opportunities when they arose and, second, the strong support of highly placed political allies. These may seem obvious points, but they are nonetheless critical: fleeting opportunities must be seized, and support from political elites is the mechanism that enables pressure for public health action to be translated into action by the state.[15] By the same token, opposition from individuals or groups in key positions or with access to allies in key positions is equally effective at preventing action, however desirable that action may seem to some, or even to a majority, of the population. The first step in explaining the active state is "to specify those policy areas in which government seems to be capable of asserting its prerogatives vis-à-vis interest groups and those policy areas in which it is dominated by them" (Vogel 1986, 268). Second, we need to identify the configurations of actors, interests, and contexts (historical, social, and political) associated with these outcomes.

State activism in public health—across all of my sixteen cases—was more the exception than the rule. Among the departmental or ministerial portfolios that constitute each of these four governments' executive branches, public health had and still has relatively low status and little power. In competition with other, more powerful interests (for example, political, economic, financial, criminal justice) and often without a vigorous constituency of their own (public health action is frequently of most benefit—or perceived as being of most benefit—to citizens who themselves have few resources and little power), advocates for public health confront significant obstacles to making their case. Thus it is important to closely examine the circumstances in which such obstacles were overcome.

The Children's Bureau was a major public health achievement of the early twentieth-century American state, the more remarkable because it was created in a period of powerful congressional aversion to expansion of executive authority (as witness the defeated proposal for a federal department of health). Recent scholarship, cited in my narrative, has focused on the importance of women's organizations both in bringing the bureau into being and supporting it once established. Less attention has been paid to the specific roles in this achievement played, first, by a close-knit network of prominent women based in Chicago and New York settlement houses and, second, by the 1904 reelection of Theodore Roosevelt to a second term, with a solid Republican Congress. The settlement house women were well connected not only with leaders of the major women's organizations but also with male civic leaders through whom they obtained access to the president and members of Congress. They exploited these connections to mobilize women in behalf of the Children's Bureau, to garner the political support essential for the bureau legislation to pass Congress and, once the bureau was established, to ensure that one of their own, Julia Lathrop, would be named as its chief. Lathrop herself was "above all, a tough, gifted politician" (Scott 2004, xix). "She knew the people whose hands were on the levers of power" (xvi), and during her tenure used this knowledge to ensure the bureau's continued political and grassroots support.

The child-welfare reform program advocated by proponents of the Children's Bureau fit directly into Roosevelt's second-term agenda.

> Roosevelt believed that the national government should be interested in a
> wide variety of social and economic problems that it had previously avoided,

and he created the machinery for such interest by convincing Congress to establish new executive agencies, by appointing special investigative commissions, and by calling for national conferences to debate and pass resolutions on specific issues. (Muncy 1991, 39)

Roosevelt met with settlement house representatives, sponsored a White House Conference on the Care of Dependent Children, and personally orchestrated pressure on members of Congress to create a federal children's bureau (42–43). "The strategic environment for state building was more favorable during the Roosevelt administration than at any other time [between 1877 and 1920]. From a position of party strength and electoral stability, Roosevelt pushed executive prerogatives to their limits" (Skowronek 1982, 171–72). Whereas grassroots mobilization is among the more stable characteristics of the American state, opportunities for the assertion of executive power are relatively rare. The Children's Bureau came about through an ephemeral conjunction of grassroots mobilization with political opportunity.

Théophile Roussel, author of the 1874 loi Roussel, which was described in chapter 3 as a marker of the entry of the French state as a major player in the protection of infant lives, was extremely well positioned as a policy entrepreneur operating in the French political context. As a member of the French Academy of Medicine and of Parliament, he belonged simultaneously to the medical and to the political elite. His successful bill to regulate the French wet-nursing industry was developed by the Academy of Medicine with the encouragement and support of the government in power. The French (and British) parliamentary systems concentrate power at the center, enabling the state to speak with one voice should it wish to do so. For reasons I have alluded to, France felt itself threatened as a state by high rates of infant mortality. Under these conditions, it chose to act with relative expedition.

There were two striking instances of autonomous state action in the late twentieth century, Britain's response to AIDS-drugs and Canada's response to smoking. These instances offer further evidence for the critical role played by relations between policy entrepreneurs and political elites.[16] In both cases, government civil servants were key players and their ability to act as stars at the center of much larger supporting casts was due to the strong support of their political masters. In the British case, the civil servant Dorothy Black took on the roles of policy entrepreneur, orchestrator, and principal conductor, and most of the action took place—in characteristic British fashion—behind closed doors. In the Canadian case, the civil servant Neil Collishaw orchestrated the relation between policy entrepreneurs outside the government and political leaders inside it to ensure that actions by each set of players were coordinated to maximum effect. In both the British and the Canadian case, once the political leaders were convinced, state action followed quickly, even (in Britain) where the policy in question was highly controversial.

In the narrative, I attributed British political leaders' response to AIDS-drugs to elements particular to the problem itself and to the history of British narcotic drugs policies. Canadian federal policy makers' embrace of tobacco control resulted, I believe, from elements of the Canadian polity both broader in their potential application and, at the same time, unique to Canada. Let me explain.

The Canadian health care system is bound together by norms or principles embodied in the Canada Health Act. Among these principles are that "the state must ensure universal coverage and equitable access" and that "the federal government belongs in the health policy arena as a guardian of the 'right' to health care" (Maioni 2002, 91). The provinces are responsible for health care. However, the central state is expected to instill a sense of unity—"a common Canadian citizenship"—and to ensure equity across the provinces and territories (92). Its leverage to accomplish these goals is, nevertheless, quite limited.[17] I alluded in the narratives both to the dominant role in health of Canada's provinces and to the sometimes tense relation between federal and provincial officials. Struggling for a role within this system, the federal government took on health promotion.[18] The much-cited Lalonde report, published in 1974 and authored by the minister of National Health and Welfare, was to all intents and purposes a mandate for federal government participation in the health arena. Health promotion was consistent with the goals of unity and equity; it was distinguishable from medical care; it was politically visible and relatively cheap, and it offered opportunities for action in arenas outside of provincial jurisdiction. Tobacco control fit these requirements perfectly. AIDS-drugs was a considerably more difficult case.

The Dilatory State

Answers to the question of why national governments fail to act in the face of widely acknowledged threats to the public's health tell at least as much about state structure and political culture as analysis of the circumstances in which they do act. I have described the systemic obstacles to public health action in France and the United States but paid considerably less attention to barriers that also exist in Canada and Great Britain. I begin by elaborating more fully a point that I made about early twentieth-century public health in the United States that applies to Canada and, with reservations, to Britain as well. In all three English-speaking countries, public health was at that time—albeit for somewhat different reasons—almost entirely a matter for municipal governments and voluntary associations.

Canada's Supreme Court in 1894 interpreted the British North America Act as giving most of the responsibility for citizens' health to the provinces

(Cassel 1994). Amid ongoing controversy about how this responsibility should be allocated, first between government and private citizens and second among the various levels of government, the provinces did very little and the federal government limited itself to questions of immigration and quarantine. Until a national health department was created immediately after World War I and the federal government began, however tentatively, to intervene in public health, how and whether Canada dealt with infant mortality and tuberculosis depended entirely on the vagaries of politics and political culture at the municipal level. These vagaries accounted for Toronto's relative success in both areas and for Montreal's abject failure— a failure due to overlapping religious, linguistic, and political divisions that rendered impossible the relation between policy entrepreneurs and political leaders that is essential to progress in public health.

Britain's circumstances were different, confirming that state inaction is more than just a matter of weak administrative capacity. By the late nineteenth century, Britain had a centrally supervised public health system that was internationally recognized for its efficiency and effectiveness. In the early twentieth century, this system remained in place but "its head [had been] severed" (Hamlin 1994, 151). Having lost political support, public health was moved from a position of relative independence within the national government to one of subordination to the Local Government Board that was in charge of local government administration (see chapter 2). "The political realities of the Local Government Board existence— its struggle against other departments for funds and staff, the discomfort of important constituencies with elements of its structure and mission— [ensured] that for the remainder of its existence [until it was abolished in 1918] it would never again aspire to medical activism" (151). With a few exceptions—tuberculosis notification was made mandatory just prior to World War I—questions of public health were left almost entirely to the ministrations of voluntary associations and local governments. Disinterest at the center was initially compensated for by partnerships between politically savvy local officials and enthusiastic medical officers of health. For much of the twentieth century (that is, after World War I), however, public health "remained an ill-unified amalgam of programmes and institutions, central and local, influenced by all manner of political, cultural, and professional concerns" (154). Central-government attention turned to curative medical care, as it did in Canada and in France as well, and Britain's public health institutions never regained the stature they had enjoyed in the late nineteenth century.

Returning to the present, why did the Canadian government delay in response to HIV in injection drug users yet act with considerable expedition to address smoking? And, in contrast, why did Britain delay in response to smoking but act expeditiously to prevent HIV in injection drug users? The answers are relatively straightforward. Canadian federalism created roadblocks in the way of centrally coordinated rapid action in response to HIV that were largely absent in response to smoking; Britain's preference for voluntary agreements between contending parties and corresponding aversion to legislative solutions created roadblocks to rapid action on the smoking front but were largely irrelevant to the problem of HIV/AIDS in injection drug users.

HIV/AIDS in injection drug users was caught in the Canadian jurisdictional thicket. Allocation of responsibility depended in theory on whether AIDS-drugs was defined as a health or a criminal justice problem and in practice on geographical location. Criminal justice is a federal responsibility, but injection drug users were in Canada's three large municipalities and their health was a matter for the provinces. Civil servants in Health Canada, however much they may have wished to intervene, and they did wish to intervene, could do so only stealthily and indirectly. Most of the 1990s was occupied in navigating and attempting to reconcile these questions of definition and responsibility. Britain as a unitary state did not confront these jurisdictional problems, and Canada largely avoided them in the case of smoking by treating the regulation of tobacco advertising as a criminal justice—and consequently a federal—question. It is ironic that Canadian tobacco-control advocates were adamant in their portrayal of smoking as a health issue whereas the government's ability to act speedily was highly dependent on its definition as a criminal justice issue.

The British approach to smoking policy—like the Canadian response to HIV/AIDS in injection drug users—was predictable from its actions in the past. State involvement in Britain's economy (tobacco control was defined by the government as an economic as much as a health issue) has been characterized historically "more by the growth of bargaining between the government and the two sides of industry [management and labor] than by the growth of unilateral state control [as in France]" (Hall 1986, 56). Noncoercive voluntary agreements between the government and economic actors, calling on the latter to regulate themselves, are normal operating procedure, and are unlikely to be associated with rapid action by the state. In negotiating tobacco control, the virtues of consensus took precedence over the virtues of speed. A second source of reluctance to take coercive action arose from the relation between smoking and social class: smoking prevalence was inversely related to class, and any legislative solution could be interpreted as favoring one class over another, something that British governments have been loath to do (Thane 1990; Crossman 1975).

Differences between the policy contexts of smoking and of HIV/AIDS in injection drug users are instructive. In the latter case there was no legitimate bargaining partner requiring protracted negotiation, no legislation was necessary to implement the state's programs, and injection drug users were a vulnerable population falling clearly within the state's social protection mandate.

Not only were the roadblocks in the way of tobacco control largely absent in the case of AIDS-drugs but the same approach to policy making that delayed vigorous tobacco-control policies also facilitated harm reduction policies in response to AIDS or drugs. Writing about British industrial policy in the nineteenth century, Frank Dobbin states that it "has been oriented to guarding citizens against harm as much as to promoting economic growth" (1994, 211). Guarding citizens against harm was construed to mean protecting individuals against industrial accidents and protecting industrial firms against destructive competition. Protections afforded to the tobacco industry through voluntary agreements, on the one hand, and to injection drug users through needle-exchange programs, on the other, are both consistent with this policy of harm minimization. Inflammatory rhetoric is decried, conflict among the contending parties is limited, and policy consensus is achieved by gentlemanly negotiation among insiders. Policy making behind closed doors may have favored the tobacco industry, delaying advertising bans and other antismoking policies, but it also favored pragmatism over ideology in response to HIV/AIDS in injection drug users, allowing effective harm-reduction policies to be adopted rather quickly.

Conclusion

The key to early and effective public health action by the state is that action be embraced by the holders of political power. Policy entrepreneurs eager to seize opportunities are thick on the ground compared with politicians eager to offer them encouragement and support. Public health policy responses by the state to disease threats were not absent, delayed, or ineffective because no one urged that these threats be addressed. Indeed, in every case, some configuration of policy entrepreneurs demanded state action. Effective responses were lacking because authorities in a position to take action did not do so. What accounts for the relatively rare instances when they did?

There is no single, simple answer to this question. In each case of early and assertive action by the state—the Roussel law, the Children's Bureau, needle-exchange programs in Britain, tobacco-control legislation in Canada—the circumstances were in large part unique, reflecting a convergence of history, politics, and opportunity unlikely to be repeated. Still, there were some commonalities. On the evidence of these cases, executive power is a sine qua non for early and assertive public health action by the state. As shown in my comparison of France and the United States, concentration of executive power is no guarantee of state action, but where the will to act is present, the power to act is greatly facilitated by a strong executive. In both of the two highly centralized parliamentary states, Britain and France, executive dominance of the political system made it possible to take potentially controversial public health actions—establish a national system for inspection of wet nurses, institute needle-exchange programs— with little fear of political repercussions. Recourse to executive power in Canada is complicated by the existence of parallel federal and provincial governments. There are, nevertheless, structural incentives for executive action by the central government to promote public health that are not present in any of the other three countries. Canada's tough tobacco-control legislation was enacted under the federal government's criminal law powers. The U.S. Children's Bureau was created during a rare and up to that point unprecedented interval of executive dominance.

Referring again to the strong state–weak state continuum displayed in table 5.1, the critical variation along this continuum is not in these states' relative aggressiveness in pursuit of public health policy but in how public health issues get on to the policy agenda and how they are managed once they arrive. In the relatively strong states of France and Britain, states that adhere to traditional hierarchies of power and access, issues got on the agenda through elite intervention and were managed by elite networks largely insulated from external political pressure by non-elite outsiders. In the weaker states of Canada and the United States, elites enjoyed less of an exclusive hold on the levers of power, and social movement organizations—the organs of civil society—played a much larger role as engines of policy innovation and policy change.

Finally, even dilatory states do, eventually, act. Who pushes them in different national contexts is the subject of the chapter that follows.

Chapter 8

Experts and Zealots

AT A SYMPOSIUM on the history of smoking and tobacco control, the medical historian Roy Porter commented on the difference between Britain and the United States in patterns of mobilization against smoking. "My suspicion [is that] relatively speaking . . . the medical profession has actually played a larger part in mobilizing anti-smoking opinion; and, relatively speaking, energetic zealots . . . have played a smaller part in Britain as compared with the United States" (1998, 226). He went on to suggest that these different patterns were of long standing, not limited to smoking but reflected in campaigns against earlier health threats as well.

> The role of populist campaigning in America, as compared and contrasted with the role of the authority of doctors in Britain is, I think, extremely interesting. It relates to things like medical charities and philanthropies, for example, to the campaigns against polio in the 1930s and 1940s where, on the whole, British activity was very much within the profession, within the hospitals, whereas in America it was very much a democratic and populist campaign. (227)

There are, indeed, systematic cross-national differences in patterns of public health advocacy along the lines Porter suggests: expert domination in Britain and France, and populist campaigning by energetic zealots in the United States and Canada. The distinction between experts and zealots is less clear, however, than Porter's comments imply. Experts took on the trappings of zealots—organizing protests and playing to the media—and zealots became experts, consulted by politicians and civil servants. The questions I address in this chapter are who advocates under what circumstances, by what means, and how these patterns might be explained.

Who Were the Actors?

Who became players in the various dramas of public health I have recounted was shaped on the one hand by relatively stable aspects of each country's political structure and culture and on the other by more transient circumstances that opened doors for one set of actors (and perhaps closed them for others).

Stable Structures

The first stable condition—state structures that open or foreclose opportunities for nonstate actors to enter policy debates—was discussed in the last chapter. A second condition—foreshadowed by Porter's observations—is the cultural authority of experts. In Britain and France, the "authority of doctors" created a culturally embedded and, therefore, largely unexamined presumption of expert credibility in matters of public health and contributed—along with these countries' closed political structures—to the muffling (and often denigration) of other voices. Credentialed expertise (along with the elite status that accompanied expertise) was a highly valuable political resource, combining in a single package recognized knowledge, exclusive authority to pronounce on danger and risk, and privileged access to the state. Neither in the United States nor in late twentieth-century Canada did experts enjoy these advantages. Last, opportunities for individuals and groups to become public health actors were affected by their location in hierarchies of prestige and power specific to each country.

The Cultural Authority of Experts   The hegemony of physicians over matters of public health in Britain and France was amply illustrated in the narratives. Even in the late twentieth century, celebrated for the emergence in Europe of new social movements focused on lifestyle change (see, for example, Pichardo 1997), tobacco-control movements in both countries were initiated and led by physicians. Lay initiatives—though they existed and had considerable impact at least in France—were belittled. Each of the four public health issues offers examples of cross-national difference in the role of experts, but perhaps most striking is the contrast between Britain's response to AIDS-drugs and that of the United States.

In all four countries, AIDS-drugs was placed on the public agenda in the mid- to late 1980s by experts in medicine and public health.[1] From the outset and across all sites, expert ownership was contested by advocates for the war on drugs. The experts' ability to sustain their ownership claims depended in large part on the culturally recognized authority of expert knowledge. In Britain, this authority is well established. Credible scientific knowledge is monopolized and deployed by closely linked experts based within and outside the government—medical civil servants, the British Medical Association, the Royal Colleges, and government-appointed advisory bodies. Of particular importance in the case of AIDS-drugs, expert consultation is closed to the media and the public. Controversial decisions arrived at behind closed doors run substantially less risk of being derailed by unaccredited outsiders than those made in full view of television and the press.

Experts in the United States enjoy no comparable authority. Sheila Jasanoff observes that in contrast with their counterparts in Europe, "powerful social actors [in the United States are reluctant] to accept 'expert' knowledge as the basis for their own political acknowledgement of risk" (1990, 72). Political authorities who are unwilling to accept experts' authority to define risk are unlikely to adopt their recommendations to mitigate risk. Routine reluctance was exacerbated in the case of AIDS-drugs by the long history of mutual mistrust between physicians and drug-enforcement bureaucrats, in contrast to the collaborative relation existing in Britain (Musto 1973). However unassailable their science, U.S. experts have been unable to persuade the federal government that harm reduction measures, such as needle-exchange and methadone maintenance, are a legitimate response to the AIDS-drugs problem.[2]

Even in Britain and France, the power of medical experts—however great their cultural authority—had its limits. When public health issues were politically or economically contentious, expert power was diluted. Tobacco control was a more politically contentious issue in Britain than harm reduction measures for injection drug users. The same closed structure of expert consultation that worked to the advantage of British expert advocates for needle-exchange worked against expert advocates for vigorous tobacco control measures. This structure is, of course, controlled by the politicians who appoint the committees. In the case of tobacco, it was the industry and more conservative physicians who were invited in and the militant doctors of the Royal College of Physicians and the British Medical Association who were kept out.

Not all experts are equally able to be heard or to have their voices counted. Since early in the twentieth century, and earlier in France, public health has taken a back seat to curative medicine. The weakness of public health in France dates from the rise of the medical syndicats in the late nineteenth century, and public health continues to be a neglected step-child in the government's administrative structure (see chapters 2, 5, and 6). By contrast, the absence of well-organized medical opposition was among the factors that made it possible for Herman Biggs to institute tuberculosis notification, segregation, and quarantine in New York City. Similar measures were impossible in France.

Hierarchies and Voices   Hierarchies of gender, race, language, ethnicity, and class have been critical in determining who would act and whose voices would be heard. In reality, of course, these hierarchies are highly interrelated. Their salience varies, however, across issues and countries. Gender hierarchies limited French and—to a somewhat lesser extent— British women's participation in early twentieth-century campaigns against infant mortality, for example. Infant and maternal health in Britain and France were questions of high politics tied to the fate of states and empires. These questions were of relatively little interest at the time to U.S. politicians or—more important in the long run—to organized medicine. Political space was open to American women, and American women were positioned to occupy that space. In the longer term, however, the structures these women created were submerged, and their intent subverted, within institutions dominated by men. America's racial hierarchy simultaneously limited collective action by blacks and prevented black voices from being heard, first in response to infant mortality and tuberculosis in the early twentieth century and more recently in response to AIDS, all conditions that disproportionately affected African Americans. Recognition of and response to public health problems in Canada has been structured by divisions of language overlaid by political divisions. The long delay before Quebec antitobacco activists found their voices was due in part to the suspicion and hostility of Québecois toward a movement initiated and led by English Canadians.

Class-based resources of education, wealth, power, political connections, and even time all influenced whether one or another set of actors would venture onto the stage. In Britain and France, elite status within the profession was virtually a requirement for recognition as a legitimate authority on public health, and physician-advocates selected themselves or were recruited (as active participants or, not infrequently, as window dressing) on that basis. In the United States, advocacy for the Children's Bureau—and for tobacco control before it became a professional subspecialty—was made possible by the existence of well-educated individuals, largely women, with secure social positions, political connections, and time and energy they could devote to the cause. At the other extreme, injection drug users are poorly positioned to act on their own behalf not only because as criminals they have no legitimate voice but also because they lack all or most of those resources.

Transient Circumstances

Among the many circumstances that create new opportunities for action and, hence, space for new actors (or old actors waiting in the wings) to speak out are shifts in local or national political structures. The prominence in late nineteenth- and early twentieth-century Britain of local medical officers of health as advocates on infant mortality and tuberculosis was associated with the gradual withdrawal of the central government's Local Government Board from the position of strong interest and involvement in public health issues it had occupied for many years under the leadership of Sir John Simon. In these circumstances, it was left to local MOHs to take up the cudgels and they responded as the narratives have described.

More broadly, the importance of local public health officials as public health actors in the early twentieth century—not only in Britain but also in major cities of North America, always with the striking exception of Montreal—was made possible by three unique circumstances: the emergence of a new and powerful causal theory of disease with which these officials were identified, political developments that made space for local public health officials to act, and the absence of organized medicine as a countervailing power. Although the first and second conditions arguably existed in France as well, the third surely did not, and neither a powerful public health establishment (as in Britain) nor individually powerful local public health officials (as in the United States and Canada) emerged in early twentieth-century France.

Actors were often moved, or pushed, into action by concerns—or opportunities—that the public health problem itself evoked. Local health officers in Vancouver, Toronto, and Montreal and local medical practitioners in Paris took action to address AIDS-drugs because the problem erupted in their own backyards, the streets and alleys of big cities. Women advocated on behalf of mothers and children out of their personal experiences as women and mothers. The founder of the (U.S.) National Tuberculosis Association himself suffered from tuberculosis. People who had a close relative die of lung cancer or who themselves were irritated by tobacco smoke formed nonsmokers' rights groups. Previously obscure physicians and epidemiologists were catapulted into prominence by the AIDS epidemic. An international conference on AIDS that brought together drug policy experts previously unknown to one another was instrumental in galvanizing AIDS-drugs activism in France.

An important distinction must be made between action on behalf of and by affected populations. Historically, most health-related mobilization fell into the latter category but in Britain and France mobilization on behalf of still dominates. However, among the more striking shifts that have occurred over the decades since the 1960s has been the move toward organization by affected groups.

The nonsmokers' rights movement was among the earliest of such groups in the United States, modeling itself on the civil rights movement. Over time, as other groups—the disabled, breast cancer survivors, persons with AIDS—adopted this model, mobilization by affected groups was transformed from an innovation into an expectation. This expectation elevates the cynical observation that only squeaky wheels get the grease into an axiom of public health policy. Little attention has been paid to the possibility that this expectation further disadvantages already disenfranchised groups—for example, injection drug users—who confront almost insuperable obstacles to organizing and advocating on their own behalf. The most effective such organization to my knowledge, the Vancouver Association of Drug Users, was the beneficiary of critical financial, logistical, and political support from local and provincial health authorities. I found no evidence of comparable organization elsewhere in Canada or in the other three countries.

When and Where? Threats and Opportunities

Public health action was triggered by perceived danger in a context of social and political opportunities that made action appear both possible and necessary. Dangers and opportunities came in various guises.

Threats

Nineteenth-century elites saw public health as an antidote to working-class rebellion, anarchy, and socialism. Later on, nationalism—instigated by defeats in war in France and Britain or by language and cultural competition in Quebec—raised fears about the numbers and (in Britain) quality of the population and thus fueled mobilization against infant deaths and (in Britain) tuberculosis. American and Anglo-Canadian elites, secure against external enemies but besieged by massive waves of immigration and urbanization, felt threatened from within. Immigrants and, in the United States, newly urbanized blacks and the diseases these populations were thought to bring with them were interpreted as dangerous to the established white population, and public health action was inspired less by the goal of preserving the nation as a whole, as in Britain and France, than of protecting one part of the nation against another.

Scientific discovery—the germ theory of disease, the relation between smoking and lung cancer—and the reinterpretation of old facts that soon followed these discoveries led at one and the same time to the recognition of new public health problems and to the opening of new opportunities for action. The enthusiastic response of the health commissioner of Providence, Rhode Island, Charles Chapin, to the germ theory made this point transparent: "Instead of an indiscriminate attack on dirt, we must learn the nature and mode of transmission of each infection, and must discover its most vulnerable point of attack" (1887, cited in Rothman 1994, 182). In the four countries studied, investigation to discover this most vulnerable point of attack led straight to "ignorant mothers." More generally, and more important in its long-term consequences, medicine's embrace of the germ theory led away from the search for environmental causes of disease—bad air, bad water, bad sewers—and toward a narrower focus on bad behavior: the insalubrious actions of individuals.

Reactions to opportunities created by the newly revealed smoking and lung cancer facts were both more variable and more uneven cross-nationally, in part because access to scientific facts was much more widely diffused, no longer controlled or controllable by physician and public health wizards with unique access to the occult.

Among the four public health problems, AIDS was the only example in which action was precipitated by a sudden and unanticipated disease threat. There was, nevertheless, enormous variation across these four countries in response to HIV/AIDS in injection drug users (see chapter 4). Public health and drug treatment specialists in Britain and, to a lesser extent and with more delay, in Canada and France, saw the AIDS-drugs nexus as an opportunity to unlock entrenched practices inimical to the health of drug users, whereas the official U.S. response was to interpret as a threat what had been seen in the other countries as an opportunity.

Opportunities

I have said that action happened in response to perceived danger and in the presence of perceived opportunities. Among those opportunities were the more or less stable openings created by divided government, as in Canada and the United States. These opportunities were exploited to advantage in both countries by women's movements of the early twentieth century (recall western Canadian women's actions against infant mortality in addition to the better-known U.S. movement), by proponents of needle-exchange and other harm reduction measures to counter the threat of AIDS and drugs, and (in the United States) by the nonsmokers' rights movement.

Opportunities arose from more fleeting circumstances and events as well, events as likely to arise under one political regime as another. Critical to state action in the cases I examined was the presence in government of key ministers or civil servants friendly to the cause. Changes in government and the comings and goings of heads of state, ministers, or civil servants created new possibilities for action or, occasionally, foreclosed those possibilities. Public health action in early twentieth-century New York City and Toronto was greatly facilitated by the election of sympathetic mayors. Changes of government in Canada that brought an anti-smoking federal health minister into office in 1984 and an equally militant provincial health minister into office in Quebec in 1994 were critical to the fortunes of antitobacco advocates. In France, the advent of a socialist government concerned about the health of its working-class constituents played a role in reviving antitobacco legislation in 1991. In Vancouver (Canada), a succession of highly supportive mayors has been instrumental to the success of VANDU.

Politicians are more often moved by political threats than by the threat of disease. If, in 1921, women's suffrage had not loomed on the horizon creating fears of a backlash from women voters, it is unlikely that Congress would have passed the Sheppard-Towner Act creating a nationwide system of maternal and infant health clinics. The highly public scandal created by France's delay in addressing the problem of HIV-contaminated blood products contributed to its quick response to AIDS and drugs once the government was forced to acknowledge a corresponding potential for political disaster (see chapter 7, note 13). The Canadian government's 1988 Tobacco Products Control Act was provoked in large part by a purely fortuitous event: the luck of the draw that led to parliamentary consideration of a private member's bill to regulate smoking in federal workplaces. Rather than be upstaged—the private bill became a lightning rod for tobacco-control activists—the government introduced its own bill.

Action Strategies

Strategies were deployed—targets selected and modes of influence (the press conference, the media event, the meeting of insiders closed to the public) designed—not because the actors were experts or zealots but because the chosen strategies made sense in the given political context. They were culturally legitimate and familiar to the actors themselves, and they were likely to resonate with the actors' intended audience. What worked in one political regime was less effective, did not work at all, or was simply unavailable in another. For example, both the Comité nationale contre le tabagisme as an organizational form (lay militants) and its tactics (litigation against the tobacco industry) were regarded as questionable by French observers, but would be familiar and legitimate in the United States. At the same time, the strategy employed by French AIDS-drugs activists— to hold an états généraux toxicomanie-sida (estates general on AIDS-drugs) using organizational forms and rhetorical constructs drawn from the French revolution—would be meaningless in the United States (and—with the possible exception of Quebec—in Britain and Canada as well).

Political scientists distinguish between insider strategies and outsider strategies—that is, between closed encounters with members of the legislature, civil servants, and ministers, and appeals to the public through mass media, staged large informational conferences, and protest demonstrations (Walker 1991, 192). My own research suggests, first, that the line between insider and outsider strategies is highly permeable, as evidenced by the numerous occasions when outsider strategies were orchestrated from the inside. For example,

> [Britain] I kept very close to the [junior] minister [in charge of smoking and health] . . . because he was such a good guy. And he knew how to use an agency like us to lobby. He'd sometimes tell me . . . publicize that you're criticizing me for this because I want to be seen under pressure to do such and such, or can you get the medical charities to do such and such? So, we'd have private meetings where we'd agree on strategy like that.

[Canada] He [civil servant] couldn't be a lobbyist but he could produce things that would be valuable . . . research that you need to move the agenda ahead. We could work very well as a team. [Further,] we could short circuit the system [that is, bypass the bureaucratic hierarchy, go directly to the minister]. A good bureaucrat would say, "Look, you know, you gotta get something pretty quick done by Tuesday." And you say, "does it have anything to do with a cabinet meeting on Wednesday?" and he says, "'yeah."

These illustrations, drawn from the smoking narratives, are from contemporary tobacco-control activists, but compare Julia Lathrop's actions as director of the U.S. Children's Bureau in the early twentieth century. Writing to a "highly placed woman in the General Federation [of Women's Clubs]," she said:

"You will understand it is very difficult for a government bureau to push legislation which would seem to increase its power and responsibility." She needed for women's organizations to lead the movement, Lathrop explained, so that the Bureau staff itself could hang back and allow the nation's women to demand an increase in the Bureau's power. (Muncy 1991, 104)

Second, the advocacy groups I studied were by no means limited to one set of tactics; they had many strings to their bows, moving back and forth between insider and outsider strategies as occasion and opportunity dictated.[3] Canadian tobacco-control activists sat down with the "good bureaucrat" one day and by the next (or at least "by Tuesday") they had placed an incendiary ad in the Toronto *Globe and Mail* attacking the prime minister. Third, strategies shifted over time. As radical demands became normative and were incorporated in institutions, insider strategies became increasingly accessible and even predominant. Among the principal— if fleeting—results of the Children's Bureau was to facilitate insider relations between women's organizations and the state.

Finally, each of these strategies has structural and symbolic implications that go beyond their tactical value. Insider strategies in particular were welcomed by some advocates and rejected by others who disbelieved in the efficacy of these strategies and were fearful of undermining their own position as uncompromising outsiders. For example,

[France] [The Health Minister] asked us to lobby the government [for tobacco control measures], that is his own administration. That's quite unusual, and we were quite uneasy with that. And, after some months, we realized that it doesn't work because you have to be silent, we were underground, official but underground, and that's not the right way.

[United States] When tobacco policy is left to the inside game played in back rooms, the outcome will favor the existing power structure. The tobacco industry is a tough, experienced inside player who has benefited from the existing power structure. In contrast, the public health groups' power is amplified in public arenas, where tobacco industry's power is sharply curtailed. (Glantz and Balbach 2000, 5)

Differences of opinion not only about tactics (the wisdom of sitting down with the devil) but also about targets (actions at the local level to advance nonsmokers' rights versus actions at the national level to regulate the tobacco industry) have led to a recent split in the American tobacco-control movement between locally oriented nonsmokers' rights groups and the major health voluntaries. The latter have been prepared to play the inside game but the former have not (Pertschuk 2001; Glantz and Balbach 2000). A parallel split exists in Canada between advocates, largely outside the government, of industry denormalization and government insiders who are prepared to be more conciliatory (Civil servant with Health Canada, personal communication).

Quantitative data would be necessary to show whether the insider tactics I have described—close and collaborative relations between advocacy group representatives and government officials—are more likely to be found in parliamentary states. This is a logical hypothesis, particularly when controversial issues are at stake, and public health issues are frequently controversial. Writing about the United States, Jack Walker observes that political mobilization led by government agencies may work in areas of low controversy but "cannot be used whenever the level of controversy rises, because the policy professionals and bureaucrats who take the lead in this process cannot count on support from the political leadership to protect their agencies against hostile critics." On the other hand, "if a single majority party . . . were firmly in control of the entire governmental system [as in parliamentary states] . . . bureaucratic leaders might enter more willingly into potentially explosive policy areas" (1991, 195). Evidence from the smoking and AIDS-drugs narratives indicates that bureaucratic leaders in parliamentary states do indeed enter more willingly into contentious policy arenas. Whether they lead (or incite) political mobilization by nonstate actors is a separate question. To engage with activist groups, government officials must recognize the existence of these groups and their legitimacy as partners in policy formation. Among the parliamentary states, recognition was least likely in Britain. The British government acted on its own, "largely untouched by arguments it [was] not disposed to hear" (Street and Weale 1992, 188). It was highly selective in France, and positively enthusiastic only in Canada. In the United States, the tactical terrain at the national level was complicated, not only by the controversial nature of tobacco and drugs, but also by the power of organized opposition to any change in the status quo. Cozy relations between insiders and outsiders—insofar as they have happened—have been limited to the state and local levels (see, for example, Wolfson 2001).

Conclusion

Public health advocacy in the countries I studied was shaped by relatively stable aspects of political structure and culture and by more dynamic processes that opened (or closed) political opportunities for particular actors at particular times and places (Meyer and Staggenborg 1996, 1633). In the former category are, first, differences in the political opportunities for nonstate actors, second, differences in the cultural authority of medical and scientific experts, and third, hierarchies of gender, race, and class. These differences are the product of each country's history and political structure and have—among three of the four countries—been relatively stable since early in the twentieth century. (The obvious exception is Canada.) These dimensions were not independent of each other. Where political opportunities for nonstate actors were low, as in France and Britain, advocacy was dominated by experts. Where these opportunities were high, experts' authority was weak and the voices of zealots were more likely to be heard.

The perhaps too pat explanation for this association is that when the political structure allows authorities to listen only to those voices they choose and to safely ignore the rest, the voices they are most likely to choose—particularly when confronted with disease threats—are voices with culturally certifiable claims to credible and relevant knowledge, that is, the voices of experts. A somewhat more elegant statement of the same point has been made by anthropologists of risk. Distinguishing between hierarchical cultures, exemplified by Britain and France, and individualistic cultures, exemplified by the United States, Mary Douglas observes that "each type of culture is based on a distinctive attitude toward knowledge" (1992, 32). In hierarchical systems, the political consensus that upholds the regime itself both guarantees the authority of accredited experts and the knowledge these experts purvey and excludes competing knowledge. In individualistic systems, experts compete in the open marketplace not only among themselves but with lay knowledge brokers, and expert knowledge must be defended at every turn. Sheila Jasanoff makes much the same point with specific reference to the credibility of statements about risk: "Differences in the societal response to risk between the United States and other nations result in part from the relatively low level of scientific pluralism in countries with a more homogenous or centralized culture of knowledge" (1990, 76).

Dynamism in public health advocacy arises from a complex set of highly nonlinear relations between, on the one hand, the opportunities and threats represented by disease and death and, on the other, the interpreters of these opportunities and threats: the actors on the ground. I use the word *opportunities* in this context advisedly: the distinction between disease as threat and disease as opportunity was fuzzy at best.

Conditions—infant mortality, tuberculosis, smoking, HIV infection—did not proclaim themselves as threats. They were so labeled by human actors intent on galvanizing public attention and political action. This casting of old facts in new lights did not require the discovery of new science or a new plague. It did require the presence of actors or groups of actors motivated and positioned to seize the opportunities these conditions presented.

Chapter 9

Political Cultures and Constructions of Risk

P UBLIC RECOGNITION of dangers to health and judgments concerning if, when and how to respond are the outcome of social processes, as I observed in chapter 1. Among the major sources of variation in recognition and response were the political cultures of nation-states. States' political practices and the ideologies associated with those practices, Frank Dobbin argues, "were socially constructed as constitutive of political order. . . . And in each state, state structure designated particular evils that threatened order" (1994, 22). Dobbin was writing about railway policy in the nineteenth century, but his point applies with equal force to public health policy, then and now.

States, Ideologies, and Geographies of Risk

Each of the four countries—France, the United States, Britain, and Canada—was attuned to different threats to political and social order and interpreted dangers to health in the light of those threats. These interpretations were critical to decisions about whether and how the dangers were met.

France

French policy makers—not surprisingly—have been less sensitive to dangers to individuals as individuals and highly sensitive to dangers to the state (la patrie en danger). These latter dangers—as they were reflected in how public health and political actors constructed the disease threats at issue in this book—took one of two forms. There were dangers to the integrity of the state itself, most clearly exemplified by the late nineteenth-century construction of high rates of infant mortality and low birth rates as threats to national survival. There were also dangers to the bonds of solidarité that linked French citizens to one another and to the state. France's legislative response to infant mortality, a response remarkable for its intrusive surveillance of women and families, was driven by a sense of crisis created by appeals to the endangered state. In the same vein, among the arguments for tobacco control and for state action to prevent HIV/AIDS in injection drug users were appeals to French pride, characterizing France as a public health laggard either in relation to neighboring states or to its own history as the country of Pasteur and calling on the state to assume its responsibilities to the French people—the collectivité.

Campaigners against tuberculosis also invoked the endangered state, but with limited success. Not only were authorities not persuaded that tuberculosis was a danger to the state comparable with infant mortality, but also measures to restrict the spread of contagious disease—notification, segregation, quarantine—were perceived by influential physician-politicians as more dangerous to the collectivité than the disease.[1] More recently, and in much the same vein, segregation of smokers from nonsmokers was conflated with racism and totalitarianism. In the French political lexicon, exclusion—the construction of barriers between one French citizen and another—is socially and politically illegitimate.[2] Exclusion is the opposite of solidarité, and promotion of solidarité was a central principle by which policies were judged. Insofar as public health protection was perceived to undermine that principle, it swam against powerful ideological currents and was extremely difficult to implement or enforce.[3]

These ideological currents go far to explain not only French reluctance to deal with tuberculosis as a contagious disease but also important aspects of the policy response to smoking and AIDS-drugs. Cigarette smoking, like enjoying a glass of wine with friends, was construed as a socially affirmative act, an expression of social solidarity. Over the past few decades, the use of narcotics came to be portrayed as the opposite, a withdrawal from social ties amounting to a rejection of the responsibilities of citizenship. Thus narcotics were dangerous and cigarettes were not. A principal strategy of French advocates of harm reduction measures (needle exchange and prescription of such oral narcotics as methadone) has been to argue that drug users are, after all, responsible citizens deserving *inclusion* in the borders of citizenship and consequently of protection from the dangers of HIV. Cigarettes, by contrast, have been redefined (not only by antitobacco campaigners but also by the state) as drugs and smokers as drug addicts.

United States

At the opposite extreme, the United States has for most of its pre-9/11 history been relatively insensitive to dangers to the state. Threats to communities and individuals have been privileged over threats to the state, and more concern has focused on drawing boundaries, often defined in moral terms, than on dissolving them. Disease—real or imagined—has long served as a boundary marker between the good and virtuous "us" and the dangerous and threatening "them," its borders defined in terms of a fluid internal geography that has shifted with time and circumstance. The "they" against whom white, middle-class, still largely rural America identified itself in the early twentieth century were immigrants from eastern and southern Europe and American blacks. Disease mapped onto those boundaries. Tuberculosis and infant mortality were construed as conditions of alien "others" and, simultaneously, as threats to the established social order: boundaries were inherently fragile and permeable. Safety was to be achieved by requiring that newcomers to the United States, the "un-American," be civilized (or constrained) to be more like Americans. There was less hope for "civilizing" African Americans, and the boundaries separating them from white America were more sharply drawn.

Boundary adjudication was always a work in progress. The villains of my late twentieth-century narratives—the "nasty, devious, predatory [disease carrying] 'them' " (Thompson 1983, 256)—were no longer immigrants from southern and eastern Europe, although the cast of villains still included blacks. Boundaries had been redrawn to place outside the moral pale, though at different distances, smokers who endangered "us" by breathing in our faces and injection drug users who threatened "us" by their existence, evoking associations (real and imagined) with violence, corruption of innocence, and (inevitably) with the stigmatized identity of blackness. The policy implications of a political culture that legitimized exclusion—drawing moral boundaries—in response to disease threats were strikingly different from the policy implications of inclusion as preached, if not always practiced, by the French. Strategies of inclusion portrayed the drug user as a member of the body politic who had strayed, not as an alien presence, and smokers as the embodiment of joie de vivre. American strategies of exclusion were little concerned with the person who used either drug other than as a foreign body to be expelled. Cigarette smokers were pushed out of doors, drug users were denied employment, and communities were happy when drug traffic moved to some other location. Dangers were portrayed as the result of *inclusion*—the smoker in your air space, the drug addict on your corner—not of exclusion.

Britain

The British have been less preoccupied than the French with dangers to the state, less concerned than the Americans with threats to individuals, and more focused on threats to vulnerable groups within the state— a concern that extended to threatened economic enterprises (for example, the tobacco industry) as well as to members of social or economic groups perceived as unable to protect themselves.

As it had somewhat earlier in France, nationalism played a major role in calling attention to infant mortality and, in Britain but not France, tuberculosis. The circumstances, however, were rather different. Britain perceived humiliation in the Boer War: "the greatest imperial power in the world [was] resisted for three years by a handful of settlers" (Speck 1993, 115). This resulted in intense anxiety among British elites about imperial decline, a threat they attributed to the poor physical condition of the lower classes, from whose ranks common soldiers were drawn.[4] In Britain as elsewhere, turn-of-the-century constructions of the so-called lower classes were contradictory and shifted over time: cannon fodder unfit for the cannon, crucibles of disorder and disease, or souls to be saved. As I suggested earlier (chapter 2), the last characterization was distinctive in its meaning and in its implications for public health. Epidemics were not interpreted as God's wrath punishing man for his sins, but as evidence that man had neglected God's injunction that the strong should look after the weak. "Sanitary reform, health care, visiting the poor, slum clearance, education of the poor in matters of health and hygiene, were all vital causes for a people inspired by both the evangelical concept of duty and, increasingly, a new secular concern for the well-ordering of society" (Wohl 1983, 6). Whereas the late nineteenth-century evangelical impulse has waned, the sense of duty—noblesse oblige—and concern for population health as fundamental to a well-ordered society have remained (Berridge 1990).

Commenting on the report of the government's Interdepartmental Committee on Physical Deterioration, appointed in response to the fears described, *The Times* of London stated that "the whole substance of its recommendations . . . turns upon the necessity for improving the health of certain strata of the population [the lower class] by the definitive application of medical science to their requirements" (cited in Brand 1965, 170). As the French had done, the British responded to their perceived peril with a spate of legislation, directed, however, not at the control of mothers and babies, but at improving the health of the working class. The principal foci of these laws were children in school and working men. The 1911 National Health Insurance Act specifically excluded these men's wives and children. Relatively little related specifically to infant mortality or tuberculosis, though the act did include a sanitarium benefit. Nevertheless, attention to these conditions was part and parcel of the concern with poverty and sickness that "arose and flourished in the early twentieth century," responding—much as in the French case—less to the germ theory of disease than to fears of national decline (Bryder 1988, 22).

Apocalyptic rhetoric—the drawing of lines and the elaboration of moral distinctions between us and them—is inseparable from a political opportunity structure where power is distrusted and interests—including public health interests—compete in the open market place. Constructions of risk have been less polarized in Britain than in the United States, in part because they were less valuable as counters in a political game that aimed at achieving consensus rather than enabling competition. AIDS and smoking generated morally tinged popular and press rhetoric about irresponsible drug users and an evil industry in Britain as elsewhere. This rhetoric had little impact on a government that wanted a national response to AIDS that would not alienate minorities or victimize those with AIDS and a response to smoking that would not alienate the tobacco industry.[5] There is a close relation between definitions of a problem and the solutions proposed. The British case suggests that causal direction may sometimes run from solutions to problems rather than the reverse. Nations vary in their preferred solutions and these preferences may be key to their definition of problems, including constructions of danger.

Canada

Throughout its history, Canada—"three civilizations and two cultures" packed uneasily into one state (Verney 1986)—has been most threatened by dissolution. This threat was much more clearly reflected in how disease problems were addressed (the solutions proposed) than in how dangers were constructed. Early twentieth-century Canadians believed in the health-giving properties of their northern environment. They were pre-occupied by economic growth, by competition with the United States, and by the problem of Quebec. The disease threats they experienced mapped onto these concerns only in the sense that they were understood very differently in English than in French Canada, as the narratives describe: disease-bearing immigrants threatened the Anglo-Saxon majority in the one case; infant mortality threatened the survival of Quebec in the other. Not coincidentally, the fears of English-Canadian elites closely resembled those of the Americans; the fears of French-Canadian elites resembled those of the French.

Canadian political culture and constructions of risk have shifted over time to the point where it is difficult to find any threads of continuity between the early and the late twentieth century. Health did not become an issue of national concern until after World War I. Its contemporary deployment by tobacco-control and AIDS activists as "a stick to beat authority, to make lazy bureaucrats sit up, to exact restitution for victims" (Douglas 1992, 25) and by the national government as an avenue to intervention in provincial and local affairs were shaped almost entirely by the political opportunities created by Canada's national health system and the centrality of that system to Canada's national identity. No argument for state action was more powerful than threats to the health of Canadians, pitted by tobacco-control advocates against industry greed and by advocates for injection drug users against the construction of drug use as a law and order problem. Invocation of these threats has the dual function, as I suggested in the Canadian tobacco-control narrative, of appealing to shared communitarian values and of allowing the federal government to intervene in its capacity as ultimate guardian of Canada's public health.

Victims and Villains

Once a credible threat had been recognized, the next acts in the drama of public health were the designation of villains and victims—who or what caused the problem and who were its victims. The basic dimensions of these scenarios were remarkably constant. Risks of a particular negative health outcome were portrayed as acquired innocently or by choice (and its victims as correspondingly innocent or culpable), as universal (we're all at risk) or particular (only they are at risk), and as arising from within the individual or from the environment. The "best" scenarios from the perspective of public health advocates were universal risks to innocent victims.

Ignorant Mothers and Contagious Consumptives

By the early years of the twentieth century, public health reformers in all four countries had shifted their causal attributions for infant mortality and tuberculosis "away from the environment [and, in the case of tuberculosis, from genetic hypotheses] and toward the individual, away from external conditions and toward personal behavior and health" (Meckel 1990, 100). Infant mortality was to be solved by educating ignorant mothers and tuberculosis by educating contagious consumptives. Writing about infant mortality, Meckel observes that "educating mothers seemed to hold promise as a panacea for infant mortality that could avoid the critical and problematic issue of poverty and make unnecessary more fundamental socioeconomic reforms and the provision of social and medical welfare" (100). In a similar vein, tuberculosis was to be controlled not by improving the living conditions of the masses but "merely . . . by confining their infective discharges" (cited in Fee 1994). Let me advance several noncompeting hypotheses to account for these shifts.

The first and perhaps most obvious hypothesis is that they occurred in response to the bacteriological revolution that followed upon the work of Pasteur, Koch, and others. The medical generation that came to power in the early twentieth century was heavily influenced, if not uniformly persuaded, by the idea that disease was caused by germs. And if each disease was caused by a germ, prevention might not require expensive intervention in the larger environment but only modifications of individual behavior to interrupt transmission of the germ (for example, educating mothers to boil milk, educating consumptives to avoid "promiscuous" spitting).

Second, although early public health activists were aware that environmental causes (poverty, inadequate living conditions, poor and insufficient food) were implicated in disease, the obstacles to addressing these causes were not only financial but—given the level of government intervention that would be required—political and philosophical as well. Reducing infant mortality and tuberculosis to questions of individual responsibility finessed these obstacles, at least temporarily. As Meckel points out, although Western industrialized countries were uniform in placing the burden of responsibility for infant mortality on the mother, "where they differed, and continue to differ, is in the amount of support they give to the mother in bearing that responsibility" (1990, 101).

Finally, this was a period of uncertainty and confusion about women's proper place and the appropriate relations between women and men. The precise terms of this debate differed from one country to another. Nevertheless, whatever their nationality, the discourses of medical and political authorities about infant mortality—holding mothers to account, proclaiming maternal ignorance, and arguing for mothers' education as the solution—were consistent in their affirmation of a patriarchal vision of gender: the conviction that mothers' place was in the home breast-feeding their babies, washing their hands, boiling their milk, and sterilizing their bottles.

Ignorant mothers were one thing, however, a relatively easy mark. Contagious consumptives were quite another. Attribution of causal responsibility to contagion—the spread of "infective discharges"—was fraught with what many physicians and politicians perceived as highly undesirable consequences: stigmatization of respectable members of society, loss of medical practice to colleagues less insistent on diagnostic precision, invasion of privacy. Alternative causal constructions were, however, equally problematic as Guillaume, writing about France, so vividly described (1990, 147).

In all four countries contagion did nevertheless become, sooner or later, the construction of choice. In all four countries, even the United States with its unique populist campaigns to educate the public on how transmission might be prevented, the result was "contagion hysteria": suspected carriers were ostracized, providers refused to treat and hospitals refused to accept tuberculosis patients, communities denied permission for sanatorium sites (McQuaig 1979; Barnes 1995; Smith 1988; Rothman 1994; Ott 1996). Voluntary associations—largely responsible in all four countries for public education on tuberculosis—were highly successful at creating fear of the disease. At the same time, their efforts produced the very response that so many physicians had warned against: stigmatization both of tuberculosis and of its victims.

Shifts in causal attribution from the environment to the individual were associated not only with new and different policy prescriptions but also with changes in the social construction of populations at risk: who was dangerous and who was endangered. In all four countries, infant mortality and tuberculosis came to be identified with groups outside the pale of middle-class respectability. In all four countries as well, the actions proposed and taken in response to these threats shaped—and were shaped by—these constructions.

For example, the measures public health authorities now believed necessary to control infant mortality and tuberculosis were regarded as highly intrusive, even by those who proposed them, and, consequently, as inappropriate to or unacceptable by ranking members of society, that is, those with the power to resist these measures. Poor mothers in Paris received free milk and other assistance at the cost of controls on their behavior unimaginable to the rich. Tuberculosis notification and other preventive measures were ultimately made possible in Britain by a "politically motivated" redefinition of tuberculosis as a disease of poverty (Hardy 1993). Hermann Biggs is reported to have assured private physicians that "their" patients would not be subjected to notification and fumigation (Winslow 1929, 135).

Although ideas about the stratification of disease were common to all four countries, there were important dissimilarities—as well as parallels—in how those ideas shaped the public health response. Real and imagined military and population crises led British and French elites to construe working-class health as a matter of national survival. Tuberculosis in Britain and infant mortality in France were problems of state and played critical roles in the evolution of national welfare policy. No comparable policy incentives at the national level existed at that period in the United States. Most American elites regarded disease among immigrants and blacks as a threat not to the nation but to white middle-class society. Immigrants were perceived as deserving of and susceptible to transformation from alien presences to good Americans through appropriate health education and exposure to middle class values. African Americans, on the other hand, were seen as undeserving and intractable, alienated less by simple ignorance of hygienic rules than by "their excessive and corrupt immorality" (Northern 1909).

Nicotine and Narcotics

My portrayal of the "victims and villains" that peopled early twentieth-century dramas of infant mortality and tuberculosis has relied, perforce, on the written word. I had the great advantage in the late twentieth century of being able to talk directly with the players. Not infrequently in the course of my interviews, actors in the two public health arenas of tobacco and AIDS/drugs would comment spontaneously on each others' domain. These comments, when they occurred, were—to my surprise—

invariably negative. A Canadian tobacco-control advocate, for example, was vehemently opposed to proposals for legalizing marijuana under active consideration in Canada at the time; a Canadian advocate on behalf of drug users referred to tobacco control as "a religious crusade against people who smoke." French actors on AIDS-drugs were similarly disdainful of their counterparts in tobacco control, and all of the former smoked, including several physicians. What to my mind had been projects with the at least implicitly shared goal of advancing public health were in the minds of my interlocutors not only opposed but even in conflict, each group seeing the other's position as injurious to its own cause: in the one case, delegitimizing a drug (nicotine) and stigmatizing its users; in the other, neutralizing (if not legitimizing) a class of drugs (narcotics), and destigmatizing its users.

Actors in these two arenas for the most part ignored each other, preferring not to confront their very different perspectives on what was essentially a common public health problem, the use and misuse of psychoactive drugs. Mutual ignorance was made easier, and more understandable, by the great differences between nicotine and narcotics in their social and economic histories, in their meaning as cultural practices, and in the historically dominant images of their users. As detailed in the narratives, in all four countries the tobacco industry had long been a respected economic actor and smokers were respectable members of society. Cigarette smoking was on a par with coffee drinking, only more glamorous. Narcotic drug addicts were, by contrast, highly stigmatized by the public and often by members of the health and political establishments as well. These background differences confronted public health actors with very different problems. For entrepreneurs of tobacco control, the problem was straightforward: to shift smoking from the positive or, at worst, neutral category it had occupied for so long to one decidedly negative. Injection drug use, on the other hand, presented activists against HIV/AIDS with the opposite (and more complex) problem: to destigmatize drug use and drug users to the point where measures for disease prevention could be instituted at all. Let me now turn to a comparative cross-national analysis of how these problems were addressed. Perhaps on no other dimension of the politics of public health as herein described has the difference between the United States and the other three countries been more marked.

Nicotine, Smoking, Tobacco   The raw materials for making the case against tobacco (for example, innocent victims, merchants of death, public health versus economic greed) were included in the discursive toolkit of antismoking advocates irrespective of nationality. Their relative emphasis in each of the four countries has depended on differences in political culture, period and circumstance, that is, on the fortunes of political opportunity. I group Canada, Britain, and France in this analysis because, though there were important differences among the three countries, actors' construction of the tobacco problem had some key elements in common that contrasted sharply with constructions prevalent in the United States. Tobacco's history, economic importance, and degree of insertion in national politics were much the same in all four countries, as I have described. Nevertheless, from very early in their campaigns, that is, beginning in the 1970s, French, British, and Canadian advocates against smoking identified corporate practices (principally advertising but also cigarette content) as primarily responsible for the harms caused by smoking. They explicitly declined to target individual smokers, holding the state wholly responsible for redress. Second, environmental tobacco smoke, though not absent as a public health concern, took second or third place behind other problems considered more pressing. Detailed evidence for each of these points was presented in the narratives.

Public health actors frame issues, allocate responsibilities, designate villains and victims that mesh with their particular political cultures and opportunities and, by the same token, appeal to their intended audiences. Common premises—based on ample precedent—of actors in the three parliamentary democracies were the legitimacy and the conceivability of government intervention both in the economy and in health. It therefore made sense to target the industry and its practices and to call on the government for redress. The United States presented a very different constellation of ideologies and opportunities. From the outset of their campaign, activists against cigarette smoking were confronted by a national ideology opposed to government intervention in the economy and by the absence of any countervailing commitment to health as an overriding public good. Aversion to government meddling with economic life has dominated Congress's approach to the tobacco industry for the past fifty years, ever since federal lawmakers' attention was first drawn to the dangers of tobacco.[6] The federal government has been equally reluctant to intervene in the health arena. Health does not trump narrow economic interests even rhetorically, as it often does in Canada, Britain, and France (Nathanson 2005).

Blocked from invoking the collective good, public health actors in the United States (regardless of the particular arena in which they operate) have turned to a culturally more resonant constellation of ideological strains, centered on protection of the individual. Commenting on her perception that "political actions to protect the environment have to be proposed as if they were to protect the personal health of individuals," Mary Douglas observed that "they look like 'political actions taken under the wrong banner,' but they are taken under the only banner that will rally support: protection of the individual" (1992, 28). This banner has two overlapping strands, one that invokes entitlement based on rights—as in gay rights, rights of the disabled, women's rights, nonsmokers' rights—

and the other grounded in entitlement based on innocence—involuntary exposure to dangers and risks (in implicit contrast to the nonentitlement of individuals who knowingly assume the risk of their circumstances or behavior—most obviously in the present context, injection drug users). In the rhetoric that inaugurated the American nonsmokers' rights movement, these two strands were seamlessly interwoven: nonsmokers, the "involuntary victims of tobacco smoke" were called upon to rise up and assert their "right to breathe clean air [that] is superior to the right of the smoker to enjoy a harmful habit" (cited in Nathanson 1999, 448). The legitimacy of the public good as a sufficient rationale for public policy in Canada, Britain, and France made the vocabularies of innocence and rights not only less necessary but also less advisable.

"Faceless corporate giants" have a history of demonization in the United States as elsewhere, but it took far more time, starker evidence of culpability, and—above all—clear demonstration of legal and political vulnerability before American public health actors adopted the anti-industry rhetoric that had become standard among advocates in Canada, Britain and, though less so, in France. Once adopted, however, this rhetoric became highly polarized. By the mid-1990s, cigarette manufacturers were openly demonized not only as "merchants of death" and drug dealers but as akin to sexual predators. "Protect our children from the tobacco companies" and "tobacco lawyers versus America's kids" appeared in public service announcements in major media outlets (for example, CNN, the *New York Times*), sponsored by mainstream health, religious, and educational organizations. Rhetorical polarization goes hand in hand with social movement–driven public health advocacy.

Narcotics, Drug Users, and HIV/AIDS   Just as cross-national differences in framing the dangers of tobacco were unrelated to the relative power of the tobacco industry, so differences in construing the dangers of AIDS-drugs were largely unrelated either to differences in the perception of drug users or to perceptions of AIDS. Drug users and drug sellers were subject to heavy—and increasing—legal penalties in all four countries and were demonized and feared by large sections of the public, not excluding politicians.[7] AIDS was widely perceived as a disease brought on themselves by people behaving badly: even Britain—the country that responded earliest and most forcefully to the AIDS-drugs problem—was no exception. Virginia Berridge cites a 1986 speech by the chief constable of Manchester to a national conference of police officers who blamed homosexuals and prostitutes and their clients—"whirling about in a human cesspit of their own making"—for the spread of AIDS (Berridge 1996, 109). The most interesting point about this speech, however, was not its intemperate language but the "massive adverse response" it evoked from the British government. Norman Fowler, the secretary of state for Health and Social

Security, "was provoked to state that the government did not have time for the luxury of a moral argument on AIDS" (109).

Again, it makes sense to group Britain, France, and Canada in this analysis and to examine how AIDS-drugs was framed as a public health and political issue in these three countries compared with the United States. I point out substantial differences among the three—particularly in the timing of government entry as a key player in shifting the discourse around AIDS-drugs toward public health and away from criminal justice— but the striking contrast with the United States remains. The key to this contrast was, indeed, the role of government, first in establishing certain ground rules for discourse on health regardless of the health problem at hand and, second, in setting the tone and the content of discussion on AIDS-drugs (as in the British example, cited earlier). First, the ground rules: in the context of AIDS-drugs, a—if not the—critical element in shaping political discourse in Canada, Britain, and France was these governments' accepted responsibility for the health of their citizens, regardless of those citizens' legal or moral standing. In principle, if not invariably in practice, innocence was irrelevant to this responsibility and rights were based on citizenship and did not have to be individually established. As a counterweight to their identities as dangerous criminals or—at best— sick addicts, drug users in these three countries had a third identity, that of citizen, on the basis of which legitimate claims to health protection could be made by users themselves or on their behalf. That counterweight did not exist in the United States.

Second, with varying alacrity each of the three parliamentary governments took deliberate steps to transform the discourse on AIDS-drugs from one dominated by the dangers of narcotics to one dominated by the dangers of HIV/AIDS. Indeed, many health ministry civil servants in both Britain and France saw the advent of HIV/AIDS as a unique opportunity to bring drug users into the mainstream of medical care: "a blessing in disguise" (Berridge 1996, 222). The earliest to effect this transformation was Britain. Canada and France, for different reasons that I describe in the narratives, moved more slowly and less publicly in the same direction. Nevertheless, by 2001, both governments had committed themselves to the proposition that injection drug use was "a health issue, as opposed to a law and order issue" (Health Canada 2001, 2), by implication privileging the identity of drug users as deserving citizens rather than as undeserving addicts and criminals.

For several reasons—in addition to the absence of an overriding commitment by the government to the health of all its citizens—no such transformation of identities was possible in the United States. First, the official position of the federal government was against any AIDS-driven change in the meaning of narcotics and, implicitly, of their users. Second, the transformative capacity of nonstate actors—the health-related social movements and interest groups that moved the tobacco-control agenda and, more generally, are key to public health action in the United States—was limited by the lack of a vocabulary suitable to the task in hand. In the United States, any advocacy grounded in protection of individual health, as opposed to the health of the collectivity, demands that the individual be portrayed not only as vulnerable but also as deserving (for example, the "involuntary victims of tobacco smoke"). Children and female partners of injection drug users could be and were so portrayed, but users were difficult to accommodate within the narrow confines of a discourse based on innocence and individual rights. Finally, any transformation to "deserving citizens" was blocked by "the boundaries of blackness" (Cohen 1997). Identified as black, injection drug users were doubly excluded from the pale of citizenship, not only by white communities but as much or more so by their own.

Conclusions

I draw three generalizations from this analysis. First, how dangers to health were portrayed depended heavily on who portrayed them and for what purpose. Collective actors outside the corridors of power (health-related social movements, political lobbies, interest groups) rattling at the gates demanding to be let in and dependent on popular and media attention and support, had the most to gain from describing dangers in apocalyptic terms and were most likely to do so. "Tobacco-control advocacy," wrote Michael Pertschuk and his colleagues in an unusually candid acknowledgment of this point, "flourishes best in an environment of fresh public outrage at the tobacco industry's wrongful behavior" (1999, 20). Public outrage—regardless of the particular villain in question—was less valuable as a forensic resource where national ideology and politics allowed outsiders to be safely ignored, as in Britain and France. In Britain, discourse on all four public health issues was dominated by the government and its designated experts. There was little opportunity for outsiders or even dissident insiders to challenge this discourse: when challenges occurred, they were rapidly defused or simply ignored. In this fashion, politicization of public health issues was minimized and policy consensus achieved. Although the French government was equally at pains to avoid politicization, its strategy was somewhat different: public health issues with the potential to cause serious contention the government did not wish to address (all except infant mortality) were simply swept under the rug and kept there until, by one means or another, the government's hand was forced. Where, as in the United States, collective action was the dominant form of advocacy, dangers were portrayed apocalyptically and public outrage was actively cultivated and has flourished.

Second, as I suggested earlier, how dangers were portrayed was by no means independent of the solutions preferred: if the cart did not come before the horse, the two often moved side by side. This is most obvious when threats to health competed with other values such as political norms that made partnership and consensus preferable to divisive political contest or when there were competing political goals such as the war on drugs. In such cases, apocalyptic portrayals of disease threats were likely to be muted. Portrayals of danger were further shaped to correspond with their promoters' preferences as to the location of responsibility for finding a solution. Thus, states invoked national peril to legitimize a national rather than a local or sectarian response to disease threats. Outside groups demanding a national response were careful to designate threats that came within the central government's jurisdiction, most obviously in Canada, where the jurisdictional split between the central government and the provinces is uniquely consequential for health advocacy.

Finally, between the early and the late twentieth century, three of these four countries—Canada, Britain, and France—experienced profound changes of institutional structure and political culture in the realms of health and disease. Each created some form of government-run national health system that guaranteed medical care to its citizens. These actions substantially changed the social and political context for advocacy around smoking and AIDS-drugs compared with infant mortality and tuberculosis. More specifically, once health was enshrined as a responsibility of government, advocates of health protection—inside the government as ministers and civil servants or outside the government as partisans—were presented not just with new strings to their rhetorical bows but with entire new bows. Far more clearly and definitively than in the early twentieth century, dangers to health were portrayed by public health actors as the responsibility of government to address and resolve.

Chapter 10

Conclusion

P UBLIC HEALTH originated as much from fear of social change—the revolutionary potential of the desperate poor huddled together in the teeming cities of the nineteenth century—as from the desire for social reform. Public health was conceived as a means to public order. Yet the social changes initiated by Edwin Chadwick, when he embarked on improvements to the sanitary environment of the poor to defray the tax rates of the rich, and by Robert Koch, when he and Pasteur and other late nineteenth-century pioneers of biomedicine, launched— perhaps unwittingly—the search for magic bullets that would target disease individual by individual, were revolutionary. The movements these men helped set in motion transformed conceptions of disease and contributed—albeit haltingly and unevenly—to a vast expansion of public responsibility for its prevention.

Change was sometimes dramatic. In 1905, the New York City health commissioner, Hermann Biggs, dumped "the entire milk supply of several large firms" into the city sewers on grounds of contamination (Winslow 1929, 194). A little less than a hundred years later, the city's health commissioner and the mayor (against objections from his staff) announced a complete ban on smoking in New York's bars and restaurants. In 1995 in Vancouver, British Columbia, the Vancouver Area Network of Drug Users was created as a political movement to pressure local politicians on behalf of injection drug users; seven years later, it took credit for the landslide election of a highly sympathetic mayor. It is these and other examples of public health action that I have sought in the preceding chapters to deconstruct and explain.

Central to the idea of social change is innovation.[1] My focus in this book has been on innovations in "community action to avoid disease and other threats to the health and welfare of individuals and the community at large" (Duffy 1990, 1). Consistent with John Duffy's definition, I have concentrated on social actors—individuals, organized groups, and states—as the principal agents of change in public health and have been interested

247

primarily in innovative forms of action. VANDU is a good example. As reflected in the examples cited, innovation has taken many forms and has occurred at different levels of organization, from social movements organized in front parlors and basement meeting rooms to legislatures and parliaments. Arguably, the most significant of these innovations in the long term were not the programmatic or policy outcomes achieved—package warnings, say, or educational brochures mailed to expectant mothers—but the recognition that public health was political and the invention of new forms of political advocacy to achieve public health goals.

At the most general level, the conclusion I draw from my work is that the obstacles to public health action, even such superficially noncontroversial action as pasteurization, are formidable. Or—stated in more positive terms—given these obstacles, it is remarkable that anything in the way of community action to avoid disease was accomplished. I begin with a brief review of the obstacles evident from the narratives and interpretation I have presented.

Obstacles

Opposition to public health action by powerful groups—economic, professional, moral, religious—that saw the measures proposed as inimical to their own interests has a long history. These groups—dairy farmers and milk dealers, tobacco manufacturers, medical syndicats, the AMA, the Catholic church—derived their power from their extensive economic and organizational resources, from their insertion (with the debatable exception of the tobacco industry) in local communities, and from their close ties with state bureaucrats and politicians. Often the principal intended beneficiaries of these same measures belonged to poor or stigmatized populations with relatively few resources and with little elite support or political access. Wherever they may have seen their interests to lie, their voices were seldom heard. The beneficiaries—intended or otherwise—of the antismoking movement are an obvious exception, helping to account for the movement's success.

With important but limited exceptions, public health as a state function was marginalized relative to other activities. Authorities with the power to override opposition to public health measures had competing priorities, did not see important political interests as threatened (or perceived the threat of action as greater than that of inaction), were ideologically committed to some form of market liberalism that precluded state action, were afraid of stirring up popular panic or incurring expenses they perceived to be unaffordable, or were simply uninterested.

Conditions for Public Health Action

Under what circumstances, then, has public health action come about? My answer is that action was made possible by some combination of three ingredients: perceived peril to the nation (la patrie en danger) or to the accepted social order, state interest and capacity, and advocacy group pressure. The relative importance of each ingredient—the amount of each in the recipe—depended on the issue at hand and was variable cross-nationally and across time. At one extreme, only the first two ingredients—perceived peril and state interest and capacity—were required for Britain to take action to protect drug injectors from HIV transmission; at the other, action to protect nonsmokers in the United States was initiated almost entirely by advocacy group pressure. More often, the ingredients were mixed. I comment briefly on each ingredient, beginning with la patrie en danger.

Fears of danger to the state or to the social order—popular revolution, national decline, the spread of disease from "them" (the stigmatized) to "us" (the general) population—have played a consistent and important role as stimuli to state action on behalf of public health, so important, in fact, that invocations of national peril are a staple in the rhetoric of public health zealots. States did not act, however, unless they had the interest and capacity to do so. Cries of "la patrie en danger" were notably ineffective in getting the early twentieth-century French state to act against tuberculosis. By the late twentieth century, all four states had the capacity to act, three of the four had an institutionalized commitment to their citizens' health in the form of a national health-care system, but in only one—Canada—did the central government have a built-in motive to be interested in public health: it paid a large portion of the bill for individual health-care services over which it had little or no formal authority or control.

It is important to emphasize that innovation in the form of laws and public policies did not always translate into energetic implementation. Public health action is a process, and the obstacles I outlined operated as strongly at the stage of implementation as they had at the innovation stage. Indeed, they operated more strongly: laws may be passed or policies announced to provide tutelary guidance (so often the case in France), as expressions of benevolent intent, or for reasons of political expedience. The true test of state interest and commitment comes at the stage of implementation. Again, the Canadian central government of the late twentieth century was—for the reasons enunciated (elaborated more fully in chapter 7)—the most likely to expend political capital overcoming obstacles to the implementation of public health measures.

The third ingredient was demand from organized advocacy groups external to the government. Advocacy group pressure was present in all four countries. Advocacy that took the form of grassroots social movements was a dominant ingredient only in America. The oft-cited political opportunities created by divided government—a distinction the United States shares with Canada—were arguably the least important of the reasons for America's exceptionalism.

More important, I believe, were the history and the corresponding legitimacy of lay advocacy as a form of public health action and the existence of clear organizational templates—in the early twentieth century the WCTU, in the late twentieth century the civil rights movement—that served as models for public health organizers to follow. Lay advocacy was delegitimized in Britain and France by the cultural authority of experts in matters of public health and, more generally, is less effective in parliamentary states where the political agenda is controlled by the party in power, allowing it to ignore interests it does not share (and, of course, to promote those it does). By the same token, U.S. advocates confronted particularly powerful obstacles to public health action initiated by the state—and corresponding incentives to take action into their own hands. First, the same government structure that created openings for groups advocating public health measures also created openings for opponents of those measures who as a rule commanded far greater economic resources and political access. Second, there was no built-in state commitment to citizens' health comparable to the commitment reflected in the national health care systems of late twentieth-century Canada, Britain, and France. Disease prevention had to be fought for, disease by disease.

Not only was there systematic cross-national variation in the balance of ingredients, but the balance peculiar to each country was also more consequential for the fate of some public health measures than for others. State capacity and interest were most critical when affected groups (for example, injection drug users) were stigmatized, lacked the resources and elite support to advocate for themselves, and were unable to attract powerful outside advocates on their behalf. In a striking example, Walter Troesken argues that the mortality from typhoid fever of U.S. blacks benefited more than white mortality from the introduction of water filtration in the early twentieth century because predominantly poor blacks, who were disadvantaged in their ability to prevent typhoid through private, household-level actions, "depended heavily on public authorities to provide clean and safe water through public water lines" (2004, 204). Britain's formula for state action—deliberation behind closed doors to which only selected guests were invited—worked well for AIDS-drugs but less well for tobacco, where the industry was among the guests. By contrast, the U.S. pattern of organized advocacy and an absent state was effective in the tobacco case not only because the organizers offered a culturally resonant message along with the resources that drug users lacked but also because their critical public health innovation—shaming or coercing their neighbors into not smoking—was inexpensive and required little in the way of state action. It goes almost without saying that the same pattern was highly ineffective for protecting injection drug users against HIV/AIDS.

Even in the best of circumstances, there were limitations to what public health—community action to avoid disease and other threats to the health and welfare of individuals and the community at large—was able to accomplish in the way of social change. The most serious threats to health and welfare in every society (not just the societies examined in this book) are the inequalities of social and economic condition perpetrated and perpetuated by national and international structures of economic and political power. These inequalities—responsible in large part for higher rates of preventable disease among poor or stigmatized populations—were only marginally visible in my narratives. The reasons are instructive. The public health actors whose words and deeds have been my subject matter were more often than not fully aware of these inequalities, though perhaps not of their origins. This is, however, a book about policy innovation and implementation, and inequalities as threats to health were seldom directly addressed, which renders all the more remarkable the early twentieth-century French anarcho-syndicalist discourse on tuberculosis. Public health actors either failed to see the role of the existing social order in creating health inequalities because they espoused medical-behavioral theories of disease causation that precluded such a role, or they understood its importance but were unwilling for reasons of ideology, prudence, or pragmatism to challenge the existing social order. Public health is an ameliorative rather than a revolutionary discipline and practice. Its founders, after all, had seen public health measures as a way not of creating revolutionary social change but of preventing it.

I wrote in chapter 1 that the public health issues I selected were important for their capacity to reveal the struggles that underlie action on behalf of the public's health. My cases, issue-and-country combinations, I argued, are cases of struggle over the definition and ownership of public problems and over the power to occupy and dominate the terrain those problems are claimed to represent. Other cases with different parameters—differences, for example, in the power of relevant actors or the political opportunities available to them—would have different trajectories, but trajectories nevertheless predictable, or at least understandable, within the framework I have presented. A couple of examples will illustrate my point. In the United States post–9/11, to frame a public health issue as an instance of potential terrorism—as was done in the fall of 2002 when cases of anthrax appeared in several widely separated locations—is immediately to engage the interest and capacity of the federal government: a classic case of la patrie en danger. In such a case, the state is likely to occupy the entire issue terrain, leaving little space for other actors. A second example is the question of anonymous HIV testing, recently revived by public health officials in New York City (see, for example, Santora 2006). The availability of treatment and the increasing concentration of the epidemic among minorities have created new political opportunities for traditional public health actors. Their power may be expected to rise relative to that of AIDS advocacy groups, leading (for better or worse) to erosion in the privacy protections established in the epidemic's early stages.

These illustrations are drawn from the United States. Both the level of engagement and the relative power of different actors in a any given public health drama will vary not only with issues and opportunities but also with political systems and political cultures, as my cases have shown. Although a different set of issues would have produced stories different in many details from the ones I have told, I have provided the tools to analyze and interpret those stories and—perhaps in a few cases—to predict the trajectories they are likely to follow.

Reflections: Where Theory Meets Data

The conceptual apparatus that framed this project served me remarkably well. Each of the elements with which I began—states, collective actions, and constructions of risk—finds its place among the ingredients for public health action outlined above. Indeed, apart from a bit of tweaking, the recipe for "low mortality countries" that I proposed in chapter 1 based on social-demographic research does not look terribly different from the recipe for social change in public health. There is, nevertheless, ample room for conceptual refinement both in theories of states and of social movements.

Weak States–Strong States

In his recent critique of the weak state–strong state dichotomy, Peter Baldwin argued that because no state is interventionist—a characterization Baldwin equated with strong—across the board, the concept itself must be abandoned: "[If comparative work is to bear fruit worth the effort] then a reconceptualization of states and statism should be the result" (2005b, 18). I make no claim to such a reconceptualization. I do think that to abandon the concept of strong and weak states altogether would be to throw out the baby with the bathwater. Strong and weak are constructs that describe polar constellations of state attributes, not state actions, interventionist or otherwise. Reading the dichotomy as an ideal-typical construct led me to ask questions about why states at different poles on the strong-weak continuum did, or did not, intervene, and to some interesting answers.

The strong state may have greater executive and administrative capacity, but it is no more likely than the weak state to take action unless its vital interests are engaged. Further, insofar as the political culture and institutions of high-capacity states restrict the opportunities, the legitimacy, and the power of nonstate actors to enter policy debates and have their voices attended to, the effect of state disengagement will be policy paralysis. At the same time, once the interests of the state are engaged, the high-capacity state is better positioned than the state with less capacity to pursue its goals independently of other groups in the society. Although the weak state affords greater opportunities and legitimacy to nonstate actors, it also depends more on them to drive public policy, a structural arrangement that tilts policy toward well-resourced groups and seriously disadvantages groups whose organizational, political and ideological resources are limited.

Fuzzy Boundaries

Conceptual distinctions that appeared self-evident on their face—between state and nonstate actors and between social movement actors and scientific or medical experts—were clearly challenged by my data. Sustained cooperation between civil servants and social movement actors was more often than not a key element in creating the political conditions necessary for innovative public health action by the state. Indeed, orchestration of outside agitation from within the state's executive or administrative arms was not uncommon. Hard and fast boundaries between nonstate actors with influence grounded in their medical expertise and those whose influence depended on the weight of their numbers or the amount of media attention they could garner were equally difficult to draw. In Britain and France, where the only legitimate zealots were experts, their strategies and tactics were only marginally distinguishable from those of lay zealots elsewhere. And among the consequences of the latter's legitimacy in Canada and the United States was that veteran lay zealots not infrequently took on the trappings of experts. The conclusion I draw from these fuzzy boundaries is that the tools of advocacy are highly fungible. Access to these tools—expertise, the media, the power of numbers—is highly variable, but no tool is the exclusive property of either states or outside actors. Individuals and groups will use whatever tools they can command that are best suited to their purposes as they see them.

The Decline of Public Health?

Book-length laments over the sorry state of public health have been published in the past fifteen years, in the United States and in Britain and France.[2] The nearest comparable work in Canada is the much earlier Lalonde report, which hardly qualifies as a lament. Public health is said to have lost its way or, in the case of France, to have never found it. It is described as weak organizationally (underfunded, fragmented in its activities, with low status relative to other functions of government and to the medical profession) and ideologically (without a clear sense of mission). Notably, the focus of these laments is on public health in its institutional form, the public health that Americans and Britons tend to associate with local health officials and health departments and the French with the Ministère de la santé on the avenue de Ségur in Paris. The sorry state of the latter has a long history that is eloquently recounted by Morelle (and that has made several appearances in the preceding pages as well). In the United States and Britain, the weak position of contemporary public health was often compared unfavorably to a supposedly halcyon past.

From the perspective adopted in this book, the situation is more complicated than these lamentations might lead one to believe. The present-day weaknesses of traditional public health are evident from my own data: in only one of the eight contemporary country-case combinations (AIDS-drugs in Canada) did leadership in recognizing and addressing a serious public health issue come from local public health officers or departments. As I stated earlier, these weaknesses are most consequential when the population at the greatest health risk is highly stigmatized and unable to speak for itself or to find representation among established elites. The systemic problems of traditional public health systems in the United States and France and the relative strength of these systems in Britain and Canada were thus highlighted by these countries' response to HIV/AIDS in injection drug users. Britain's recognition and timely implementation of measures to address the AIDS-drugs connection was initiated by public health officials at the national level strongly and openly supported by their political masters. In Canada, though their power was limited by jurisdictional conflicts with the police and other officials, local health officers in major urban centers, quietly encouraged and abetted by federal civil servants, were the vanguard of the response. No comparable leadership existed—or was politically possible—in the United States and France, and action was absent or delayed. On the other hand, energetic public health action in the smoking–tobacco control arena depended far less on traditional public health actors.

Stepping back from these late twentieth-century laments, the picture of public health I have presented is one of continuity rather than decline. In the United States, public health action was rarely initiated by the state on behalf of the collectivity and, with certain exceptions, local public health institutions (where formal responsibility for this activity lies) have been poorly supported politically and financially. At the same time, geographically widespread collective action by lay groups and organizations not identified with traditional public health was a major source of public health innovation in the early as well as the late twentieth century. This arrangement has important strengths but also serious limitations, as I have explained. The weakness of public health in France—where both state and civil society can be equally paralyzed—is rooted in long-standing aspects of that country's society and culture. Action, when it came, was precipitated by political crises. Public health in Britain was dominated by medical elites in and outside of government who made their voices heard or had them silenced through well-established channels—old-boy networks and government-appointed committees of the great and the good. As I have pointed out, the British system worked well in some circumstances, less well—or more slowly—in others. Canada's approach to public health has long been characterized by a pattern of institutionalized buck-passing between levels of government and by the federal government's efforts to create a unique role for itself in the health domain.

Public Health, Disease Prevention, and the Decline of Mortality

My analysis of the sociology and politics of public health was grounded on the premise that these policies, hence the processes that underlie their being adopted and implemented, make a difference—that, as I stated in chapter 1, they play a major role in disease prevention and in the decline of mortality. This premise drove the actions of public health reformers. My own conviction of its truth drove this book.

Among Thomas McKeown's principal contributions to the study of mortality has been as a stimulus to sophisticated social-demographic research on mortality decline in developed countries during the nineteenth and early twentieth centuries. This work makes a strong case for the importance of human agency in the form of public health measures—principally protection of the water supply and regulation of the built environment—to overall mortality decline in England and Wales (Szreter 1988; Hardy 1993; Millward and Bell 2000), France (Preston and van de Walle 1978), and the United States (Troesken 2004; Cutler and Miller 2005). With specific reference to infant mortality, the two recently published analyses just cited present persuasive quantitative evidence to support their separate conclusions that the major factor in the decline of infant deaths was the provision of clean water supplies. Indeed, David Cutler and Grant Miller attribute 74 percent of the reduction in infant mortality between 1900 and 1930 in the thirteen large U.S. cities where they had complete data to the introduction of water protection technologies. There is, to my knowledge, no comparable quantitative support for the impact (in isolation from other variables) of clean milk or the education of mothers—the preventive measures stressed by public health actors at the time. Infant feeding was critical, but babies may have benefited more from public health interventions over which their mothers had little control—water filtration plants and pasteurization—than from changes in mothers' behavior (see, for example, Woods 2000; Woods, Watterson, and Woodward 1988, 1989; Ewbank and Preston 1990; Fairchild and Oppenheimer 1998).

Tuberculosis is more controversial. Multiple post-McKeown hypotheses have been advanced to account for its decline in the late nineteenth and early twentieth centuries, focused primarily on the decline in England and Wales, but extending to a few other European countries and to locations in the United States where adequate mortality time series exist: general improvement in the sanitary environment, more salubrious housing, decreased virulence of the disease, and the notification and isolation of cases (McFarlane 1989; Wilson 1990; Fairchild and Oppenheimer 1998; Woods 2000). No quantitative analyses to evaluate the relative plausibility of these hypotheses have been completed and, indeed, such analyses may not be possible, given the limitations of data for the period in question. Nevertheless, a strong argument can be made for the critical importance of case notification and the subsequent isolation of individuals with the disease—public health measures that were at the center of early twentieth-century conflict between medicine and public health (Fairchild and Oppenheimer 1998). This argument was first advanced based on an ingenious series of analyses carried out in the early twentieth century by Arthur Newsholme, medical officer of health for Brighton and subsequently Britain's chief medical officer (Wilson 1990). Newsholme's central thesis was that "the segregation of consumptives with active disease [in British Poor Law infirmaries and workhouses], by diminishing the transmission of infection, must have had a significant effect on TB incidence and mortality rates" (Fairchild and Oppenheimer 1998, 1108). Based on review of this and subsequent studies, Amy Fairchild and Gerald Oppenheimer conclude that "both original data and the quantitative analyses of earlier historians strongly suggest that [notification and] patient isolation did make a difference" (1109–10).

The relation of cigarette smoking to the risk of lung cancer and other diseases and of drug injection with nonsterile equipment to the risk of HIV transmission are clear. The question here is whether the manner in which these threats were addressed in each of the four countries had different consequences for the rates at which these risks declined. (Although this question is equally appropriate in relation to infant mortality and tuberculosis, the absence of national mortality data for Canada and the United States in the late nineteenth and early twentieth centuries places severe limitations on comparative demographic analysis.) Data presented earlier on patterns of decline in smoking (figures 5.1 and 5.2) and lung cancer (figure 5.4) suggest, first, that there is more than one way to skin a cat. The different policy regimes followed by the United States, Canada, and the UK were equally effective in bringing down cigarette consumption among men, and in all three countries male lung cancer mortality rates have declined. Second, though cigarette consumption rates in France at the beginning of the antismoking campaign were much lower than in the other three countries, the hesitancy of France's policy response was associated both with a slower rate of decline in smoking (indeed, by the year 2000 cigarette consumption in France was higher than in the UK) and with a rise in male lung cancer mortality rates to the highest among the four countries. Women present a different and more complicated picture (for an analysis of these complications, see Nathanson 1995).

Central to the public health strategy for preventing HIV among injection drug users is ensuring access to clean needles and to oral forms of narcotic drugs. Where this strategy was put in place early and enthusiastically, as in Britain, an HIV epidemic in the drug-using population was averted. Where the strategy was delayed, as in France, complicated by interjurisdictional conflicts, as in Canada, or sidelined by the war on drugs, as in the United States, the percentage of injection drug users relative to other exposure categories (as described in each country's surveillance reports) has fluctuated in recent years but remained considerably higher than comparable rates in Britain.

Let me return in conclusion to John Walton's injunction that cases—however they are selected—must be "shown to be [cases] of something important" (1992, 125). The sixteen cases on which my analysis is based are important because public health stands or falls depending on the outcome of these and comparable struggles between antagonists with very different amounts of social, economic, and political power. In these struggles, public health often holds the short end of the stick. Although opportunities and constraints will vary across countries and issues, and advocates need to be alert to the particular circumstances they confront, there are nevertheless a few simple lessons to be drawn from this research. To win, public health advocates need elite allies in and out of government, and they need a well-crafted message that resonates with their intended audience. Given those resources, seemingly unsuperable obstacles can be overcome, as shown by the recent success of New York City in reversing an entrenched epidemic of HIV/AIDS in injection drug users (Des Jarlais et al. 2005). The politics of public health are—as I hope this book has demonstrated—fundamental to the conquest of disease.

Notes

Chapter 1

1. McKeown's thesis was adopted enthusiastically by some social scientists, primarily for its scathing critique of Big Medicine's claims to responsibility for declining death rates (McKinlay and McKinlay 1977; McKinlay, McKinlay, and Beaglehole 1989). Although these authors make no bones about the political implications of their position, the lesson drawn in the publications cited is somewhat inconsistent with McKeown's essential rejection of human agency. In the view of McKinlay and colleagues, to refute the claims of Big Medicine was to make the case for social reform. In more recent work, McKinlay has joined the advocates of public health (McKinlay and Marceau 2000).

2. In work that harks back to McKeown, Link and Phelan have identified socioeconomic status as a fundamental cause of disease and death (Phelan et al. 2004, 265; see also Link and Phelan 1995). I would argue that public policies are critical in potentiating or mitigating the impact of socioeconomic status on public (as well as individual) health.

3. Comparative work on the environment includes Mary Douglas and Aaron Wildavsky (1982), David Vogel (1986), and Howard Kunreuther and Joanne Linerooth (1983). On HIV-AIDS, it includes David Kirp and Ronald Bayer (1992), Eric Feldman and Bayer (1999), and Peter Baldwin (2005a). On tobacco, it includes Donley Studlar (2002), Feldman and Bayer (2004), and Roddy Reid (2005).

4. In the words of its inventor, Max Weber, the function of the ideal type "is the comparison with empirical reality in order to establish its divergence or similarities, to describe them with the *most unambiguously intelligible concepts,* and explain them causally" (1949, 43, emphasis in original). The strong and weak state constructs are just such ideal types. (As should be self-evident from this explanation, "ideal" as used by Weber is not intended to be evaluative: one may construct ideal types of dictators or saints.)

Chapter 2

1. Greater knowledge of causes and cures has not, of course, eliminated the politicization of disease, as the subsequent narratives will amply illustrate.

2. Public health historians of both countries are in agreement on this point (see La Berge 1992; Pickstone 1982; Cooter 1983). Anthony Brundage describes how in 1840 a House of Commons Select Committee on the Health of Towns was deflected away from an inquiry into "the discontents of the working classes in populous districts" into the safer topic of working class public health (1988, 81).

3. To trace the origins of the highly pragmatic evangelism that characterized British public health reformers in the nineteenth century is beyond the scope of this project. It is important to note, however, that even before the 1860s and later, when this movement spread to the mayors and city councils of industrial towns, it had inspired the closely allied network of men whose writings and public appeals laid the groundwork for later events. Anthony Wohl writes,

> [the] opening phase of sanitary reform [in the 1840s] was . . . infused with the enthusiasm and moral fervour of a small group of men, well-known to one another, and approaching the work ahead of them with optimism and proselytizing zeal. Typical was the Metropolitan Health of Towns Association, which was formed in 1844. Inspired by Dr. Southwood Smith, a Benthamite and close associate of [Edwin] Chadwick's, it brought together political leaders and aspiring politicians . . . and [prominent] doctors. . . . The purpose of the Association was principally propaganda [for public health]. (1983, 144–45)

4. The story of how this happened—from Edwin Chadwick's landmark report *The Sanitary Condition of the Labouring Population of Great Britain* published in 1842 to the resignation of John Simon in 1876 as medical officer to the Privy Council—has been often and well told (see, for example, Flinn 1965; Lewis 1952; Wohl 1983; Brundage 1988). My purpose is limited to establishing the historical setting for the narratives that follow and highlighting the contrast between public health in Britain and France.

5. The Local Government [Board] Act of 1871 merged the activities of several existing bodies (the Poor Law Board, the Local Government Act Office, the Registrar-General's Office, and the Medical Office of the Privy Council) to create a centralized authority for public health in Britain. Subsequent acts, in 1872 and 1875, further refined and clarified the Board's responsibilities. The Local Government Board's (LGB) effectiveness in practice, however, was substantially limited by the act's placement of medical civil servants under lay authority (Brand 1965, 22). Local officials fearful of central government interference could—and sometimes did—refuse the LGB's money.

6. From about 1858, when John Simon—"the greatest of the Victorian medical officers" (Wohl 1983, 8)—assumed the post of medical officer to the Privy Council until Simon resigned in 1876 (an internal reorganization had substantially reduced his authority and political access), the role of the central government in public health increased continually. Simon was far more diplomatic than Chadwick had been and was able to nudge local governments into public health action without offending their well-developed sensitivities to any compromise of local autonomy. His tenure is described by Anthony Wohl as " 'the heroic age' of state medicine" in Britain (155). Although Simon

was something of a one-man show, the structure he left in place remained—
at least for a time. For a detailed account of Simon's career, see Royston
Lambert's *Sir John Simon, 1816–1904, and English Social Administration* (1963).

7. I am indebted to Gerald Oppenheimer for helping me articulate this point.

8. *Bulletin du syndicat de l'association des médecins du Rhône,* [May 1, 1901] (cited
in Hildreth 1987, 52).

9. Antagonism between elite, hospital-based consultants and general practitioners existed in Britain as well as France (Abel-Smith 1964, 101–18). British
consultants, however, were not identified with public health, as they were in
France. Support for public health among British practitioners was considerable, as I observe, and any antagonism was muted, at least relative to France.
British physicians' "thirst for professional unity . . . spread widely and encouraged compromises that everyone could live with" (Weisz 2003, 573).

10. Griscom met his fate in the 1840s, but the vulnerability of health officers to the
winds of local politics is a continuing story (see, for example, Leavitt 1976;
Anderson 1991).

11. This hypothesis does not help in accounting for U.S. differences with France,
of course. Nineteenth-century public health in France was more intellectual
than pragmatic, however, and it was in its religiously inspired pragmatism
that British public health was unique.

12. Other hypotheses advanced by Duffy are the very low status of American
physicians in the first half of the nineteenth century and the absorption of
reformers' energies by the abolition movement. The relatively low status of
French local practitioners in the early part of the nineteenth century did not
prevent public health ideas from appearing there, and to call on the abolition
movement as an explanation for the absence of other movements begs the
question. The comparative role of religious movements in nineteenth-century
public health is a large topic which I do little more here than open for further
investigation.

13. The subordination of economic expansion and (European) settlement to all
other considerations was especially devastating to the health of Canada's
native peoples, amounting to a policy not simply of disinterest but of deliberate and cynical neglect (Lux 2001).

14. The Canadian founding fathers could not, of course, have anticipated that by
the mid-twentieth century health—which they had dismissed as sufficiently
unimportant to be left to the provinces—was to become perhaps the greatest
subject of legislation.

15. My account of the evolution of public health activity in Toronto is very much
indebted to the work of Heather MacDougall (1990).

16. Without more detailed information it is impossible to know the role that
Hastings may have played in bringing about the political changes that strengthened his position. Had he done so, it would not be a surprise. More generally,
the history of Victorian and Progressive era public health offers other examples of individuals who, through fortuitous combinations of contemporary

ideology and politics with personal qualities of energy, ambition, and political savvy, advanced their own careers in parallel with the cause of public health. John Simon (England) and Hermann Biggs (United States) are examples.

17. The following description is based on a number of sources, principally Terry Copp (1974), Claudine Pierre-Deschênes (1981), and Martin Tétreault (1983). Given the enormous disparities in mortality between Toronto and Montreal in this period, it is striking how little has been written either to describe or explain them.

18. The principal authors of this critique appear to have been the francophone physicians of Montreal, organized into la Societé médicale de Montréal (Pierre-Deschênes 1981).

19. A recent history of the Montreal City Health Department by Benoit Gaumer and his colleagues states that the highly critical appraisals I have cited—along with a scathing evaluation by officials of the New York City Health Department published in 1917—are valid (Gaumer, Desroisers, and Keel 2002, 100–1). At the same time they argue—somewhat unconvincingly—that the health department did manage to accomplish a great deal in the face of enormous obstacles. These accomplishments were not reflected, however, in the city's death rates.

Chapter 3

1. The phrase "massacre of the innocents" is drawn from the title of chapter 2 of *Endangered Lives in Victorian Britain* by Anthony Wohl. *The New York Times* editorialized in 1876 on "the annual slaughter of little children" (Meckel 1990, 11). Although the status of infant mortality as an emotionally evocative "public problem" has waxed and waned over the past 150 years, it continues to be a principal indicator of social and economic development, particularly in developing countries (Masuy-Stroobant and Gourbin 1995, 63). The article cited is critical of this use, particularly in countries where new technologies allow increasing numbers of very small babies to survive. Increased survival in these cases, as they point out, does not necessarily mean better health.

2. Samuel Preston and Michael Haines offer a considered evaluation of the Massachusetts data: "By 1860, the Massachusetts death registration data were quite good . . . [However,] the population of Massachusetts was . . . more urban and industrial and had a higher percentage born abroad than the population of the country as a whole" (1991, 50). For these reasons, its "representativeness [of the United States as a whole] has been seriously questioned" (50). Preston and Haines estimate the U.S. IMR in 1900 at 150:1,000, higher than Massachusetts (141:1,000) but lower than England and Wales (154:1,000) or France (160:1,000).

3. As would be expected, infant mortality was associated inversely with income and social class; the difference between social class I and VIII was about 36 percent in 1895 and 1897 and 55 percent in 1910. Robert Woods and colleagues argue, however, that these differences "do not appear to have been of critical

importance in influencing either the timing of decline or the rate of change of infant mortality" (Woods, Watterson, and Woodward 1988, 365). Contemporaries clearly regarded infant mortality as a problem of the poor (Lambert 1963; Wohl 1983).

4. As Woods and colleagues point out, very similar arguments are "used by demographers who are studying Africa and Asia today, especially those relating to fertility and the education of women" (1989, 132).

5. Preston and Haines make the important point that mortality among the children of rural blacks in the South, where the majority of the black population then lived, was considerably more favorable than that of highly urbanized northern blacks (1991, 95). Overall, however, the mortality of black children was higher than that of the children not only of native-born but also of foreign-born white women, regardless of size of place.

6. Woods and his colleagues do not subject their data to multivariate analysis. It is possible that, had they done so, social class would have loomed larger as a predictor of infant mortality in late nineteenth-century England. Comparative analysis by Preston and Haines indicates that social class differentials in child mortality were substantially larger in England and Wales (1911) than in the United States (1900) (1991, 196–97).

7. Terry Copp presents a graph for the period 1897 to 1930 based on figures from the Annual Report of the Montreal Board of Health, 1900 to 1930 showing infant mortality rates through 1910 that are consistently above 250:1,000 (1974, 167).

8. The role of wealthy philanthropists (Nathan Strauss, for example, to whom I refer later) in actively supporting the campaign against infant mortality and other public health causes had no parallel in the other countries.

9. From at least the mid-nineteenth century on public health developments in England were "widely reported in the [U.S.] popular and medical press" (Meckel 1990, 16).

10. There is a large literature on the U.S. campaigns against infant mortality in the late nineteenth and early twentieth centuries. The principal sources for my own account are Richard Meckel (1990), Alisa Klaus (1993), Theda Skocpol (1992), and Seth Koven and Sonya Michel (1993).

11. American physicians had long been concerned with infants' high death rates from digestive disorders, particularly during the summer months. Yet bacterial contamination of the milk supply did not become an issue until the end of the nineteenth century. The new focus on infant feeding and the quality of milk was not driven primarily by the discoveries of Koch and Pasteur.

12. Meckel places little emphasis on the significant role of women in the campaign against infant mortality, and the comments he does make are decidedly patronizing, for example, women's entry into the public sphere is attributed to "a profound restlessness among turn-of-the-century middle-class women" (1990, 149).

13. Abraham Jacobi, an eminent U.S. pediatrician, had recommended milk stations as early as 1881. It took him eleven years, however, to find anyone willing to fund them.

14. Paul Starr observes that "the AMA itself agitated for a Cabinet-level department of health throughout the Progressive era" (1982, 185).

15. In these respects Biggs's career pattern closely follows that of John Simon, the most influential public health official in England in the latter part of the nineteenth century. Simon also maintained his elite private practice and his teaching appointments and moved among London's political and social elite.

16. Although New York City may have been in the forefront of public health reform, it was not so far ahead that it could not pave the way for the rest of the country. In a case originating in New York City, the right of boards of health to regulate the sale of milk within their jurisdictions was upheld by the U.S. Supreme Court in 1905. By 1921, 90 percent of U.S. cities over 100,000 had mandated pasteurization of their milk (Meckel 1990, 89).

17. Seth Koven and Sonya Michel argue that "the power of women's social action movements was inversely related to the range and generosity of state welfare benefits for women and children" (1990, 1079–80). Other scholars disagree with this analysis (see, for example, Thane 1991).

18. Demonstrating the cross-national reach of this emphasis on the education of mothers, the internal quotation is from George Newman, chief medical officer of the British Ministry of Health.

19. The American Association for the Study and Prevention of Infant Mortality was founded in 1909, about the same time as parallel associations in Britain and France. In addition, many existing organizations (for example, the National Conference on Charities and Corrections) moved to include mothers' education within their purview.

20. The Sheppard-Towner Act provided matching funds to states for maternal and infant "well-baby" clinics for education and disease prevention. States responded favorably, and Sheppard-Towner was responsible for the first such services in most of the South and the West.

21. For an excellent analysis of the effort to institute maternity insurance in the United States just before the end of World War I, and of the reasons for its failure, see Richard Meckel (1990, 178–99).

22. The principal source for this narrative is *La politique à l'égard de la petite enfance sous la IIIe République* by Catherine Rollet-Echalier (1990). Additional important sources include *Gender and the Politics of Social Reform in France, 1870–1914,* edited by Elinor Accampo, Rachel Fuchs, and Mary Lynn Stewart (1997) and *Every Child a Lion* by Alisa Klaus (1993).

23. Between 1870 and 1914, the percent of physicians in parliament ranged between 10 percent and 12 percent (forty-three to seventy-one individuals). Thirteen physicians served as cabinet ministers (Ellis 1990, 3–4). Many more were mayors, town and department council members, and other local officials.

24. Rollet estimates that between 1898 and 1914 approximately 10 percent of infants per year were placed with wet nurses (Rollet-Echalier 1990, 500). George Sussman's estimate is virtually identical, a little over 10 percent (1982, 167).

25. Data presented to the Academy of Medicine indicated that "in all departments, the mortality rate of children placed out to nurse was 55 to 70 percent" (Klaus 1993, 55). Whatever the reliability of these figures in detail, their impact on physicians and public officials was profound.

26. Sterilization of milk by boiling preceded the somewhat different process that came to be known as pasteurization (Steele 2000).

27. A detailed account of the larger political and social context surrounding the passage of the loi Roussel goes beyond the scope of this narrative. It was non-controversial, first, because it appeared to address the population crisis, second, because deputies could not agree on pro-natalist measures, and, third, because it did not engage much more fraught political, social, and religious issues that underlay the depopulation debate (Klaus 1993, 57).

28. Strauss was one of the few nonphysician politicians engaged in the campaign against infant mortality. As if to rectify this anomaly, he was elected to the Academy of Medicine in 1909.

29. Roussel and his compatriots were wholly focused on the rural countryside as the site of infant mortality and—in sharp contrast to their colleagues in the other three countries—virtually ignored the high mortality of infants in big cities.

30. The vast majority of Breton babies were bottle-fed (Rollet-Echalier 1990, 360).

31. Catherine Rollet describes the scale as a symbol of medical objectivity. It was also, of course, a way to measure, and critique, maternal compliance with doctors' orders.

32. Any attempt to summarize the story of public health action to combat infant mortality in Britain based on secondary sources is significantly complicated by the very different perspectives of this story's historians. There are marked (and often explicit) disagreements among these authors in emphasis, in interpretation, and—in a few cases—even in adduced facts. I have drawn principally on three books: Jane Lewis's *The Politics of Motherhood* (1980), Deborah Dwork's *War is Good for Babies and Other Young Children* (1987), and Lara Marks's, *Metropolitan Maternity: Maternal and Infant Welfare Services in Early Twentieth Century London* (1996), along with articles by Seth Koven (1993) and Pat Thane (1991). I have tried to thread my way through these conflicting arguments to produce as close to a fact-based narrative as possible.

33. The Boer War was not disastrous because the British lost; they did not lose. Winning, however, took three years, at a terrible financial and human cost. More important, it "jolted Victorian confidence in progress" and exacerbated fears of imperial decline (Speck 1993, 115).

34. As noted, evidence recently adduced suggests that working-class mothers in Britain at the time were considerably more likely than mothers on the continent to breast-feed their babies (see, in addition to references cited earlier, Thompson 1984).

35. Dwork observes that "the anti-tuberculosis campaign and the drive to reduce infant mortality from all causes intersected at one particular point: the milk supply" (1987, 62). Despite physicians' awareness that contaminated milk

posed the threat of diarrhea, discussions about cleaning up the milk supply took place almost entirely in the context of concern about tuberculosis transmission from cows to human infants (59–90).

36. Sanitary inspectors (invariably male) employed by the central government or by local authorities to investigate disease outbreaks, inspect the state of water and sewage systems, and investigate housing conditions were a prominent feature of British public health in the nineteenth century. The biographers of Edwin Chadwick and John Simon discuss the latter's concerns about how inspectors would be received by the tenants of Britain's urban slums. They appear, in fact, to have been surprisingly well received. In any case, the precedent they set for government-authorized "inspection" at the household level may have helped to pave the way for lady "health visitors."

37. The Midwives Act, passed in 1902, established a system of training and certification of midwives, which was to be compulsory for all new practitioners. An act to provide for the early notification of births so that arrangements could be made for the infant to be visited by a health visitor was first introduced in 1907. It was strongly opposed by the *BMA* and although the profession ultimately lost this fight, the Notification of Birth Act did not become compulsory until 1915.

38. French authorities had no such scruples despite their adherence to classic liberalism in other contexts.

39. In Britain "significant number[s] of women . . . could vote and hold office at the local level from the mid-nineteenth century" (Thane 1993, 350).

40. Relevant British legislation—for example, the Notification of Births Act—was often permissive rather than mandatory (at least initially). Thus, local government action was required for implementation, and women could play an important role in pushing local governments to take action.

41. "Highly organized feminist movements" existed in Britain before World War I—the Fabian Women's Group, the Women's Cooperative Guild, and the Women's Labour League (Pedersen 1993, 55). The primary focus of these movements, however, was on obtaining benefits for mothers, not on saving babies.

42. Cynthia Comacchio describes the "Canadian response to infant mortality" prior to "the years immediately preceding World War One" as "one of resignation, at times even Darwinian, grounded in the notion of 'survival of the fittest' " (1993, 17).

43. A poster displayed at an exposition devoted to infant welfare held in Montreal in 1912 read as follows: "le voix de l'enfant s'élève contre vous! L'année dernière 5,355 enfants sont décédés à Montréal. Les deux tiers de ces morts auraient pu être évitées. Que ferez-vous pour enrayer ce fléau? [The voice of the baby is raised against you! Last year 5,355 babies died in Montreal. Two-thirds of these deaths could have been prevented. What will you do to prevent this tragedy?]"

44. Following the same pattern, in 1912 the Toronto chapter of the Canadian Association for the Prevention of Tuberculosis gave up its charter on the grounds that its work could now be done by the health department.

45. Among the most prominent were Dr. E. P. Lachapelle, who directed the provincial Bureau de médecine from 1877 to 1907 and in 1887 founded the Conseil d'hygiène de la province de Québec, which he directed until his death in 1918 (Pierre-Deschênes 1981, 360–61). Dr. Louis Laberge, as I noted earlier, headed the Montreal Health Department from 1885 until 1913. Note that these physicians' tenures straddled the shift from miasmas to germs as dominant theories of disease causation.

46. From the first, in 1900, the city health department published infant mortality rates by a combination of religion and ethnicity: French-Canadian, other Catholic, Protestant, and Jewish.

47. For example, conditions were sometimes imposed—for example, mothers without their babies in tow could not get milk—and evening hours when fathers might be available to stay with the children were disallowed in deference to middle-class women reformers' belief that a woman's place in the evening was at home with her family (Baillargeon 1996, 43).

Chapter 4

1. The only country with reasonably reliable mortality data for the nineteenth century is the United Kingdom. Gillian Cronje reports that over one-third of deaths from tuberculosis in England and Wales between 1851 and 1910 were in the fifteen to thirty-four age group (1984, 83). The ages of peak pulmonary tuberculosis mortality rose from twenty to twenty-four for males and twenty-five to thirty-four for females from 1851 to 1860 to forty-five to fifty-four for males and thirty-five to forty-four for females from 1901 to 1910 (90).

2. These commonalities do not, of course, represent independent developments. There was substantial communication among medical professionals in the form of cross-national visits by medical delegations, international meetings, journal subscriptions, study abroad (for example, elite American doctors studying in Germany), and the like.

3. Other preventive measures adopted at various stages in each country included preventing transmission of bovine tuberculosis and BCG vaccination. However, notification and quarantine were the most salient issues at the turn of the century and well illustrate the important cross-national differences.

4. The apparent difference between British and North American TB mortality rates does not reflect the limitation of the North American rates to large cities. The reported tuberculosis mortality rate for London in the period from 1891 to 1900 was 180/100,000 (Hardy 1993, 218).

5. Starr points out that New York City "was no microcosm of America" and that public health overall was underdeveloped in the United States. Nevertheless, he argues and I agree that, "The experience in New York is significant precisely because, as an exceptional case, it discloses some of the political constraints limiting public health at its boldest" (Starr 1982, 185). New York served as a model for the rest of the country and is important as well for its striking contrast with the experience of other European cities, including London and Paris.

6. There is disagreement among medical historians on the extent to which an attack on "the germ" replaced social reform in the goals of antituberculosis workers (see Lerner 1998, 3). Feldberg states that "by 1915, medical reformers repeatedly argued that it was useless to treat tuberculosis independently of poverty" (1995, 104). Richard Harrison Shryock's history of the National Tuberculosis Association suggests that though poverty and the need for social reform (for example, replacement of crowded tenements, provision for health insurance) were surely discussed by antituberculosis campaigners, no effort was made to confront these problems in any serious way: the association "continued to carry on within the existing social order" (1957, 99).

7. Biggs's remarks were entirely consistent with the thinking of major leaders of the Progressive movement. Jane Addams, for example, stated that: "A new form of social control is slowly establishing itself on the principle, so widespread in contemporary government, that the state has a responsibility for conditions which determine the health and welfare of its own members; that it is in the interests of social progress itself that hard-won liberties must be restrained by the demonstrable needs of society" (Addams 1913, 206). Lest it be thought that this thinking has disappeared, newspaper reports of arrests for noncompliance with TB medication regimes appeared as recently as 1994 (*Baltimore Sun,* "It's Medicine or Jail Time for Those with TB," November 26, 1994, p. 3A).

8. The foregoing quotation is from a letter from Lawrence Flick to one of his colleagues, cited in Richard Shryock (1957, 112). Nancy Tomes quotes from a physician's 1909 address on TB prevention to a group in Pennsylvania: "The antituberculosis campaign has in it much of the fervor of a new religion" (1998, 114).

9. This was far from an unusual pattern. Some of the most active advocates against tuberculosis in the United States had themselves been diagnosed with the disease.

10. Tomes quotes the popular writer Samuel Hopkins Adams as saying, "How any citizen of Wisconsin, unless he is a real badger and lives in a burrow, can escape getting his chance to purchase a seal and thus contribute his cent to the cause is difficult to imagine" (1998, 122).

11. The social constructions I describe are, more accurately, social constructions of social constructions. They are social and medical historians' readings of what is undoubtedly a highly selective historical record. Thus, nineteenth-century accounts undoubtedly overrepresent the experience of "interesting" middle-class and literate invalids, whereas twentieth-century accounts may overrepresent the poor who came to the attention of public clinics, hospitals, and sanatoria.

12. The enormity of the gap between blacks and whites was recognized by authorities at the time (McBride 1991; Ott 1996; Smith 1995; Gamble 1989; Brandt 1903). In the death "registration area," which excluded the South, where nearly 80 percent of the black population lived, the rate for blacks was 485:100,000 compared to 174:100,000 for whites. Although, as I have observed, tuberculosis came to be perceived as a disease of the immigrant and the poor, there

were no comparable data on tuberculosis death rates by social class. Indeed, insofar as data were available, they indicated that the "relative mortality of different immigrant elements could not be correlated with poverty" (Shryock 1957, 64). Race rather than (as in England, for example) social class became the defining demographic identifier, regularly attached to patient records and to public health reports of mortality and morbidity.

13. Villemin's conclusion that tuberculosis was contagious was rejected first in 1865, as I have stated, and again in 1889 (post-Koch). Mandatory notification of tuberculosis cases to public health authorities was rejected by the academy in 1902 and again in 1913. In 1919 mandatory notification was proposed by Premier Georges Clemenceau and was rejected by the National Assembly.

14. Following America's entry into World War I, considerable alarm about France's high rates of tuberculosis and the lack of action to address the problem was voiced by observers from the United States. The result was organization by the Rockefeller Foundation's International Health Board of an antituberculosis mission to France. During the period of its activity in France (1917 to 1923), the foundation vastly increased the infrastructure for tuberculosis management—dispensaries, sanatorium and hospital beds, health visitors (an innovation in France). Guillaume presents data indicating, for example, that the number of sanatorium beds increased from 1,162 in 1917 to nearly 20,000 in 1923! (Guillaume 1986, 195–96). The period following the Foundation's departure in 1923 is outside my chronological purview. A British historian of tuberculosis observes, however, that the "French ethical dilemma on the infectivity of tuberculosis effectively paralysed prevention action until the 1960s" (Hardy 1993, 257, fn. 228).

15. Reactions of Academy of Medicine physicians to the publicity in the lay press that surrounded the first international conference on tuberculosis held in Paris in 1888 are striking evidence of French medical paternalism. Academicians regarded the publicity as unwanted interference in medical debate, fraught with danger to the status of the medical profession as the sole arbiter of medical knowledge (Guillaume 1986, 121). After heated debate, a set of instructions warning of TB's contagiousness and recommending a series of precautions was published in 1890, but only in the academy's weekly *Bulletin,* not for public consumption (Mitchell 1988, 218).

16. Calmette is best known for his role in the invention of B.C.G. (Bacille Calmette Guérin), the only vaccine available against tuberculosis.

17. The most famous of these endeavors was l'oeuvre Grancher. Grancher, a physician, undertook to send unaffected children from families with tuberculosis into homes or institutions in the country. Between 1903 and 1923 2,500 Parisian children were so placed. The program proved popular in other parts of the country as well (Guillaume 1986, 189). Other such efforts targeted children with tuberculosis or appear to have been directed simply at children considered vulnerable by virtue of poverty, living conditions, or for other reasons.

18. Reflecting the many ideological splits among French doctors at the time, the main tenets of the syndicalist argument were developed by radical physicians.

19. Note the striking contrast with Biggs's remarks, cited in the U.S. TB narrative. Libertarian rhetoric depends very much on whose ox will be gored when the state intervenes. It seems very likely that Russell had in mind notification's impact on the patients of private physicians, whereas Biggs was thinking of poor and voiceless immigrants to New York City.

20. Both income relief (welfare) and medical care were provided to the indigent under the Poor Law system. Local boards of guardians operating under the authority of the central Local Government Board appointed district medical officers with the responsibility of treating the sick poor at home or in dispensaries. Poor Law relief was highly stigmatized—the Poor Laws "reflected the view that poverty demonstrated a personal failing and alms were likely to contribute to the shortcomings of the poor." Recipients had little power to influence their treatment (Hollingsworth 1986, 14).

21. It is worth noting that neither sexually transmitted infections nor AIDS are reportable diseases in Britain: "there are no requirements for quarantine or public notification" (Street and Weale 1992, 191–92; UK Health Protection Agency 2005). Voluntary reporting, however, appears to be fairly complete.

22. The full history of tuberculosis sanatoria is well beyond the scope of this book. Their value as a so-called cure for tuberculosis or even as a preventive measure to isolate individuals with tuberculosis from the larger population is thought to have been extremely limited (Smith 1988; McFarlane 1989). Neil McFarlane states that the sanatorium entitlement remained largely on paper; it was rescinded in 1921, leaving tuberculosis prevention and treatment in the hands of local authorities. The National Health Insurance (NHI) plan, pushed through by Lloyd George in 1911 against considerable opposition from the medical profession, insured manual workers between the ages of sixteen and sixty-five, but not their dependents, against the costs of general practitioner (GP) but not hospital services (Hollingsworth 1986). Francis Smith maintains that the addition of the sanatorium benefit to the NHI plan "pacified" insured workers who might otherwise have agitated for social reform instead of sanatoria (1988, 245).

23. Smith argues that "a coterie of medical practitioners captured the tuberculosis specialty in the late 1880s and thereafter set the terms by which the disease was comprehended" (1988, 245). The leader of this coterie, Sir Robert Philip, was influential in the NAPT's failure to endorse either pasteurization or BCG vaccination until after World War II.

24. Jay Cassel asserts that "no lay people . . . had a major influence on the development of ideas about health reform in this period" and that "the promoters of public health measures were first and foremost physicians and other specialists" (1994, 284). Katherine McQuaig's detailed analysis of the antituberculosis campaign in Canada after 1900 would seem to contradict these assertions, unless Cassel is referring exclusively to the development of ideas rather than to advocacy and social action.

25. Canadian perspectives on the role of government were and are driven more by pragmatic than by ideological considerations. In the late nineteenth century, economic development was viewed by Canadian political and business

elites as an urgent necessity; a strong central government prepared to underwrite railroad building, immigration, and related economic activity was the key to realization of this project. Health and welfare were distinctly secondary, left to private initiative. Once the prevalence of tuberculosis and other diseases was recognized as a major public problem, however, the ideological obstacles to government intervention were relatively few, certainly as compared with the United States.

26. The highest recorded rates of tuberculosis were among French-Canadians in Quebec and, in particular, in Montreal (Tétreault 1983) and among Canadian Indians (Grygier 1994). Rates among immigrants were virtually impossible to determine. Toward the end of the period I cover, around 1920, Canadian public health authorities as well as interested laity began to recognize that high rates also existed in rural areas (Baldwin 1990).

Chapter 5

1. From a political and policy perspective, the relationship between what we now refer to as passive smoking or environmental tobacco smoke and lung cancer has been at least as important as the direct relationship between smoking and disease; this relationship plays a major role in my subsequent analysis. However, the relationship was accepted by advocates and by some policy makers considerably before it was established scientifically, although it is now widely accepted (U.S. Department of Health and Human Services 2006). The relationship is statistically weak, however, and there continue to be dissenting voices (see, for example, Barnes and Bero 1998; Dockery and Trichopoulos 1997; Hackshaw, Law, and Wald 1997).

2. For a comprehensive history of tobacco focused primarily on the seventeenth through the late nineteenth and early twentieth centuries, see Jordan Goodman (1993). All four countries had transient antitobacco movements around the turn of the century. The U.S. movement was the most long-lived and politically influential, leading to laws prohibiting the sale of cigarettes to minors and to laws against the manufacture and sale of cigarettes in at least eleven states (Troyer 1984). By 1927, however, the laws banning cigarettes had been repealed and even the U.S. movement was dead.

3. Catherine Hill gives a considerably higher underreporting estimate for France, from 15 to 45 percent (1998). An analysis published in 2000 in the *Bulletin Épidémiologique Hebdomadaire* suggests that sales figures may also underestimate consumption. These figures take no account of accommodation to increased cigarette prices such as black market purchases and the use of roll-your-own cigarettes.

4. Given the evidence that smoking is underreported in surveys, there are two alternative explanations for the observation: that French men now smoke substantially more than their counterparts in the other three countries or that French men are more willing to report that they smoke. Although reporting may play some role, the consumption data suggest that there is a real difference in smoking patterns between France and the other countries.

5. Survey data underreport overall consumption, but they remain the best available source of information on within-country variation in smoking habits by sociodemographic characteristics.

6. The sources cited present data on smoking prevalence by education in the United States and Canada, by occupation in the UK, and by education and occupation in France. By 2004 there was relatively little variation by education in Canada except relative to the "completed university" level, where prevalence was down to 14 percent.

7. Trends in lung cancer mortality are the principal determinants of overall cancer mortality trends in developed countries (Lopez 1995). Cardiovascular disease is responsible for nearly twice as many deaths as lung cancer, and while it is clear that smoking plays an important role in CVD, the relative contribution of smoking is far less clear in the case of CVD than of lung cancer (Hunink et al. 1997). Consequently, I have chosen to focus on lung cancer as the principal marker for smoking's danger to the public health.

8. This narrative is a much revised and abbreviated version of material that appeared in an earlier paper, "Social Movements as Catalysts for Policy Change: The Case of Smoking and Guns" (1999).

9. The surgeon general was also required to issue legislative recommendations. There is little evidence of these recommendations in the reports. Richard Kluger tells us that recommendations to ban smoking in enclosed public places inserted by Surgeon General Jesse Steinfeld were "regularly removed by Nixon's Office of Management and Budget" (1996, 366).

10. Between 1966 and 1976, Congress specifically excluded tobacco from regulation under five different statutes: the Fair Packaging and Labeling Act (1966); the Controlled Substances Act (1970); the Consumer Product Safety Act (1972); the Federal Hazardous Substances Act (1976); and the Toxic Substances Control Act (1976).

11. For a far more detailed and very lively account of these events, see Martha Derthick's book, *Up in Smoke* (2005). There is much in her analysis with which I disagree, but the book is an excellent resource on the tobacco dramas of the 1990s.

12. The Interagency Council on Smoking and Health, formed in 1964, was a loose grouping of public and private organizations interested in the smoking-and-health issue (the health voluntaries, professional societies, the Public Health Service, the Children's Bureau). The council was the forerunner to CDC's Office on Smoking and Health, established in the early 1980s.

13. The contrast between the government's reaction and that of the public was sharp. Jesse Steinfeld states that "this call for a nonsmokers' rights movement was not looked upon approvingly within the Office of the Secretary of HEW [but] it brought forth a blizzard of mail with an overwhelmingly favorable response" (1983, 1258).

14. Duke did not confine his activities to the United States. He was active and highly successful in opening overseas markets, first in China and later in India. By 1898, "according to one estimate, one-third of Duke's production of

cigarettes was exported," over half of it to China (Goodman 1993, 234). Marketing cigarettes to developing countries is by no means a recent industry innovation.

15. In his 2001 book, *The Fight Against Big Tobacco*, Mark Wolfson raises—and answers affirmatively—the question of whether tobacco-control efforts can still, in the twenty-first century, be described as a social movement. What was surely a grassroots social movement for nonsmokers' rights at its inception has become institutionalized within the public health establishment and, as Wolfson points out, "interpenetrated" by the state (2001, 7). I question, however, whether, as Wolfson argues, this latter phase represents a new model of state-movement relations. Apart perhaps from the passion of its advocates, tobacco control in the United States is now no more a social movement than such other accepted public health activities as venereal disease control or maternal and child health, or than state-centered tobacco control as practiced in, say, France.

16. Michael Pertschuk observes that Lane Adams, the CEO of ACS during much of the period in question, decreed "a flat ban on *any* activist advocacy" (2001, 54).

17. Between 1960 and 1975, the lung cancer mortality rates of white males born between 1901 and 1910 quadrupled and those for white males born between 1911 and 1920 increased by a factor of eight (HHS 1991, 92).

18. Of the seven early nonsmokers' rights activists I interviewed, three had close relatives who died from causes the activists attributed to smoking, and two had previously been active in related social movement or public interest organizations.

19. "Maybe part of the secret of [GASP's] success," Clara Gouin observed when I interviewed her in 1995, "was that it was never thoroughly organized. Sometimes you have a good idea and in the beginning stages there is great enthusiasm, and then once the idea gets structured into rules, regulations, formal dues, offices, and all of that, it loses a bit of its initial impetus. . . . [People in the movement now] didn't have to join a group and carry a banner. When you feel you're alone, you have to join a group. You don't need little organizations when everybody's doing it."

20. This is a revised and condensed version of my chapter, "*Liberté, Egalité, Fumée:* Smoking and Tobacco Control in France," originally published in *Unfiltered: Conflicts Over Tobacco Policy and Public Health,* edited by Eric Feldman and Ronald Bayer (Nathanson 2004).

21. This sequence of events was described to me by Professor Tubiana and confirmed by other accounts.

22. The official title is *Loi no 76-616 du 9 juillet 1976 relative à la lutte contre le tabagisme.*

23. The sensitivity of the price issue was reflected in the 1976 parliamentary debate on the Veil law. Mme. Veil noted that the government had rejected an increase in tobacco prices, observing that a massive increase in prices would amount to "shocking" discrimination based on wealth. In his response, a member noted the "illogic" of condemning tobacco while at the same time selling cigarettes

at "dumping" prices and distributing an even cheaper monthly cigarette ration to members of the military (France 1976).

24. The official title is *Loi no 91-32 du 10 janvier 1991 relative à la lutte contre le tabagisme et l'alcoolisme*.

25. Cinq sages was a label initially applied to these five doctors by the media. It may be translated as five wise men, but sage also means well behaved: a good child is sage. Thus, the term has a perhaps intentional double meaning when used in the context of alcohol and tobacco control.

26. The loi Evin called for evaluations of the law's operation to be prepared by the government and presented to Parliament in 1993 and 1995. This was not done. However, a full-scale evaluation was initiated in 1997 and completed in October 1999. In the course of this evaluation testimony was received from a very wide range of interested parties, existing research was reviewed, and additional research was commissioned. This evaluation, authored by the Commissariat général du plan, Conseil national de l'évaluation, was published in 2000 under the title *La loi relative à la lutte contre le tabagisme et l'alcoolisme*. It is an authoritative source for French perspectives on tobacco control in France.

27. The very different perspectives on these points of three knowledgeable French observers whom I consulted suggests that extreme caution should be exercised in jumping to interpretive conclusions.

28. Claude Got was a professor of anatomy at one of the Paris hospitals and frequent consultant to the French government on a wide range of public health issues. Some indication of his stature is the fact that he was invited by the government to do the first overall report on AIDS in France, just after the French blood scandal broke (Got 1989). He has also published a wide-ranging book on the current state of public health in France (1992). Got had a brief stint as a civil servant in the Office of the Minister of Health in the early 1980s. Dubois was a professor of public health in Amiens and advisor to the French system of national health insurance. Based outside of Paris and in public health rather than one of the medical specialties, he ranks considerably below Got on the French scale of medical prestige. Dubois received his public health training in the early 1970s at the Johns Hopkins School of Hygiene and Public Health.

29. Hirsch saw this report as the French equivalent of the Royal College and Surgeon General's reports: "Nothing new, of course, but new in this country. [It was] the first one in France and in French." Interestingly, the report had almost nothing to say about what was essentially non-implementation of the Veil law's provisions on smoking in places open to the public.

30. There is a dual problem here because though French scientists are reluctant to address the issue of smoking and health in their own research, they were for many years unwilling to accept the results of research from other countries as being applicable to France.

31. In a bow to French sensibilities, the president of CNCT has always been a physician. But the organization is run by its executive director who, during the period of my observation, was a lay militant with no medical training.

32. That CNCT had been burned is reflected in Hirsch's statement to the commission evaluating the Evin law: "C'est au Parquet, et non plus aux associations, à faire respecter l'inderdiction de la publicité et des promotions en faveur du tabac [It is up to the Justice Ministry, not to associations, to ensure respect for (the law's) advertising prohibitions]" (Commissariat général du plan 2000, 371). Industry representatives' submissions to the commission uniformly suggested that CNCT's primary interest was in feathering its own nest (see, for example, 533).

33. The quote is from an interview with Luc Bihl, one of the lawyers for CNCT and a smoker, conducted by a member of the CNCT staff ("Entretien avec Luc Bihl realisé par Lise Mingasson le 15 avril 1995," *Tabac et Santé* 135[1995], n.p.). This interpretation of the meaning of cigarettes and smoking is by no means unique to M. Bihl, however. I suggested this characterization of the contrast between French attitudes about illegal drugs and the "legal drug" tobacco, to a meeting of French demographers, including at least one highly respected expert on French smoking practices, Alfred Nizard. These scholars confirmed my interpretation.

34. The state's responsibility for individual medical care in the case of illness is, of course, taken for granted.

35. In a striking instance of smoking's political positioning on the left, an article in the journal *Libération* explained the failure of legislation to ban smoking in all public places on the grounds that if the (conservative) party in power had allowed this (private) bill on the floor, it would have risked 13 million smokers "a fag in one hand, a ballot in the other" electing a "left wing president in 2007" (Ecoiffier 2006).

36. Among the notable aspects of this debate is its elevated philosophical tone. Both sides draw on central themes in French political thought: on the one hand, the necessity for individuals to resist the encroachment of an oppressive, authoritarian state; on the other, the state's responsibilities to act on behalf of the common good, to protect its citizens and to erase—or at least address— social inequalities. The contradictory nature of these ideas—the state as oppressive authority vs. the state as benevolent parent—should be self-evident. Steven Lukes has a highly relevant discussion of the problematic nature of the concept of individualisme in French social and political thought (1973).

37. The quote is from an essay by a young woman fired from her job for complaining about environmental tobacco smoke. It was reprinted in *Tabac et santé*.

38. This report, *Smoking and Health Now*, was unsparing in its condemnation of the government: "Ministers, without reference to the fatal effects of cigarette smoking or to the economic loss it occasions, have stated that the large revenue from taxation provided by undiminished sales of cigarettes is indispensable" (Royal College of Physicians of London 1971, 2).

39. "I do not believe that the agreement with the tobacco industry is entirely voluntary," said one member of Parliament in debate. "When a Minister goes to an industry and says that he wants an understanding, that he wants some progress . . . the industry knows that he has in his pocket proposals for

legislation, or rules, or regulations which in effect, say that if the industry does not do what the Government wants, the result will be achieved by the use of compulsory powers" (United Kingdom 1976, 866). The industry knows with equal certainty that the minister does not want to legislate.

40. The British commitment to depoliticizing potentially explosive policy issues through gentlemanly negotiation among insiders may have protected the demon tobacco industry; however, it protected injection drug users as well, creating an environment that made possible the emergence of "harm minimization" policies relatively early in the AIDS epidemic, as I describe in chapter 6.

41. It is striking that in parliamentary debate, no defender of smoking as a working-class pleasure ever raised this question of the differential impact on the rich and the poor of what is essentially a flat tax. Alan Marsh and Stephen McKay, authors of *Poor Smokers*, an analysis and interpretation of this differential impact based on a government-funded sample survey of 2,200 low income families, commented: "It is easy to put up the price of cigarettes, within reason. Governments always like to be seen to be 'doing something' about a national health problem, and they have no objection to a course that also increases short term tax revenues" (1994, 81). They argued, however, that "if the purpose of tobacco taxation is to stop smoking most effectively among those who really cannot afford to smoke and who have most to gain by giving up, this policy is not working" (81).

42. Richard Doll was the lead author on the British doctor studies demonstrating the association between smoking and lung cancer (see Doll and Hill 1950, 1954).

43. Implicit in Fletcher's comments is that public response is conditional on government action. This belief shapes British advocacy, directing it far more exclusively toward the government than is the case of health-related advocacy in the United States.

44. Simpson described ASH's relationship with the Health Education Authority as that of a "manoeuvrable frigate, with limited firepower but able to move in and out of various issues [with a] more ponderous capital ship, much better armed with money for media programmes, but less manoeuvrable" and more responsive to the whims of government ministers (Simpson 1998, 209).

45. I remind the reader that in the British system funding appropriations are the prerogative of the executive not, as in the United States, the legislative branch. Parliament may raise objections in various forms, but it has no veto over these decisions.

46. A former civil servant in the Ministry of Health suggested to me that caution on the part of pressure groups was the intended effect of giving them money. "From the government point of view it's a good idea to give pressure groups money because it cuts them off from the more radical constituency, which we don't have to deal with, and it keeps them a little bit careful" (Interview, May 1995).

47. The BMA's actual power in the early 1980s is subject to conflicting accounts. On the one hand, Margaret Thatcher's reorganization of the National Health Service to become more market-driven compromised the profession's authority

both substantively and symbolically. Neither the BMA nor the Royal Colleges were consulted in a reorganization that put substantially greater power in the hands of lay health managers (Wilsford 1995). On the other hand, these actions on the part of the government had a powerful effect in radicalizing and mobilizing the BMA. There was a rapid increase in membership from 47 percent of active physicians in 1977 to 72 percent in the 1980s, and an increase in collective action, including strikes and demonstrations (Grant 1995; Kingdom 1991).

48. The reasons for this delay, and for the BMA's change of heart are not wholly clear. However, they appear to bear close resemblance to a pattern also exemplified by the American Cancer Society. The BMA's representative body had passed antitobacco resolutions regularly since 1965. However, its directors clearly regarded the tobacco issue as a highly sensitive one, and were unprepared to take direct action until it was perceived to be relatively safe to do so. "Now, with the British cigarette market in decline, public opinion perceptibly changing and BMA leaders more receptive to the idea of campaigning, [the BMA's press officer and parliamentary lobbyist] thought the balance was swinging in favour of a major campaign" (British Medical Association 1986, 4).

49. The word "appears" is used advisedly. Given the British government's secretive modus operandi it is difficult to know what goes on behind the scenes (see, for example, my earlier description of the genesis of the first RCP report on smoking).

50. The Independent Scientific Committee on Smoking and Health, for example, met throughout the 1970s, focusing primarily on the development of a safer cigarette—an approach strongly opposed by the RCP and ASH, which took the position that the only safe smoking was no smoking.

51. This account of Phase One would be incomplete without reference to the publication in 1974 of the Lalonde report under the auspices of the Canadian federal Minister of Health Marc Lalonde (1974). In its focus on lifestyle behaviors (including smoking) as causes of ill health this report was highly influential in fueling, at least in the United States, a turn by health policy experts away from environmental (for example, poverty) and structural (for example, unequal access to medical care) models of disease causation to models that emphasized personal habits thought to be under the individual's control (Nathanson 1999). This was something of a distortion of the report. It stressed environmental as well as lifestyle factors and, more importantly, was a call for greater federal involvement in the health arena. In Canada, Christopher Manfredi and Antonia Maioni observed, the report "inspired a new focus on health promotion within the federal government, including life-style changes like smoking cessation that would enhance health outcomes" (2004, 79). It did not, however, immediately inspire new legislation. As finance minister in 1983, Lalonde himself opposed tax increases to reduce smoking (cited in Cunningham 1996, 122).

52. As is the usual practice in parliamentary government, most bills are introduced by the government and are, in effect, proposed laws (Forsey 1988). Although any MP may introduce a bill, private bills have much less chance of making it through the Parliamentary system.

53. A Canadian civil servant who has followed the tobacco story from its inception argues that the alleged increases in consumption following the tax rollback have been considerably exaggerated and were, in any case, temporary.

54. Cunningham observes that federal aid to help farmers exit from tobacco farming was "easily the most expensive part of the government's comprehensive tobacco-control policy announced in 1987" and "was critical in assisting passage of the TPCA [Tobacco Products Control Act]" (Cunningham 1996, 187). This aid allowed the agricultural minister to stand by quietly while the health minister promoted advertising bans and other regulatory measures.

55. *Webster's Unabridged Dictionary* defines zealot as "one who engages warmly in any cause and pursues his object with earnestness and ardor." This is a fair description of lay tobacco control advocates I interviewed in the United States and Canada. A zealot may be a fanatical partisan (and some were), but the term is not limited to fanatics. A common characteristic of the lay zealots with whom I spoke was single-mindedness.

56. In 1974, the membership list of the U.S.-based GASP (Group Against Smokers' Pollution) included two Canadian affiliates. Rob Cunningham states that in the early 1970s "dozens of local antismoking groups" sprouted up across the country (1996, 110).

57. The Canadian medical profession has neither the political power nor the cultural authority of its British and French counterparts. This difference is due in part to the structure of Canadian federalism that assigns responsibility for medical care to the provinces and in part to a sixty-year history of state-professional battles over questions of professional autonomy and authority, battles which the profession almost invariably lost (Cassel 1994).

58. Insider strategies focus on members of the government: MPs, members of Congress, civil servants, administrative agencies, the judiciary. Outsider strategies focus on appeals to the public through the mass media, staged large informational conferences open to the public, speakers at conventions and other events, and protest demonstrations (Walker 1991, 192).

59. In a celebratory photograph following passage of Canada's major tobacco-control legislation in 1988 not a single physician is shown or listed as being present.

60. Canadian tobacco legislation is explicit in giving provinces this "ratcheting up" power (Grossman and Price 1992, 3–8). This is in sharp contrast to the United States, where federal tobacco statutes explicitly preempt stronger state action.

61. Rochon is a physician with training in public health. He had worked in WHO with Neil Collishaw, and so was well-versed in Canadian tobacco politics before coming to office.

62. As described by coalition staff, Rochon went directly to their member organizations and said, "Attack me, please!"

63. Heidi Rathjen, former head of the gun-control coalition, was brought in to co-direct the antitobacco coalition by its co-founder, Louis Gauvin, who was

and continues to be employed by the Quebec Department of Health. The gun-control coalition had worked well with the provincial health authorities.

64. The coalition adopted a "kinder, gentler" approach for two reasons: first, it operated initially in a far more hostile political and media environment than that experienced by the national NSRA; second, it acts as the representative of 750 provincial organizations that have signed on to its mission. It should be emphasized that the local representative of the NSRA works very closely with the small (three-person) coalition staff. Essentially, these four individuals are the tobacco-control movement in Quebec.

65. Neil Collishaw, the civil servant who worked most closely with Epp on the TPCA, states that "The Catalogue of Deception" was among the most powerful lobbying tools he had ever seen. Indeed, Collishaw had encouraged NSRA to produce the report and supplied some of the information it contained. (Interview, March 6, 2002).

66. The first quotation is from the *Catalogue of Deception*. The second is from a report dated June 1996, and titled simply *Prime Minister*. Besides the NSRA, the signatories of the second report include the Canadian Council on Smoking and Health, the Canadian Dental Association, the Canadian Medical Association, the Canadian Pharmaceutical Association, the Ontario Medical Association, Physicians for a Smoke-Free Canada, and The Lung Association.

67. This quotation is from debate in the Ontario parliament on the Smoking in the Workplace Act of 1989. Much the same arguments privileging the fetus as the victim of secondhand smoke had been put forward on behalf of the federal Non-Smokers' Health Act.

Chapter 6

1. In his *Histoire du sida*, Mirko Grmek (1995) cites thirteen scientific publications between June and December, 1981, the majority in journals with wide international circulation (these included, besides *MMWR*, *Lancet*, and *The New England Journal of Medicine*). Eight of these articles were by American and five by European investigators. Grmek further confirms the instant attention these communications received in France (58).

2. The *New York Times* published its first account, by its medical reporter, physician Lawrence K. Altman, on July 3, 1981, one day before the second CDC report in *MMWR*.

3. To avoid constant repetition, I now and then shorten the phrase "HIV/AIDS in injection drug users" to "AIDS-drugs."

4. One of these early reports describes half (seven) of the cases seen by the authors as "drug abusers," but this connection was lost in later 1981 reports. The reasons for this nearly exclusive initial focus on male homosexuals has been extensively analyzed and discussed (for example, Oppenheimer 1988; Epstein 1996).

5. It is instructive to read these early reports. The human immunodeficiency virus (HIV) that attacks immune-system cells and thus allows opportunistic

infections to take hold was not discovered until 1983, and these authors were largely baffled by what they were seeing: neither Kaposi's sarcoma nor Pneumocystis pneumonia were expected to occur in young, previously healthy, individuals. Death rates among these individuals were "fearfully high" (Durack 1981, 1465). With the exception of one group, who did suggest that what they were seeing was "the tip of the iceberg . . . the evolution of a new syndrome of epidemic proportions" (Friedman-Kien 1981, 470), there was more evidence of curiosity than alarm.

6. The original case definition for AIDS developed by CDC was rather narrow and has broadened considerably over time: however, the definition currently used in Europe is somewhat different from that in the United States. Further, "under-recognition of AIDS cases by the healthcare system and the completeness and timeliness of reporting of identified cases by the surveillance system" are significant problems (Low-Beer et al. 1998, 298). These authors estimate that in industrialized countries about 80 percent of AIDS cases are reported. The accuracy and completeness of reporting of AIDS as a cause of death is lower: "Even in the United States, reported deaths may underestimate current AIDS related mortality by 15–35 per cent in young men and 20–45 per cent in young women" (310).

7. This figure shows the incidence of AIDS relative to the total population. To show the incidence of AIDS among injection drug users would require data on the size of the drug using population in each country. These data do not exist in any form useful for cross-national comparison.

8. In principle, incidence of HIV infection would better measure the progress of the epidemic. Much as was the case with tuberculosis reporting, however, and for similar reasons, HIV reporting has been highly controversial and has only recently begun to be implemented on any scale. In none of the four countries are reports of HIV infection sufficiently complete or reliable over time to make them useful measures for comparative purposes.

9. In reality, AIDS is not a disease, but a constellation of opportunistic infections. For ease of exposition, I follow most earlier work (for example, IOM 1986) in referring to this constellation as a disease.

10. Blood and perinatal transmission as a percentage of total cases were and have remained relatively low. The relative importance of heterosexual transmission, some of which is due to intravenous drug use by a sexual partner, is increasing in all four countries.

11. As early as 1986, an international conference sponsored by the World Health Organization concluded that "initiatives of this kind (exchange of sterile needles and syringes) could have an important role to play in stopping the spread of HIV" (cited in Anderson 1991, 1508). Additional preventive measures recently proposed include safe injection sites, which have been implemented in Australia, and heroin maintenance under controlled conditions.

12. These findings were confirmed two years later in a report for the secretary of Health and Human Services by the U.S. surgeon general (Office of the Surgeon General 2000).

13. A web search in June 2006 found no current references to the National AIDS Commission.

14. In the United States, the terms *needle-exchange* and *syringe-exchange* to describe the exchange of used for sterile needles and syringes are used interchangeably.

15. Tacoma is usually given priority (see, for example, Burris, Strathnee, and Vernick 2003, 817), but Barbara Tempalski asserts that the National AIDS Brigade started the first underground needle exchange program in New Haven in 1986 (2005, 9).

16. The most recent CDC report suggests that these numbers are probably underestimates of the actual number of programs but compare the UK with more than 2000 such programs (CDC 2005b; Parsons et al. 2002).

17. This aspect of the New York City story has not so far received the research attention that it fully deserves, attention that was well beyond the scope of the present project.

18. In New York City, 60 percent of cases reported before 1982 were among white gay men. This figure dropped to 39 percent in 1982 and by 1988 was down to 25 percent (CDC 2005d). Particularly in the epidemic's early years, AIDS in white gay men had a relatively high probability of being diagnosed and reported (see, for example, Epstein 1996, 49–50).

19. The chair of the commission, Robert Henrion, was an obstetrician-gynecologist, and relatively few of the commission's members were specialists in the treatment of drug addiction. However, four of the seventeen members were part of the criminal justice system. The omission of drug-treatment specialists was deliberate and the cause of some grumbling in the ranks of that profession (Follea 1995).

20. My account of French drug treatment professionals' ideology and its implications for their confrontation with AIDS is based on published sources and on my interviews with several of the actors involved. Published sources include *Le double recontre: Toxicomanie et sida*, edited by Jean Claude Rouchy (1996) and *Toxicomanies et lois: Controverses*, by Robert Boyer and his colleagues (2002).

21. Among many examples of and reflections on this ideological perspective, see the compilation of articles and brief statements from a symposium titled *Santé publiques et libertés individuelles* (Malet 1993) and a lengthy interview with Claude Got that appeared in *Le Monde* on June 17, 1992 (Nau and Nouchi 1992).

22. Certainly not the most important, but one factor in Coppel's ability to take a leadership role was the fact that she read English. For the most part, French drug treatment specialists, including the most eminent psychiatrists, do not read or speak English.

23. The name états généraux, with its echoes of the French Revolution, was specifically intended to call attention to the status of the drug user as citoyen, a point to which I will return.

24. AIDES is the largest organization in France on behalf of persons with AIDS or affected by the AIDS epidemic. There are many published accounts of its

emergence and evolution, ideology and activities (see for example, Hirsch 1991; Rosman 1994; de Busscher and Pinell 1996). Médecins du Monde is a humanitarian medical organization that had previously worked primarily in developing countries.

25. During an interview I conducted at Médecins du Monde in Paris with the physician responsible for AIDS prevention programs among injection drug users, he spent much of his time on the telephone attempting to retrieve arrangements made for parking a bus that would provide interim methadone treatment. A monkey wrench had been suddenly thrown into arrangements put in place over the course of the previous year involving negotiations with multiple levels of local (at the level of the arrondissement), city (Paris), and national hierarchies in both the health and criminal justice systems. A civil servant who had been heavily involved in the early development of needle distribution programs told me that the prospect of such negotiations had been a principal deterrent to the rapid development of these programs. The 2004 report of the Conseil national du sida indicates that implementation problems continue, their extent highly variable from one region of the country to another.

26. The quote is from Jeffrey Weeks, *Sexuality and its Discontents*, describing the British policy making style (1985, 30).

27. The Advisory Council on the Misuse of Drugs (ACMD) is a statutory body required to be set up under the 1971 Misuse of Drugs Act, and thus pre-existed AIDS. Its members are appointed by the Home Office on advice of civil servants, including civil servants in the Department of Health. The parent ACMD was responsible for setting up the working group that produced the ACMD report on drugs and AIDS. The government created a number of advisory groups in response to the AIDS crisis. However, the ACMD working group was the only one to focus exclusively on the problem of HIV/AIDS in injection drug users.

28. The following account draws heavily on my interview with Dr. Black, a psychiatrist and senior medical officer in the Department of Health between 1981 and 1994. Dr. Black was a key participant in all of the critical events surrounding the development of British policy in the AIDS–drugs arena. She was invited to testify before the McClelland committee and was present as a Department of Health representative during the deliberations of the ACMD working group. Published accounts of these events and information from interviews with other individuals involved are wholly consistent with Dr. Black's description. Quotes not otherwise attributed are from this interview.

29. The chief medical officer (CMO) is medical advisor to all government departments as well as to the minister of health. The post has its origins in the late nineteenth century with positions held by Sir John Simon at the Privy Council Office and the Local Government Board, and "can have a lot of influence if [the occupant] chooses to use it." Virginia Berridge comments that "the status of public health was lower than ever" in 1983 when Acheson took on the job and that part of his brief was "to restore public health to some of its nineteenth-century glory" (1996, 67).

30. From parliamentary debate on the AIDS (Control) Bill, a modest bill requiring health authorities to produce annual reports on AIDS. This is representative of many similar comments. In the course of two debates on this bill, only one member of parliament is recorded as having raised any serious questions, asking why a "self-inflicted" condition should receive so much attention (and resources). Response to his remarks was forceful: "That is a shameful statement. The hon. Gentleman should be thoroughly ashamed of himself" (UK 1987b, 693).

31. Although there are some points of disagreement, the two major British commentators on these policies, Virginia Berridge and Gerry Stimson, generally agree on the continuity of contemporary with past drugs policies, at least through the late 1980s. It may be that this continuity appears even more striking to an observer from another country.

32. The existence of these programs was acknowledged in a report written in 1989 at the suggestion of Health Minister Perrin Beatty (Canada: Parliamentary Ad Hoc Committee on AIDS 1990, 44).

33. There is an interesting parallel between the Hankins-Beatty television encounter and that of Maurice Tubiana and Simone Veil over smoking in France. The circumstances were slightly different in the two cases, but the effect—galvanizing a minister into action—was much the same.

34. My description of the Toronto history is based on interviews with Health Department staff, with the director of an off-site needle exchange program that subcontracts with the Department, and with an AIDS researcher at the University of Toronto who has observed developments in Toronto over the past ten years.

35. These comments are based on a review of all relevant articles in *The Vancouver Sun* from 1997, when the data associating HIV with needle-exchange attendance were first published, through March 2001.

36. Over the past several years, Steffanie Strathdee has spent much of her time countering the negative impact of her original article, responding to the inference, drawn with some glee by opponents and with fury by proponents of needle exchange, that she believed these programs had failed. A recent paper by an unusual combination of authors—authorities (including Strathdee) on HIV/AIDS prevention among injection drug users, policymakers and a state legislator—reflects on the politicization of epidemiologic data that these controversies represent (Vlahov et al. 2001).

Chapter 7

1. Monica Prasad, comparing recent economic policy making in France with that in the United States, confronted a similar paradox, less aggressive policy making by France and more aggressive by the United States than would have been anticipated from widely accepted views of these two states. As she points out, such "anomalies show us that there is something else going on which we need to understand" (2005, 368).

2. At both federal and provincial levels, the Canadian civil service, like that of Britain and France, is composed overwhelmingly of career officials who retain their positions independently of shifts in the political party in power, further increasing the state's capacity to act.

3. Arguably, this increase in nongovernmental collective action began earlier, in the late 1960s and early 1970s, strongly encouraged under the prime ministry of Pierre Trudeau (Pal 1993).

4. Amplifying this conclusion based on further data analysis, Mebs Kanji and Neil Nevitte conclude that "Canadian and American values toward authority are more similar than different" and that "where there are discernible differences, it is Canadians, not Americans, who consistently appear to be the least deferential" (2000, 135).

5. For a Boolean analysis to explain advanced industrial countries' adoption of national health insurance, Charles Blake and Jessica Adolino constructed variables to measure two institutional characteristics hypothesized to be predictive of adoption—executive dominance and a unitary state—and one cultural variable, "a culture favorable to government activity in this sphere," which they measured as simply "not Anglo-American" (2001, 694). France was positive on all three characteristics, Britain on two, Canada on one, and the United States on none. Blake and Adolino's variables capture—however simplistically—several dimensions of the strong state–weak state construct, and their ordering of the four countries along this continuum is identical with my own.

6. Material in quotes and otherwise unattributed is taken from the narratives.

7. Pasteurization was delayed in Britain as well. It was opposed by the highly influential National Association for the Prevention of Tuberculosis whose physician leaders were committed to sanitariums as the solution to tuberculosis and regarded pasteurization as competitive with their interests, and also (as in France) by dairymen.

8. The following analysis corresponds very closely to that of Aquilino Morelle in his book on the current state of French public health, *La défaite de la santé publique*, with the exception that Morelle makes no reference to the weaknesses of civil society in France. Indeed, as is characteristic of French scholars, he perceives activity by the organs of civil society (associations) as undesirable and a reflection of state weakness (1996).

9. It is important to be aware that the French interpretation of "private interests" includes not only economic and political interests, but also the interests of advocates for causes such as tobacco control, people with disabilities, the environment, and so on.

10. Monica Prasad observes that for the period she studied, from 1974 to 1981, "trust in government [was] actually *lower* in France than in other countries" including the United States (2005, 379).

11. Many French intellectuals are remarkably hostile to the idea of public health. There are at least two strands to this hostility. First, public health is identified

with state interference in the individual's liberty to dispose of his or her body as he or she sees fit. Second, public health is seen as a form of state paternalism: the individual is to be denied bodily pleasures for his or her "own good." This ideologically based opposition from a class with substantial influence in French society has played an important role in inhibiting the development of public health.

12. "The foundation of all [France's] modern regimes on one version or another of a revolutionary tradition has, paradoxically, justified the government's taking on of exceptional powers when it could declare *la patrie en danger*" (Tilly, Tilly, and Tilly 1975, 85).

13. Delay by French authorities in confronting the problem of HIV in the blood supply erupted in 1991 into a full-blown public scandal fanned by a highly competitive press (Steffen 1999). The government was ultimately forced to establish an extremely generous, and expensive, compensation program for victims of blood-borne HIV infection. Fear that this experience might be repeated for HIV-infected injection drug users was among the factors that led to creation of the Henrion commission and rapid acceptance of its recommendations.

14. In striking parallel, French elite reformers had in the late nineteenth century mounted a similar effort (that is, to create a Ministry of Health) with equal lack of success. This was due in the French case, however, to opposition from private medical practitioners. American practitioners at the time, that is, before World War I, supported reform efforts.

15. The key role played by allies within the polity in advancing the political agenda of outsiders, whether these outsiders are individual policy entrepreneurs, interest groups, or social movements, has been strongly asserted in recent work by social movement scholars (for example, Tarrow 1998) and by students of public policy (for example, Oliver 2004).

16. The narratives contain two instances of how a close relation between policy entrepreneurs and political insiders may influence policy outcomes at the local level. Hermann Biggs's draconian approach to tuberculosis notification and pasteurization was powerfully facilitated by his own elite status combined with his close relation to New York's political bosses. Similarly, Toronto's Charles Hastings was able to create a forceful, active health department where his predecessors had failed, and where Montreal continued to fail, because of support from reform mayors who "shared his views and supported his efforts."

17. Historically, "the federal government used its spending power in areas of provincial jurisdiction to build social programs" (Rocher and Smith 2002, 16). Its financial leverage in the health care system has eroded over time, however, as a result of declines in the amount contributed and of changes in the formula by which that amount is calculated (Gray 1991; Maioni 2002). It plays a significant role in ensuring financial equity between richer and poorer provinces, however, through "equalization payments" (Maioni 2002, 92).

18. The quote is from a former health official in the government of Saskatchewan, currently a consultant on Canadian health policy. It reflects the consensus of

Canadian health policy activists and analysts I interviewed for this project. The problem is apparently longstanding. When Canada's federal Department of Health was created in 1919, a member of the House of Commons commented acidly that it was a department "all dressed up [with] no place to go" (cited in McQuaig 1980, 494) The search for places to go appears to have occupied the department ever since.

Chapter 8

1. Gay men (again, in all four countries) played an important role in bringing the larger problem of HIV-AIDS to political and public attention but were less committed to or effective in drawing attention to HIV-AIDS in injection drug users.

2. Monica Prasad would argue that the difference in expert power between the United States and (at least) France is less a question of cultural authority than the fact that in France experts "control the state" as a consequence of how state bureaucrats and politicians are recruited (2005, 397). The relative impacts of culture and social structure on this and other cross-national differences are, of course, extremely difficult to disentangle.

3. Social movements organized on the bad cop–good cop model may divide tactical responsibilities: the respectable good cops engage in insider tactics and the militant bad cops agitate from the outside.

Chapter 9

1. There are important similarities between the difficulties France experienced responding to tuberculosis and to HIV-AIDS (Steffen 1992). In both cases, the potential gains from a targeted response to interrupt transmission of an infectious disease conflicted with the commitment to solidarité.

2. Exclusion is defined in *Larousse* as "to put outside." As my observations may suggest, French public health authorities have difficulty with the notion of risk groups and consequently with the idea of public health programs targeted to these groups. This aversion surfaces in a wide variety of public health settings.

3. For example, a poll conducted in 1994 showed that majorities of the public believed the loi Evin was not respected, except in public transport (*Le Monde*, February 26, 1994). The exact proportions were: not respected in cafes (78 percent), in workplaces (61 percent), in restaurants (58 percent). The 1999 evaluation of the law's operation indicated that little had changed.

4. The military threat was not, however, as perceived in France, to the state directly but to Britain's position as an imperial power and was not, even then, central to the country's political culture: "War on land, even in the Crimea and South Africa, had been seen as a marginal matter, to be fought by professionals and a few volunteers . . . military matters seldom impinged on the thinking of government and society" (Matthew 1984, 580).

5. The government's primary concern in the early days of the smoking and health controversy was not to alienate a working class fond of its addiction to smoking and whose votes were necessary to the Labour Party (Crossman 1975).

6. Federally funded subsidies to tobacco farmers are, of course, a glaring exception.

7. The United States plays a major—and influential—role internationally in pushing countries to impose increasingly severe penalties for drug trafficking. At the same time, ironically, the image of the United States in the 1960s as home to a wild teenage drug scene was an important influence pushing France and Britain toward more severe policies in the early 1970s.

Chapter 10

1. Innovation has been variously defined by sociologists. Fifty-five years ago, William Fielding Ogburn defined invention (which he used interchangeably with innovation) as "a combination of existing and known elements of culture . . . or a modification of one to form a new [element]" (1950, 378). He made clear that he meant his definition to include social (the League of Nations is his example) as well as mechanical inventions. I prefer the term innovation as more clearly encompassing this broader meaning.

2. These works include the Institute of Medicine report *The Future of Public Health*, published in 1988, *What Price Community Medicine?* by Jane Lewis, published in 1986, and Aquilino Morelle's 1996 publication, *La défaite de la santé publique* (The Defeat of Public Health). Two 1997 articles, both of which refer to the 1988 IOM report, suggest that, in the United States at least, little had changed in the intervening nine years (Burris 1997; Lee and Paxman 1997). Laurie Garrett's book *Betrayal of Trust*, published in 2000, takes a global purview but is particularly scathing about the United States.

References

Abel-Smith, Brian. 1964. *The Hospitals 1800–1948*. Cambridge, Mass.: Harvard University Press.

Accampo, Elinor A. 1997. "Gender, Social Policy, and the Formation of the Third Republic." In *Gender and the Politics of Social Reform in France, 1870–1914*, edited by Elinor A. Accampo, Rachel G. Fuchs, and Mary L. Stewart. Baltimore, Md.: Johns Hopkins University Press.

Accampo, Elinor A., Rachel G. Fuchs, and Mary L. Stewart, eds. 1997. *Gender and the Politics of Social Reform in France, 1870–1914*. Baltimore, Md.: Johns Hopkins University Press.

Addams, Jane. 1913. *A New Conscience and an Ancient Evil*. New York: Macmillan.

Ahmed, Shukoor. 1999. "Needle Exchange Programs Not the Way to Stop HIV/AIDS." *Prince Georges Journal* (Maryland), December 12, 1999, Editorial.

amfAR. 2002. "Public Policy: Syringe Exchange" New York: The Foundation for AIDS Research. http://www.amfar.org.

Amick, Benjamin C. I., Sol Levine, Alvin R. Tarlov, and Diana C. Walsh. 1995. *Society and Health*. New York: Oxford University Press.

Anderson, Norman B. 1999. "Solving the Puzzle of Socioeconomic Status and Health: The Need for Integrated, Multilevel, Interdisciplinary Research." In *Socioeconomic Status and Health in Industrial Nations: Social, Psychological, and Biological Pathways*, vol. 896, edited by Nancy E. Adler, Michael Marmot, Bruce S. McEwen, and Judith Stewart. New York: The New York Academy of Sciences.

Anderson, Warwick. 1991. "The New York Needle Trial: The Politics of Public Health in the Age of AIDS." *American Journal of Public Health* 81(11): 1506–17.

Avert.org. 2005. "United Kingdom HIV & AIDS Statistics by Year" [Web Page]. Available at: http://www.avert.org/statsyr.htm.

Avery, Donald. 1979. *"Dangerous Foreigners": European Immigrant Workers and Labour Radicalism in Canada 1896–1932*. Toronto: McClelland and Stewart.

Baillargeon, Denyse. 1996. "Fréquenter Les Gouttes De Lait: L'Expérience Des Mères Montréalaises, 1910–1965." *Revue D'Histoire De L'Amérique Française* 50(1): 29–68.

———. 1998. "Gouttes De Lait Et Soif De Pouvoir. Les Dessous De La Lutte Contre La Mortalité Infantile à Montréal, 1910–1953." *Canadian Bulletin of Medical History* 15:27–57.

———. 2002. "Entre La 'Revanche' Et La 'Veillée' Des Berceaux: Les Médecins Québécois Francophone, La Mortalité Infantile Et La Question Nationale,

1910–1940." *Canadian Bulletin of Medical History/Bulletin Canadien D'Histoire De La Médecine* 19(1): 113–37.

Baldwin, Douglas O. 1990. "Volunteers in Action: The Establishment of Government Health Care on Prince Edward Island, 1900–1931." *Acadiensis* 19(2): 121–47.

Baldwin, Peter. 2005a. *Disease and Democracy: The Industrialized World Faces AIDS.* Berkeley: University of California Press.

————. 2005b. "Beyond Weak and Strong: Rethinking the State in Comparative Policy History." *The Journal of Policy History* 17(1): 12–33.

Barnes, D. E., and L. Bero. 1998. "Why Review Articles on the Health Effects of Passive Smoking Reach Different Conclusions." *Journal of the American Medical Association* 279(19): 1566–70.

Barnes, David S. 1995. *The Making of a Social Disease: Tuberculosis in Nineteenth-Century France.* Berkeley: University of California Press.

Barrick, E. J. 1899. "How to Deal with the Consumptive Poor." *The Canadian Journal of Medicine and Surgery* October: 1–8.

Bayer, Ronald, and David L. Kirp. 1992. "The U.S.: At the Center of the Storm." In *AIDS in the Industrialized Democracies: Passions, Politics, and Policies,* edited by David L. Kirp and Ronald Bayer. New Brunswick, N.J.: Rutgers University Press.

Beauchamp, Dan E. 1988. *The Health of the Republic: Epidemics, Medicine, and Moralism as Challenges to Democracy.* Philadelphia, Pa.: Temple University Press.

Benford, R. D., and D. Snow. 2000. "Framing Processes and Social Movements: An Overview and Assessment." *Annual Review of Sociology* 26: 611–39.

Bensaïd, Norbert. 1993. "Les illusions de la mobilisation: Ou comment informer les citoyens." In *Santé publique et libertés individuelles,* edited by Emile Malet. Paris: Passages Tirer Profit.

Berger, Carl. 1986. "The True North Strong and Free." In *Interpreting Canada's Past,* vol. 2, edited by J. M. Bumsted. Toronto: Oxford University Press Canada.

Berridge, Virginia. 1990. "Health and Medicine." In *The Cambridge Social History of Britain 1750–1950,* vol. 3, *Social Agencies and Institutions,* edited by F. M. L. Thompson. Cambridge: Cambridge University Press.

————. 1993. "AIDS and British Drug Policy: Continuity or Change?" In *AIDS and Contemporary History,* edited by Virginia Berridge and Philip Strong. Cambridge: Cambridge University Press.

————. 1996. *AIDS in the UK: The Making of Policy, 1981–1994.* Oxford: Oxford University Press.

————. 1997. "Two Histories of Harm Reduction; Opium and Tobacco." *8th International Conference on the Reduction of Drug Related Harm.* Paris (March 23–27, 1997).

————. 1998. "Science and Policy: The Case of Postwar British Smoking Policy." In *Ashes to Ashes: The History of Smoking and Health,* edited by S. Lock, L. A. Reynolds, and E. M. Tansey. Amsterdam: Editions Rodopi.

————. 1999. "Passive Smoking and Its Pre-History in Britain: Policy Speaks to Science?" *Social Science and Medicine* 49: 1183–95.

————. 2004. "Militants, Manufacturers, and Governments: Postwar Smoking Policy in the United Kingdom." In *Unfiltered: Conflicts over Tobacco Policy and Public Health,* edited by Eric A. Feldman and Ronald Bayer. Cambridge, Mass.: Harvard University Press.

Berridge, Virginia, and Griffith Edwards. 1981. *Opium and the People: Opiate Use in Nineteenth Century England.* London: Allen Lane/St. Martin's Press.

Bertram, Eva, Morris Blachman, Kenneth Sharpe, and Peter Andreas. 1996. *Drug War Politics: The Price of Denial.* Berkeley: University of California Press.

Bienvault, Pierre. 2004. "La Lutte Contre Le Cancer." *La Croix* (Paris), April 29, p. 3.

Blake, Charles L., and Jessica R. Adolino. 2001. "The Enactment of National Health Insurance: A Boolean Analysis of Twenty Advanced Industrial Countries." *Journal of Health Politics, Policy and Law* 26(4): 679–708.

Blatherwick, John. 1989. "How to 'Sell' a Needle Exchange Program." *Canadian Journal of Public Health* 80(May/June): S26–S27.

Blum, Alan, Eric Solberg, and Howard Wolinsky. 2004. "The Surgeon General's Report on Smoking and Health 40 Years Later: Still Wandering in the Desert." *The Lancet* 363(January 10): 97–98.

Blumer, Herbert. 1971. "Social Problems as Collective Behavior." *Social Problems* 18:298–307.

Bluthenthal, Ricky. 1998. "Syringe Exchange as a Social Movement: A Case Study of Harm Reduction in Oakland, California." *Substance Use and Misuse* 33(5): 1147–71.

Booth, Christopher C. 1998. "Smoking and the Royal College of Physicians." In *Ashes to Ashes: The History of Smoking and Health,* edited by S. Lock, L. A. Reynolds, and E. M. Tansey. Amsterdam: Editions Rodopi.

Boris, Eileen. 1993. "The Power of Motherhood: Black and White Activist Women Redefine the 'Political.' " In *Mothers of a New World: Maternalist Politics and the Origins of Welfare States,* edited by Seth Koven and Sonya Michel. New York: Routledge.

Boseley, Sarah. 1998. "Dobson Declares War on Tobacco." *The Guardian* (London), December 11, 1998, p. 4.

Bourgeois–Pichat, J. 1965. "The General Development of the Population of France Since the Eighteenth Century." In *Population in History: Essays in Historical Demography,* edited by D. V. Glass and D. E. C. Eversley. Chicago: Aldine Publishing.

Boyer, Robert, Carry Chantal, Patrick Chailonick, Jeanine Friess, Nicole Gerey, Michel Lecamp, Alain Oddou, Gilles Raguin, and Isabelle Rome. 2002. *Toxicomanies et lois: Controverses.* Paris: L'Harmattan.

Braden, Christopher R., Ida M. Onorato, and Joseph H. Kent. 1996. "Tuberculosis—United States." In *Tuberculosis,* edited by William N. Rom and Stuart M. Garay. Boston, Mass.: Little, Brown.

Brand, Jeanne L. 1965. *Doctors and the State: The British Medical Profession and Government Action in Public Health, 1870–1912.* Baltimore, Md.: Johns Hopkins University Press.

Brandt, Allan M. 1992. "The Rise and Fall of the Cigarette: A Brief History of the Antismoking Movement in the United States." In *Advancing Health in Developing Countries,* edited by Lincoln C. Chen, Arthur Kleinman, and Norma C. Ware. New York: Auburn House.

Brandt, Lillian. 1903. "Social Aspects of Tuberculosis." *Annals of the American Academy* 21:407–18.

British Medical Association. 1986. *Smoking Out the Barons: The Campaign Against the Tobacco Industry.* Chichester: John Wiley & Sons.

British Medical Journal. 1991. "Indoor Pollution: Restricting Smoking." *British Medical Journal* 303:669–70.

Brundage, Anthony. 1988. *England's "Prussian Minister": Edwin Chadwick and the Politics of Government Growth, 1832–1854*. University Park: Pennsylvania State University Press.

Bruneau, Julie, François Lamothe, Eduardo Franco, Natalie Lachance, Marie Désy, Julio Soto, and Jean Vincelette. 1997. "High Rates of HIV Infection among Injection Drug Users Participating in Needle Exchange Programs in Montreal: Results of a Cohort Study." *American Journal of Epidemiology* 148(12): 994–1002.

Bryder, Linda. 1988. *Below the Magic Mountain: A Social History of Tuberculosis in Twentieth-Century Britain*. Oxford: Clarendon Press.

Bula, Frances. 2000. "Activists, Drug Users Seek Funds for Safe-Injection Rooms" *The Vancouver Sun*, November 24, 2000, p. B1.

———. 2001. " Safe–Injection Site a Go If B. C. Wants It, Rock Says" *The Vancouver Sun*, November 15, 2001, p. A1.

Buning, E., R. A. Coutinho, and G. H. A. van Brussel. 1986. "Preventing AIDS in Drug Addicts in Amsterdam." *Lancet* 1: 1435–36.

Burney, Leroy E. 1959. "Smoking and Lung Cancer: A Statement of the Public Health Service." *Journal of the American Medical Association* 171(13): 1829–37.

Burris, Scott. 1997. "The Invisibility of Public Health: Population-Level Measures in a Politics of Market Individualism." *American Journal of Public Health* 87(10): 1607–10.

Burris, Scott, Kim Blankenship, Martin Donoghoe, Susan Sherman, Jon S. Vernick, Patricia Case, Zita Lazzarini, and Stephen Koester. 2004. "Addressing the Risk Environment for Injection Drug Users: The Mysterious Case of the Missing Cop." *The Milbank Quarterly* 82(1): 125–56.

Burris, Scott, Steffanie A. Strathdee, and Jon S. Vernick. 2003. "Lethal Injections: The Law, Science, and Politics of Syringe Access for Injection Drug Users." *University of San Francisco Law Review* 37(4)(Summer): 813–85.

Burton, Michel. 1995. "Justiciers ou rapaces?" *Revue des tabacs* (408):3, 25–27.

Caldwell, John C. 1986. "Routes to Low Mortality in Poor Countries." *Population and Development Review* 12(2): 171–220.

Calnan, M. 1984. "The Politics of Health: The Case of Smoking Control." *Journal of Social Policy* 13(3): 279–96.

Canada. F/P/T Advisory Committee on Population Health. 2001. *Reducing the Harm Associated with Injection Drug Use in Canada*. Working Document for Consultation. Ottawa: Public Health Agency of Canada.

Canada. House of Commons. 2001. "Allotted Day—Drugs." *House of Commons Debates*, 37th Parliament, 1st Session (17 May 2001). http://www.parl.gc.ca/37/1/parlbus/chambus/house/debates/064_2001-05-17/HAN064-E.HTM#LINK24.

Canada. Minister of National Health and Welfare [Canada Health and Welfare]. 1990. *Building an Effective Partnership: The Federal Government's Commitment to Fighting AIDS*. Ottawa: Minister of Supply and Services Canada.

Canada. NAC-AIDS Working Group on HIV Infection and Injection Drug Use [Canada NAC-AIDS]. 1994. "HIV Infection and Injection Drug Use." In *Second National Workshop on HIV, Alcohol, and Other Drug Use—Proceedings*.Edmonton, Alberta: Canadian Centre on Substance Abuse. http://www.hc-sc.gc.ca/ahc-asc/pubs/drugs-drogues/second_hiv-deuxieme_vih/index_e.html.

Canada. Parliamentary Ad Hoc Committee on AIDS. 1990. *Confronting a Crisis: The Report of the Parliamentary Ad Hoc Committee on AIDS*. Toronto: Canadian Public Health Association.

Canada. Senate. 1995. "Proceedings of the Standing Senate Committee on Legal and Constitutional Affairs" (12 December 1995). Ottawa: Canadian Public Health Association. Available at: http://www.cfdp.ca/70ev-e.html.

———. 1996. "Proceedings of the Standing Senate Committee on Legal and Constitutional Affairs" (29 May 1996). Ottawa: Canadian Public Health Association. Available at: http://www.cfdp.ca/960529 html.

Canada. Task Force on HIV, AIDS and Injection Drug Use. 1997. *HIV, AIDS and Injection Drug Use: A National Action Plan*. Ottawa: Canadian Public Health Association and Canadian Centre on Substance Abuse.

Canadian HIV/AIDS Legal Network. 1999. *Injection Drug Use and HIV/AIDS: Legal and Ethical Issues*. Montreal: Canadian HIV/AIDS Legal Network.

Cassel, Jay. 1994. "Public Health in Canada." In *The History of Public Health and the Modern State*, edited by Dorothy Porter. Amsterdam: Editions Rodopi.

Chen, David W. 2006. "No Compromise in Sight on Plan to Fight H.I.V." *The New York Times*, June 4, 2006, n.p.

Clemens, Elizabeth S. 1997. *The People's Lobby: Organizational Innovation and the Rise of Interest Group Politics in the United States, 1890–1925*. Chicago: University of Chicago Press.

Cohen, Cathy J. 1997. *The Boundaries of Blackness: AIDS and the Breakdown of Black Politics*. Chicago: University of Chicago Press.

Cohen-Tanugi, Laurent. 1987. *Le droit sans l'état: Sur la démocratie en France et en Amérique*. Paris: Presses universitaires de France.

Cole, Joshua. 1996. " 'A Sudden and Terrible Revelation': Motherhood and Infant Mortality in France, 1858–1874." *Journal of Family History* 21(4): 419–45.

Cole, P., and B. Radu. 1996. "Declining Cancer Mortality in the United States." *Cancer* 78(10): 2045–48.

Coleman, Michel P., Jacques Estève, Philippe Damiecki, Annie Arslan, and Hélène Renard. 1993. "Lung." In *Trends in Cancer Incidence and Mortality*. IARC Scientific Publication No. 121. Lyon, France: International Agency for Research on Cancer.

Coleman, William. 1982. *Death Is a Social Disease: Public Health and Political Economy in Early Industrial France*. Madison: University of Wisconsin Press.

Colgrove, James. 2002. "The McKeown Thesis: A Historical Controversy and Its Enduring Influence." *American Journal of Public Health* 92(5): 725–29.

Comacchio, Cynthia R. 1993. *Nations Are Built of Babies: Saving Ontario's Mothers and Children, 1900–1940*. Montreal: McGill-Queen's University Press.

Commissariat général du plan. 2000. *La loi relative à la lutte contre le tabagisme et l'alcoolisme: Rapport d'évaluation*. Paris: La documentation française.

Conrad, Peter, and Joseph W. Schneider, eds. 1980. *Deviance and Medicalization: From Badness to Sickness*. St. Louis, Mo.: C. V. Mosby.

Conseil national du sida. 2004. *Éthique, sida et société*. Paris: La Documentation Française.

Cook, Michelle. 2000. "Drug Users to Get 'Safe Site' for Fixes: Downtown Eastside Rally Mourns Death of 2,000 Addicts Over 10 Years." *The Vancouver Sun*, July 12, 2000, p. B1.

Cooter, Roger. 1983. "Anticontagionism and History's Medical Record." *The Problem of Medical Knowledge*, edited by P. I. Wright and A. Treacher. Edinburgh: Edinburgh University Press.

Copp, Terry. 1974. *The Anatomy of Poverty: The Condition of the Working Class in Montreal, 1897–1929.* Toronto: McClelland and Steweart.

———. 1981. "Public Health in Montreal, 1870–1930." In *Medicine in Canadian Society. Historical Perspectives,* edited by E. D. Shortt. Montreal: McGill-Queen's University Press.

Coppel, Anne. 1996. "Les intervenants en toxicomanie, le sida et la réduction des risques en France." In *Vivre Avec Les Drogues.* Paris: Seuil.

Crain, Robert L., Elihu Katz, and Donald B. Rosenthal. 1969. *The Politics of Community Conflict: The Fluoridation Decision.* Indianapolis, Ind.: Bobbs-Merrill.

Crampton, Thomas. 2006. "Smoking Ban in France Faces a Host of Questions." *International Herald Tribune.* October 10. Available at: http://www.iht.com/articles/2006/10/10/news/smoke.php.

Cronje, Gillian. 1984. "Tuberculosis and Mortality Decline in England and Wales, 1851–1910." In *Urban Disease and Mortality in Nineteenth Century England,* edited by Robert Woods and John Woodward. London: Batsford Academic and Educational and St. Martin's Press.

Crossman, Richard. 1975. *The Diaries of a Cabinet Minister,* vol. II. New York: Holt, Rinehart and Winston.

———. 1978. *The Diaries of a Cabinet Minister,* vol. III. New York: Holt, Rinehart and Winston.

Crozier, Michel. 1964. *The Bureaucratic Phenomenon.* Chicago: University of Chicago Press.

Cunningham, Rob. 1996. *Smoke & Mirrors: The Canadian Tobacco War.* Ottawa: International Development Research Centre.

Cutler, David, and Grant Miller. 2005. "The Role of Public Improvements in Health Advances: The Twentieth-Century United States." *Demography* 42(1): 1–22.

de Busscher, Pierre-Olivier, and Patrice Pinell. 1996. "La naissance de la lutte contre le sida en France (1981–1988)." *Bulletin de l'ANEF* 19(Printemps): 62. http://www.anef.org/telechargement/20-MARS_96.pdf.

de Peretti, Christine, Nelly Leselbaum, Sadika Benslimane, and Christine Piorier. 1995. *Tabac, alcool, drogues illicites: Opinions et consommations des lycéens.* Paris: Institut National de Recherche Pédagogique.

Derthick, Martha A. 2005. *Up in Smoke: From Legislation to Litigation in Tobacco Politics,* 2nd ed. Washington, D.C.: CQ Press.

Des Jarlais, Don C., Courtney McKnight, Karen Eigo, and Patricia Friedmann. 2002. "2000 United States Syringe Exchange Program Survey." Presented at the 12th North American Syringe Exchange Convention. Albuquerque, New Mexico (April 24, 2002). http://www.harmreduction.org.

Des Jarlais, Don C., Theresa Perlis, Kamyer Arasteh, Lucia V. Torlan, Sara Beatrice, Judith Milliken, Donna Mildvan, Stanley Yancovitz, and Samuel R. Friedman. 2005. "HIV Incidence Among Injection Drug Users in New York City, 1990 to 2002: Use of Serologic Test Algorithm to Assess Expansion of HIV Prevention Services." *American Journal of Public Health* 95(8): 1439–44.

Dessertine, D., and Olivier Faure. 1988. *Combattre La Tuberculose, 1900–1940.* Lyon: Presses Universitaires de Lyon.

Dobbin, Frank. 1994. *Forging Industrial Policy: The United States, Britain, and France in the Railway Age.* Cambridge: Cambridge University Press.

Dockery, Douglas W., and Dimitrios Trichopoulos. 1997. "Risk of Lung Cancer from Environmental Exposures to Tobacco Smoke." *Cancer Causes and Control* 8: 333–45.

Doll, Richard. 1998. "The First Reports on Smoking and Lung Cancer." In *Ashes to Ashes: The History of Smoking and Health,* edited by S. Lock, L. A. Reynolds, and E. M. Tansey. Amsterdam: Editions Rodopi.

Doll, Richard, and Austin B. Hill. 1950. "Smoking and Carcinoma of the Lung: Preliminary Report." *British Medical Journal* 2(4682): 739–48.

———. 1954. "The Mortality of Doctors in Relation to Their Smoking Habits: A Preliminary Report." *British Medical Journal* 1: 1071–6.

Douglas, Mary. 1992. *Risk and Blame: Essays in Cultural Theory.* London: Routledge.

Douglas, Mary, and Aaron Wildavsky. 1982. *Risk and Culture: An Essay on the Selection of Technological and Environmental Dangers.* Berkeley: University of California Press.

Drucker, Ernest. 1999. *Drug Prohibition and Public Health: 25 Years of Evidence. Public Health Reports* 114(1): 14–29.

Dubos, René, and Jean Dubos. 1952/1987. *The White Plague: Tuberculosis, Man, and Society,* 2nd ed. New Brunswick, N.J.: Rutgers University Press.

Duchesne, Sophie. 1997. *Citoyenneté à la Française.* Paris: Presses de Sciences Po.

Duffy, John. 1990. *The Sanitarians: A History of American Public Health.* Urbana: University of Illinois Press.

Dufour, A. 1978. "Centenaire du comité national contre le tabagisme." *Tabac et santé* 29:3–4.

Durack, D. T. 1981. "Opportunistic Infections and Kaposi's Sarcoma in Homosexual Men." *New England Journal of Medicine* 305(24): 1465–67.

Dwork, Deborah. 1987. *War Is Good for Babies & Other Young Children: A History of the Infant and Child Welfare Movement in England, 1898–1918.* London: Tavistock.

Ecoiffier, Matthieu. 9 Jan 2006. "L'UMP intoxiquée par le lobby du tabac." *Libération* (Paris).

Ehrenberg, Alain. 1995. *L'Individu incertain.* Paris: Calmann-Lévy.

Ellis, Jack D. 1990. *The Physician-Legislators of France: Medicine and Politics in the Early Third Republic, 1870–1914.* Cambridge: Cambridge University Press.

Epstein, Steven. 1996. *Impure Science: AIDS, Activism, and the Politics of Knowledge.* Berkeley: University of California Press.

Evans, Peter B., Dietrich Rueschemeyer, and Theda Skocpol, eds. 1985. *Bringing the State Back In.* Cambridge: Cambridge University Press.

Ewbank, Douglas C., and Samuel H. Preston. 1990. "Personal Health Behaviour and the Decline in Infant and Child Mortality: The United States, 1900–1930." In *The Cultural, Social and Behavioral Determinants of Health,* vol. 1, edited by John Caldwell. Canberra: Australian National University.

Fairchild, Amy L., Ronald Bayer, James Colgrove, and Daniel Wolfe. 2007. *Searching Eyes: Privacy, the State, and Disease Surveillance in America.* Berkeley: University of California Press.

Fairchild, Amy L., and Gerald M. Oppenheimer. 1998. "Public Health Nihilism vs. Pragmatism: History, Politics, and the Control of Tuberculosis." *American Journal of Public Health* 88(7): 1105–17.

Fee, Elizabeth. 1991. "The Origins and Development of Public Health in the United States." In *Oxford Textbook of Public Health*, 2nd ed., vol. 1, edited by Walter W. Holland, Roger Detels, and George Knox. Oxford: Oxford University Press.

———. 1994. "Public Health and the State: The United States." In *The History of Public Health and the Modern State*, edited by Dorothy Porter. Amsterdam: Editions Rodopi.

Fee, Elizabeth, and Daniel M. Fox. 1988. *AIDS and the Burdens of History*. Berkeley: University of California Press.

Fee, Elizabeth, and Dorothy Porter. 1991. "Public Health, Preventive Medicine, and Professionalization: Britain and the United States in the Nineteenth Century." In *A History of Education in Public Health*, edited by Elizabeth Fee and Roy M. Acheson. Oxford: Oxford University Press.

Feldberg, Georgina D. 1995. *Disease and Class: Tuberculosis and the Shaping of Modern North American Society*. New Brunswick, N.J.: Rutgers University Press.

Feldman, Eric A., and Ronald Bayer, eds. 1999. *Blood Feuds: AIDS, Blood, and the Politics of Medical Disaster*. New York: Oxford University Press.

———. 2004. *Unfiltered: Conflicts over Tobacco Policy and Public Health*. Cambridge, Mass.: Harvard University Press.

Fernando, M. D. 1993. *AIDS and Intravenous Drug Use*. Westport, Conn.: Praeger.

Fiellin, David A., Patrick G. O'Connor, Marek Chawarski, Juliana P. Pakes, Michael V. Pantalon, and Richard S. Schottenfeld. 2001. "Methadone Maintenance in Primary Care: A Randomized Controlled Trial." *Journal of the American Medical Association* 286(14): 1724–31.

Fischer, Benedikt. 1999. "Prescriptions, Power and Politics: The Turbulent History of Methadone Maintenance in Canada." *Journal of Public Health Policy* 21(2): 187–210.

Fletcher, Charles. 1998. "The Story of the Reports on Smoking and Health by the Royal College of Physicians." In *Ashes to Ashes: The History of Smoking and Health*, edited by S. Lock, L. A. Reynolds, and E. M. Tansey. Amsterdam: Editions Rodopi.

Flinn, Michael W. 1965. "Introduction." In *The Sanitary Condition of the Labouring Population of Great Britain*, by Edwin Chadwick. Edinburgh: Edinburgh University Press.

Follea, Laurence. 1995. "Simone Veil écarte une dépénalisation de l'usage de drogue." *Le Monde* February 6: n.p.

Forsey, Eugene A. 1988. *How Canadians Govern Themselves*. Ottawa: Minister of Supply and Services Canada.

Foucault, Michel. 1963. *The Birth of the Clinic*. New York: Vintage Books.

Fowler, Norman. 1991. *Ministers Decide*. London: Chapmans.

Fox, Daniel M. 1975. "Social Policy and City Politics: Tuberculosis Reporting in New York City, 1889–1900." *Bulletin of the History of Medicine* 49(Summer): 169–95.

———. 1986. *Health Policies, Health Politics: The British and American Experience, 1911–1965*. Princeton, N.J.: Princeton University Press.

France. 1976. "Débats parlementaires, assemblée nationale." *Journal officiel de la république Française*. Seconde session ordinaire de 1975–76.

———. 1990. "Débats parlementaires, assemblée nationale." *Journal officiel de la république Française*. Seconde session ordinaire de 1989–1990 (1re séance du lundi, 25 juin 1990).

Friedman, Kenneth M. 1975. *Public Policy and the Smoking-Health Controversy*. Lexington, Mass.: Lexington Books.

Friedman–Kien, A. E. 1981. "Disseminated Kaposi's Sarcoma Syndrome in Young Homosexual Men." *Journal of the American Academy of Dermatology* 5(4): 468–71.

Fritschler, A. Lee. 1989. *Smoking and Politics*, 4th ed. Englewood Cliffs, N.J.: Prentice-Hall.

Fuchs, Rachel G. 1997. "The Right to Life: Paul Strauss and the Politics of Motherhood." In *Gender and the Politics of Social Reform in France, 1870–1914*, edited by Elinor Accampo, Rachel G. Fuchs, and Mary L. Stewart. Baltimore, Md.: Johns Hopkins University Press.

Gagnon, Eugène. 1910. "Comment diminuer la mortalité infantile." *Union médicale du Canada* 39(12): 713–20.

Gamble, Vanessa N. 1989. *Germs Have No Color Line: Blacks and American Medicine, 1900–1940*. New York: Garland Publishing.

Garrett, Laurie. 2000. *Betrayal of Trust: The Collapse of Global Public Health*. New York: Hyperion.

Gaumer, Benoit, Georges Desrosiers, and Othmar Keel. 2002. *Histoire du Service de santé de la ville de Montréal, 1865–1975*. Sainte-Foy, Québec: Les Presses de l'Université de Laval.

Gerth, H. H., and C. W. Mills. 1946. *From Max Weber: Essays in Sociology*. New York: Oxford University Press.

Gilmore, Anna, and Martin McKee. 2004. "Tobacco-Control Policy in the European Union." In *Unfiltered: Conflicts over Tobacco Policy and Public Health*, edited by Eric A. Feldman and Ronald Bayer. Cambridge, Mass.: Harvard University Press.

Givel, M., and S. A. Glantz. 2004. "The 'Global Settlement' With the Tobacco Industry: 6 Years Later." *American Journal of Public Health* 94(2): 218–24.

Glantz, Stanton A., and Edith D. Balbach. 2000. *Tobacco War: Inside the California Battles*. Berkeley: University of California Press.

Glantz, Stanton, John Slade, Lisa Bero, Peter Hanauer, and Deborah E. Barnes. 1996. *The Cigarette Papers*. Berkeley: University of California Press.

Godt, Paul J. 1987. "Confrontation, Consent, and Corporatism: State Strategies and the Medical Profession in France, Great Britain, and West Germany." *Journal of Health Politics, Policy and Law* 12(3): 459–80.

Goodlatte, Robert. 1999. "Scientific Evidence Proves Failure of Needle Exchange Programs." House of Representatives, 6th District, Virginia. Letter to members of Congress (March 30, 1999).

Goodman, Jordan. 1993. *Tobacco in History: The Cultures of Dependence*. London: Routledge.

———. 1998. "Webs of Drug Dependence: Towards a Political History of Tobacco." In *Ashes to Ashes: The History of Smoking and Health*, edited by S. Lock, L. A. Reynolds, and E. M. Tansey. Amsterdam: Editions Rodopi.

Gordon, Diana R. 1994. *The Return of the Dangerous Classes: Drug Prohibition and Policy Politics*. New York: W. W. Norton.

Gostin, Lawrence O., Zita Lazzarini, T. S. Jones, and Kathleen Flaherty. 1997. "Prevention of HIV/AIDS and Other Blood-Borne Diseases among Injection Drug Users." *Journal of the American Medical Association* 277(1): 53–62.

Got, Claude. 1989. *Rapport sur le sida*. Paris: Flammarion.

———. 1992. *La santé*. Paris: Flammarion.

Gouin, Clara. 1977. "Nonsmokers and Social Action." In *Proceedings of the ACS/ NCI Conference*. DHEW Publication No. [NIH] 77–1413. Washington: U.S. Department of Health, Education and Welfare.

Grant, W. 1995. *Pressure Groups, Politics and Democracy in Great Britain*. London: Harvester Wheatsheaf.

Gray, Charlotte. 1997. "Tobacco Wars: The Bloody Battle between Good Health and Good Politics." *Canadian Medical Association Journal* 156(2): 237–40.

Gray, Gwendolyn. 1991. *Federalism and Health Policy: The Development of Health Systems in Canada and Australia*. Toronto: University of Toronto Press.

Grmek, Mirko. 1995. *Histoire du sida*. Paris: Payot.

Grossman, Michael, and Philip Price. 1992. *Tobacco Smoking and the Law in Canada*. Toronto and Vancouver: Butterworths.

Grygier, Pat S. 1994. *A Long Way from Home: The Tuberculosis Epidemic among the Inuit*. Montreal and Kingston: McGill-Queen's University Press.

Guillaume, Pierre. 1986. *Du désespoir au salut: Les tuberculeux aux 19e et 20e siècles*. Paris: Aubier.

Gusfield, Joseph R. 1981. *The Culture of Public Problems: Drinking-Driving and the Symbolic Order*. Chicago: University of Chicago Press.

Haas, François, and Shiela S. Haas. 1996. "The Origins of *Mycobacterium tuberculosis* and the Notion of Its Contagiousness." In *Tuberculosis*, edited by William N. Rom and Stuart M. Garay. Boston, Mass.: Little, Brown.

Haas, Michael. 1992. *Polity and Society: Philosophical Underpinnings of Social Science*. New York: Praeger.

Hackshaw, A. K., M. R. Law, and N. J. Wald. 1997. "The Accumulated Evidence on Lung Cancer and Environmental Tobacco Smoke." *British Medical Journal* 315: 980–88.

Hall, Peter. 1986. *Governing the Economy: The Politics of State Intervention in Britain and France*. New York: Oxford University Press.

Ham, Christopher. 1992. *Health Policy in Britain: The Politics and Organisation of the National Health Service*, 3rd ed. London: Macmillan.

Hamlin, Christopher. 1994. "State Medicine in Great Britain." In *The History of Public Health and the Modern State*, edited by Dorothy Porter. Amsterdam: Editions Rodopi.

Hammond, E. Cuyler, and D. Horn. 1954. "The Relationship between Human Smoking Habits and Death Rates: A Follow-Up Study of 187,766 Men." *Journal of the American Medical Association* 155(15): 1316–27.

Hanauer, P., G. Barr, and S. Glantz. 1986. *Legislative Approaches to a Smoke-Free Society*. Berkeley, Calif.: American Nonsmokers' Rights Foundation.

Hankins, Catherine A. 1998. "Syringe Exchange in Canada: Good but Not Enough To Stem the HIV Tide." *Substance Use & Misuse* 33(5): 1129–46.

Hardy, Ann. 1993. *The Epidemic Streets: Infectious Disease and the Rise of Preventive Medicine, 1856–1900*. Oxford: Clarendon Press.

Harris, José. 1990. " Society and the State in Twentieth-Century Britain." In *The Cambridge Social History of Britain 1750–1950*, vol. 3, *Social Agencies and Institutions*, edited by P. L. Thompson. Cambridge: Cambridge University Press.

Hays, Samuel P. 1995. *The Response to Industrialism 1885–1914*, 2nd ed. Chicago: University of Chicago Press.

Health Canada. 2001. *Injection Drug Use and HIV/AIDS: Health Canada's Response to the Report of the Canadian HIV/AIDS Legal Network. H39-581/2001.* Ottawa: Health Canada.

———. 2004. "HIV/AIDS in Canada. Surveillance Report to December 31, 2003." Surveillance and Risk Assessment Division, Centre for Infectious Disease Prevention and Control, Health Canada. Available at: http://www.phac-aspc. gc.ca/publicat/aids-sida/haic-vsac1203/pdf/haic-vsac1203.pdf.

———. 2005. "Canadian Tobacco Use Monitoring Survey, February-December 2004." Ottawa: Health Canada. http://www.hc-sc.gc.ca/hl-vs/pubs/tabac-tabac/ctums-esutc-2004/tabl08_e.html.

Heimann, Robert K. 1960. *Tobacco and Americans.* New York: McGraw-Hill.

Henrion, Roger. 1995. *Rapport de la comission de réflexion sur la drogue et la toxicomanie.* Paris: La Documentation Française.

Hildreth, Martha. 1987. *Doctors, Bureaucrats, and Public Health in France, 1888–1902.* New York: Garland Press.

Hill, Catherine. 1998. "Trends in Tobacco Smoking and Consequences on Health in France." *Preventive Medicine* 27: 514–19.

Hilts, Philip J. 1996. *Smokescreen: The Truth behind the Tobacco-Industry Cover-Up.* New York: Addison-Wesley.

Hirsch, Albert, Catherine Hill, Michel Frossart, Jean-Pol Tassin, and Madeleine Pechabrier. 1987. *Lutter contre le tabagisme.* Paris: La documentation Française.

Hirsch, Albert, and Serge Karsenty. 1992. *Le prix de la fumée.* Paris: Editions Odile Jacob.

Hirsch, Emmanuel. 1991. *AIDES solidaires.* Paris: Les editions du cerf.

HM Revenue and Customs. 2005. Annual Report 2004–05 and Autumn Performance Report 2005. Presented to Parliament by the Paymaster General by Command of Her Majesty. London, Crown Copyright 2005. Available at: http://customs. hmrc.gov.uk/channelsPortalWebApp/channelsPortalWebApp.portal?_nfpb= true&_pageLabel=pageVAT_ShowContent&id=HMCE_PROD1_025022& propertyType=document.

Hofstadter, Richard. 1955. *The Age of Reform.* New York: Vintage Books.

Hollingsworth, J. R. 1986. *A Political Economy of Medicine: Great Britain and the United States.* Baltimore, Md.: Johns Hopkins University Press.

Huettner, Steven. 1998. "Statement of the Presidential Advisory Council on HIV/AIDS." *Drug War Chronicle,* April 22, 1998. Washington, D.C.: Stop the Drug War (DRCNet).

Hunink, M. G., L. Goldman, A. N. Tosteson, M. A. Mittleman, P. A. Goldman, L. W. Williams, J. Tsevat, and M. C. Weinstein. 1997. "The Recent Decline in Mortality from Coronary Heart Disease, 1980–1990: The Effect of Secular Trends in Risk Factors and Treatment." *Journal of the American Medical Association* 277(7): 535–42.

Immergut, Ellen M. 1992. *Health Politics: Interests and Institutions in Western Europe.* Cambridge: Cambridge University Press.

Institute of Medicine, Committee on a National Strategy for AIDS [IOM]. 1986. *Confronting AIDS: Directions for Public Health, Health Care, and Research.* Washington, D.C.: National Academy Press.

Institute of Medicine, Committee for the Study of the Future of Public Health [IOM]. 1988. *The Future of Public Health.* Washington, D.C.: National Academy Press.

Institut de veille sanitaire. 2005. "Données épidémiologiques (tableaux et figures)." *Maladies à déclaration obligatoire: Infection à VIH et sida.* Saint-Maurice: Institut de Veille Sanitaire. http://www.invs.sante.fr/surveillance/vih-sida.

Irvine, Ian J., and William A. Sims. 1997. "Tobacco Control Legislation and Resource Allocation Effects." *Canadian Public Policy—Analyse De Politiques* 23(3): 259–73.

Jacobson, Peter D., and Jeffrey Wasserman. 1999. "The Implementation and Enforcement of Tobacco Control Laws: Policy Implications for Activists and the Industry." *Journal of Health Politics, Policy, and Law* 24: 567–98.

Jacobson, Peter D., Jeffrey Wasserman, and Kristiana Raube. 1992. *The Political Evolution of Anti-Smoking Legislation.* Santa Monica, Calif.: Rand.

Jacobson, Peter D., and Lisa M. Zapawa. 2001. "Clean Indoor Air Restrictions: Progress and Promise." In *Regulating Tobacco,* edited by Robert L. Rabin and Stephen D. Sugarman. New York: Oxford University Press.

Jasanoff, Sheila. 1990. "American Exceptionalism and the Political Acknowledgement of Risk." *Daedalus* (Fall): 61–81.

Johansson, S. R., and Carl Mosk. 1987. "Exposure, Resistance and Life Expectancy: Disease and Death during the Economic Development of Japan, 1900–1960." *Population Studies* 41:207–35.

Jordan, Grant, and Jeremy Richardson. 1982. "The British Policy Style or the Logic of Negotiation." In *Policy Styles in Western Europe,* edited by Jeremy Richardson. London: George Allen and Unwin.

Kagan, Robert A., and David Vogel. 1994. "The Politics of Smoking Regulation: Canada, France, the United States." In *Smoking Policy: Law, Politics, and Culture,* edited by Robert L. Rabin and Stephen D. Sugarman. New York: Oxford University Press.

Kanji, Mebs, and Neil Nevitte. 2000. "Who Are the Most Deferential—Canadians or Americans?" In *Canada and the United States: Differences That Count,* edited by David M. Thomas. Peterborough, Ont.: Broadview Press.

Katz, Michael. 1996. *In the Shadow of the Poorhouse: A Social History of Welfare in America.* New York: Basic Books.

Katznelson, Ira. 1985. "Working-Class Formation and the State: Nineteenth-Century England in American Perspective." In *Bringing the State Back In,* edited by Peter B. Evans, Dietrich Rueschemeyer, and Theda Skocpol. Cambridge: Cambridge University Press.

Kearns, Gerry. 2000. "Town Hall and Whitehall: Sanitary Intelligence in Liverpool, 1840–63." In *Body and City: Histories of Urban Public Health,* edited by Sally Sheard and Helen Power. Aldershot, Hampshire: Ashgate Publishing.

Kessler, David. 2001. *A Question of Intent.* New York: Public Affairs.

Kingdom, John. 1991. *Government and Politics in Britain.* Cambridge: Polity Press.

Kirp, David L. 1997. "Look Back in Anger: AIDS, Tainted Blood, and the Hemophilia Movement." *Dissent* 44(3): 65–70.

———. 1999. "The Politics of Blood: Hemophilia Activism in the AIDS Crisis." In *Blood Feuds: AIDS, Blood, and the Politics of Medical Disaster,* edited by Ronald Bayer and Eric Feldman. New York: Oxford University Press.

Kirp, David L., and Ronald Bayer. 1992. *AIDS in the Industrialized Democracies: Passions, Politics, and Policies.* New Brunswick, N.J.: Rutgers University Press.

————. 1993. "The Politics." In *Dimensions of HIV Prevention: Needle Exchange,* edited by Jeff Stryker and Mark Smith. Menlo Park, Calif.: Henry J. Kaiser Family Foundation.

Kitschelt, Herbert P. 1986. "Political Opportunity Structures and Political Protest: Anti-Nuclear Movements in Four Democracies." *British Journal of Political Science* 16: 57–85.

Klaus, Alisa. 1993. *Every Child a Lion: The Origins of Maternal and Infant Health Policy in the United States and France, 1890–1920.* Ithaca, N.Y.: Cornell University Press.

Kluger, Richard. 1996. *Ashes to Ashes: America's Hundred-Year Cigarette War, the Public Health, and the Unabashed Triumph of Philip Morris.* New York: Alfred A. Knopf.

Koop, C. Everett. 1989. "Preface." In *Reducing the Health Consequences of Smoking: Twenty-Five Years of Progress, A Report of the Surgeon General.* Publication No. (CDC) 89–8411. Rockville, Md.: U.S. Department of Health and Human Services.

Koven, Seth. 1993. "Borderlands: Women, Voluntary Action, and Child Welfare in Britain, 1840–1914." In *Mothers of a New World: Maternalist Politics and the Origins of Welfare States,* edited by Seth Koven and Sonya Michel. New York: Routledge.

Koven, Seth, and Sonya Michel. 1990. "Womanly Duties: Maternalist Politics and the Origins of Welfare States in France, Germany, Great Britain, and the United States." *American Historical Review* 95(October): 1076–1108.

————. 1993. *Mothers of a New World: Maternalist Politics and the Origins of Welfare States.* New York: Routledge.

Kunreuther, Howard C., and Joanne Linerooth, eds. 1983. *Risk Analysis and Decision Processes: The Siting of Liquified Energy Gas Facilities in Four Countries.* Berlin: Springer-Verlag.

La Berge, Ann F. 1992. *Mission and Method: The Early-Nineteenth Century French Public Health Movement.* Cambridge: Cambridge University Press.

Lalonde, Marc. 1974. *A New Perspective on the Health of Canadians.* Ottawa: Health and Welfare Canada.

Lambert, Royston. 1963. *Sir John Simon, 1816–1904, and English Social Administration.* London: Macgibbon and Kee.

Landes, Ronald G. 1995. *The Canadian Polity: A Comparative Introduction.* Scarborough, Ont.: Prentice-Hall Canada.

Langford, Nanci. 1995. "Childbirth on the Canadian Prairies, 1880–1930." *Journal of Historical Sociology* 8(3): 278–302.

Latour, Bruno. 1986. "Le théâtre de la preuve." In *Pasteur et la révolution Pastorienne,* edited by Claire Salomon-Bayet. Paris: Payot.

Laxton, Paul. 2000. "Fighting for Public Health: Dr. Duncan and His Adversaries, 1847–63." In *Body and City: Histories of Urban Public Health,* edited by Sally Sheard and Helen Power. Aldershot, Hampshire: Ashgate Publishing.

Leavitt, Judith W. 1976. "Politics and Public Health: Smallpox in Milwaukee, 1894–1895." *Bulletin of the History of Medicine* 50: 553–68.

Lécuyer, Bernard P. 1986. "L'Hygiène en France avant Pasteur." In *Pasteur et la révolution Pastorienne,* edited by Claire Salomon–Bayet. Paris: Payot.

Lee, P., and D. Paxman. 1997. "Reinventing Public Health." *Annual Review of Public Health* 18:1–35.

Leman, Christopher. 1980. *The Collapse of Welfare Reform: Political Institutions, Policy, and the Poor in Canada and the United States.* Cambridge, Mass.: MIT Press.

Lerner, Barron H. 1993. "New York City's Tuberculosis Control Efforts: The Historical Limitations of the War on Consumption." *American Journal of Public Health* 83(5): 758–66.

———. 1998. *Contagion and Confinement: Controlling Tuberculosis along the Skid Road.* Baltimore, Md.: Johns Hopkins University Press.

Lewis, Jane. 1980. *The Politics of Motherhood.* London: Croom Helm.

———. 1986. *What Price Community Medicine? The Philosophy, Practice and Politics of Public Health since 1919.* London: Wheatsheaf Books.

Lewis, Richard A. 1952. *Edwin Chadwick and the Public Health Movement, 1832–1854.* London: Longman, Green.

Link, Bruce G., and Jo Phelan. 1995. "Social Conditions as Fundamental Causes of Disease." *Journal of Health and Social Behavior* 35 (Extra Issue): 80–94.

Litfin, Karen T. 1994. *Ozone Discourses: Science and Politics in Global Environmental Cooperation.* New York: Columbia University Press.

Lock, S., L. A. Reynolds, and E. M. Tansey. 1998. *Ashes to Ashes: The History of Smoking and Health.* Amsterdam: Editions Rodopi.

Lopez, Alan D. 1995. "The Lung Cancer Epidemic in Developed Countries." In *Adult Mortality in Developed Countries: From Description to Explanation,* edited by Alan D. Lopez, Graziella Caselli, and Tapani Valkonen. Oxford: Clarendon Press.

Low–Beer, Daniel, Rand Stoneburner, Thierry Mertens, Anthony Burton, and Seth Berkley. 1998. "HIV and AIDS." In *Health Dimensions of Sex and Reproduction,* edited by Christopher J. L. Murray and Alan D. Lopez. Cambridge, Mass.: Harvard School of Public Health.

Lukes, Steven. 1973. *Individualism.* Oxford: Blackwell

Lux, Maureen K. 2001. *Medicine That Walks: Disease, Medicine, and Canadian Plains Native People, 1880–1940.* Toronto: University of Toronto.

MacDougall, Heather. 1990. *Activists and Advocates: Toronto's Health Department 1883–1983.* Toronto and Oxford: Dundern Press.

MacGregor, Susanne. 1989. "The Public Debate in the 1980s." In *Drugs and British Society,* edited by Susanne MacGregor. London: Routledge.

———. 1995. "Drugs Policy, Community and the City." Occasional paper. London: School of Sociology and Social Policy, Middlesex University.

MacGregor, Susanne, Betsy Ettore, Rose Coomber, and Adam Crosier. 1990. *Drugs Services in England and the Impact of the Central Funding Initiative.* London: Department of Politics and Sociology, Birkbeck College, University of London.

Mahoney, James. 2004. "Comparative-Historical Methodology." *Annual Review of Sociology* 30: 81–101.

Maioni, Antonia. 1994. "Divergent Pasts, Converging Futures? The Politics of Health Care Reform in Canada and the United States." *Canadian-American Public Policy* 18: 1–34.

———. 2002. "Health Care in the New Millennium." In *Canadian Federalism,* edited by Herman Bakvis and Grace Skogstad. Oxford: Oxford University Press.

Malet, Emile, ed. 1993. *Santé publique et libertés individuelles.* Paris: Passages Tirer Profit.

Manfredi, Christopher P., and Antonia Maioni. 2004. "Rights and Public Health in the Balance: Tobacco Control in Canada." In *Unfiltered: Conflicts Over Tobacco Policy and Public Health,* edited by Eric A. Feldman and Ronald Bayer. Cambridge, Mass.: Harvard University Press.

Marks, Lara V. 1996. *Metropolitan Maternity: Maternal and Infant Welfare Services in Early Twentieth Century London.* Amsterdam: Editions Rodopi.

Marsh, Alan, and Stephen McKay. 1994. *Poor Smokers.* London: Policy Studies Institute.

Masuy-Stroobant, Godelieve, and Catherine Gourbin. 1995. "Infant Health and Mortality Indicators." *European Journal of Population* 11: 63–84.

Matthew, H. C. G. 1984. "The Liberal Age (1851–1914)." In *The Oxford History of Britain,* edited by Kenneth O. Morgan. Oxford: Oxford University Press.

McAdam, Doug. 1994. "Culture and Social Movements." In *New Social Movements,* edited by Enrique Larana, Hank Johnston, and Joseph R. Gusfield. Philadelphia, Pa.: Temple University Press.

McBride, David. 1991. *From TB to AIDS: Epidemics Among Urban Blacks Since 1900.* Albany: State University of New York Press.

McCormack, A. R. 1977. *Reformers, Rebels, and Revolutionaries: The Western Canadian Radical Movement 1899–1919.* Toronto: University of Toronto Press.

McFarlane, Neil. 1989. "Hospitals, Housing, and Tuberculosis in Glasgow." *Social History of Medicine* 2: 59–85.

McInnis, Marvin. 1997. "Infant Mortality in Late Nineteenth Century Canada." In *Infant and Child Mortality in the Past,* edited by Alain Bideau, Bertrand Desjardins, and Hector P. Brignoli. Oxford: Clarendon Press.

McKeown, Thomas. 1965. "Medicine and World Population." In *Symposium on Research Issues in Public Health and Population Change,* edited by Mindel C. Sheps and Jeanne C. Ridley. Pittsburgh, Pa.: University of Pittsburgh.

———. 1976. *The Modern Rise of Population.* London: Edward Arnold.

McKeown, Thomas, and R. G. Brown. 1955. "Medical Evidence Related to English Population Changes in the Eighteenth Century." *Population Studies* 9(2): 119–41.

McKeown, Thomas, R. G. Record, and R. D. Turner. 1975. "An Interpretation of the Decline of Mortality in England and Wales during the Twentieth Century." *Population Studies* 29: 391–422.

McKinlay, John B., and Lisa D. Marceau. 2000. "Upstream Healthy Public Policy: Lessons From the Battle of Tobacco." *International Journal of Health Services* 30(1): 49–69.

McKinlay, John B., and Sonja M. McKinlay. 1977. "The Questionable Contribution of Medical Measures to the Decline of Mortality in the United States in the Twentieth Century." *Milbank Memorial Fund Quarterly* 55(Summer): 405–28.

McKinlay, John B., Sonja M. McKinlay, and Robert Beaglehole. 1989. "Trends in Death and Disease and the Contribution of Medical Measures." In *Handbook of Medical Sociology,* 4th ed., edited by Howard E. Freeman and Sol Levine. Englewood Cliffs, N.J.: Prentice-Hall.

McNaught, Kenneth. 1982. *The Pelican History of Canada.* Toronto: Penguin Books.

McQuaig, Katherine. 1979. "The Campaign against Tuberculosis in Canada, 1900–1950." Unpublished Ph.D. diss. McGill University, Montreal, Canada.

———. 1980. "From Social Reform to Social Service. The Changing Role of Volunteers: The Anti–Tuberculosis Campaign, 1900–1930." *Canadian Historical Review* 61: 480–501.

————. 1984. "Tuberculosis: The Changing Concepts of the Disease in Canada 1900–1950." In *Health, Disease, and Medicine,* edited by Charles G. Roland. Toronto: Hannah Institute for the History of Medicine.

Meckel, Richard A. 1990. *Save the Babies: American Public Health Reform and the Prevention of Infant Mortality, 1850–1929.* Baltimore, Md.: Johns Hopkins University Press.

Meier, Barry. 1999. "Philip Morris to Publish Statement Saying Smoking Causes Cancer." *The New York Times,* October 13, 1999, p. A1.

Meier, Kenneth J. 1994. *The Politics of Sin: Drugs, Alcohol, and Public Policy.* Armonk, N.Y.: M. E. Sharpe.

Meyer, David S., and Suzanne Staggenborg. 1996. "Movements, Countermovements, and the Structure of Political Opportunity." *American Journal of Sociology* 101(6): 1628–60.

————. 1998. "Countermovement Dynamics in Federal Systems: A Comparison of Abortion Politics in Canada and the United States." *Research in Political Sociology* 8: 209–40.

Millward, Robert, and Frances Bell. 2000. "Choices for Town Councillors in Nineteenth-Century Britain: Investment in Public Health and Its Impact on Mortality." In *Body and City: Histories of Urban Public Health,* edited by Sally Sheard and Helen Power. Aldershot, Hampshire: Ashgate Publishing.

Mintz, Morton. 1990. "No Ifs, Ands, or Butts." *Washington Monthly* July/August: 30–37.

Mitchell, Allan. 1988. "Obsessive Questions and Faint Answers: The French Response to Tuberculosis in the Belle Epoque." *Bulletin of the History of Medicine* 62: 215–35.

Mitchell, Brian R. 1992. *International Historical Statistics: Europe, 1750–1988.* New York: Stockton Press.

Mitchell, Chester N. 1991. "Introduction: A Canadian Perspective on Drug Issues." *The Journal of Drug Issues* 21(1): 9–16.

Moore, Barrington, Jr. 1993. *Social Origins of Dictatorship and Democracy.* Boston, Mass.: Beacon Press.

Morelle, Aquilino. 1996. *La Défaite De La Santé Publique.* Paris: Flammarion.

Morone, James A. 2003. *Hellfire Nation: The Politics of Sin in American History.* New Haven, Conn.: Yale University Press.

Morton, Desmond. 2000. "Strains of Affluence 1945–1996." In *The Illustrated History of Canada,* edited by Craig Brown. Toronto: Key Porter Books.

Muncy, Robyn. 1991. *Creating a Female Dominion in American Reform, 1890–1935.* New York: Oxford University Press.

Musto, David F. 1973. *The American Disease: Origins of Narcotic Control.* New Haven, Conn.: Yale University Press.

Nadeau, Jean B. 1995. "L'Ayatollah Du Tabac." *L'Actualité* 20(13): 26–30.

Nag, Moni. 1985. "The Impact of Social and Economic Development on Mortality: Comparative Study of Kerala and West Bengal." In *Good Health at Low Cost,* edited by Scott B. Halstead, Julia A. Walsh, and Kenneth S. Warren. New York: Rockefeller Foundation.

Nathanson, Constance A. 1995. "Mortality and the Position of Women in Developed Countries." In *Adult Mortality in Developed Countries: From Description to Explanation,* edited by Alan D. Lopez, Graziella Caselli, and Tapani Valkonen. Oxford: Clarendon Press.

———. 1996. "Disease Prevention as Social Change: Toward a Theory of Public Health." *Population and Development Review* 22(4): 609–37.

———. 1999. "Social Movements as Catalysts for Policy Change: The Case of Smoking and Guns." *Journal of Health Politics, Policy and Law* 24(3): 421–88.

———. 2004. "Liberté, Egalité, Fumée: Smoking and Tobacco Control in France." In *Unfiltered: Conflicts over Tobacco Policy and Public Health,* edited by Eric A. Feldman and Ronald Bayer. Cambridge, Mass.: Harvard University Press.

———. 2005. "Collective Action and Corporate Targets in Tobacco Control: A Cross-National Comparison." *Health Education & Behavior* 32(3): 337–54.

National Consensus Development Panel on Effective Medical Treatment of Opiate Addiction [National Consensus Development Panel]. 1998. "Effective Medical Treatment of Opiate Addiction." *Journal of the American Medical Association* 280: 1936–43.

Nau, Jean Y., and Franck Nouchi. 1992. "La 'retraite' du professeur Got, défenseur acharné de la santé publique." *Le Monde,* June 17, 1992.

Nettl, John Peter. 1968. "The State as a Conceptual Variable." *World Politics* 20(4): 559–92.

Newman, Katherine. 1999. "Summary: What Is to Be Done?" In *Socioeconomic Status and Health in Industrial Nations: Social, Psychological, and Biological Pathways,* vol. 896, edited by Nancy E. Adler, Michael Marmot, Bruce S. McEwen, and Judith Stewart. New York: The New York Academy of Sciences.

New York City Department of Health and Mental Hygiene. 2005a. "New York City HIV/AIDS Surveillance Statistics 2001." New York: Department of Health and Mental Hygiene. http://www.nyc.gov/html/doh/html/ah/hivtables2001.shtml.

———. 2005b. "HIV Surveillance Statistics 2004." New York: Department of Health and Mental Hygiene. http://www.nyc.gov/html/doh/downloads/pdf/ah/surveillance 2004_tabl3.6.1_to_3.6.5.pdf.

New York Times. 2005. "Playing AIDS Games in New Jersey."*New York Times.* June 30, 2005. Editorial.

Nicolaides–Bouman, Ans, Nicholas Wald, Barbara Forey, and Peter Lee, eds. 1993. *International Smoking Statistics: A Collection of Historical Data From 22 Economically Developed Countries.* Oxford: Oxford University Press.

Non-Smokers' Rights Association. 1986. *A Catalogue of Deception: The Use and Abuse of Voluntary Regulation of Tobacco Advertising in Canada.* A Report for Submission to the Honourable Jake Epp, Minister of Health, Health and Welfare Canada. Toronto: Non-Smokers' Rights Association.

Normand, Jacques, David Vlahov, and Lincoln E. Moses. 1995. *Preventing HIV Transmission: The Role of Sterile Needles and Bleach.* Washington, D.C.: National Academy Press.

Northern, W. J. 1909. "Tuberculosis Among Negroes." *Journal of the Southern Medical Association* 6: 407–19.

O'Conner, Michael. 1995. "Smoking and Health in Britain." Unpublished paper.

Office of the Surgeon General. 2000. "Evidence-Based Findings on the Efficacy of Syringe Exchange Programs: An Analysis from the Assistant Secretary for Health and the Surgeon General of the Scientific Research Completed since April 1998." Washington: U.S. Department of Health and Human Services. http://www.harmreduction.org/research/surgeongenrev/surgeonintro.html.

Ogburn, William F. 1950. *Social Change*. New York: Viking Press.

Oliver, Thomas R. 2004. "Policy Entrepreneurship in the Social Transformation of American Medicine: The Rise of Managed Care and Managed Competition." *Journal of Health Politics, Policy and Law* 29(4–5): 701–34.

Oppenheimer, Gerald M. 1988. "In the Eye of the Storm: The Epidemiological Construction of AIDS." In *AIDS and the Burdens of History*, edited by Elizabeth Fee and Daniel M. Fox. Berkeley: University of California Press.

Orloff, Ann S., and Theda Skocpol. 1984. "Why Not Equal Protection? Explaining the Politics of Public Spending in Britain, 1900–1911, and the United States, 1880s–1920." *American Sociological Review* 49(December): 726–50.

Oscapella, Eugene, and Richard Elliott. 1999. "Injection Drug Use and HIV/AIDS: A Legal Analysis of Priority Issues." In *Injection Drug Use and HIV/AIDS: Legal and Ethical Issues. Background Papers*. Montreal: Canadian HIV/AIDS Legal Network.

Ott, Katherine. 1996. *Fevered Lives: Tuberculosis in American Culture Since 1870*. Cambridge, Mass.: Harvard University Press.

Pal, Leslie A. 1993. *Interests of State: The Politics of Language, Multiculturalism, and Feminism in Canada*. Montreal and Kingston: McGill-Queen's University Press.

Palloni, Alberto. 1985. "An Epidemio-Demographic Analysis of Factors in the Mortality Decline of 'Slow-Decline' Developing Countries." *International Population Conference*. Liege: International Union for the Scientific Study of Population.

Parsons, James, Matthew Hickman, Paul Turnball, Timothy McSweeney, Gerry V. Stimson, Ali Judd, and Kay Roberts. 2002. "Over a Decade of Syringe Exchange: Results from 1997 UK Survey." *Addiction* 97(7): 845–50.

Patrick, David M., Steffanie A. Strathdee, Christopher P. Archibald, Marianna Offner, Kevin J. P. Craib, Peter G. A. Cornelisse, Martin T. Schecter, Michael L. Rekart, and Michael V. O'Shaugnessy. 1997. "Determinants of HIV Seroconversion in Injection Drug Users during a Period of Rising Prevalence in Vancouver." *International Journal of STD & AIDS* 8: 437–45.

Pedersen, Susan. 1993. *Family, Dependence, and the Origin of the Welfare State: Britain and France, 1914–1945*. New York: Columbia University Press.

Penner, Norman. 1992. *From Protest to Power: Social Democracy in Canada 1900–Present*. Toronto: James Lorimer.

Pernick, Martin S. 1972. "Politics, Parties, and Pestilence: Epidemic Yellow Fever in Philadelphia and the Rise of the First Party System." *William and Mary Quarterly* 29: 559–86.

Perrow, Charles, and Mauro F. Guillén. 1990. *The AIDS Disaster: The Failure of Organizations in New York and the Nation*. New Haven, Conn.: Yale University Press.

Pertschuk, Michael. 1986. *Giant Killers*. New York: W. W. Norton.

———. 2001. *Smoke in Their Eyes: Lessons in Movement Leadership from the Tobacco Wars*. Nashville, Tenn.: Vanderbilt University Press.

Pertschuk, Mike, Karla Sneega, Kay Arndorfer, Stephen Bobb, Theresa Gardella, and Joel Papo. 1999. *A Movement Rising: A Strategic Analysis of U.S. Tobacco Control Advocacy*. Washington, D.C.: Advocacy Institute.

Pfeiffer, J. E. 1965. "A Visit With Cuyler Hammond." *Think* 31(March-April): 11–14.

Phelan, Jo C., Bruce G. Link, Ana Diez-Roux, Ichiro Kawachi, and Bruce Levin. 2004. " 'Fundamental Causes' of Social Inequalities in Mortality: A Test of the Theory." *Journal of Health and Social Behavior* 45(3): 265–85.

Pichardo, Nelson A. 1997. "New Social Movements: A Critical Review." *Annual Review of Sociology* 23: 411–30.

Pickstone, John V. 1982. "Establishment and Dissent in Nineteenth-Century Medicine: An Exploration of Some Correspondence and Connections between Religious and Medical Belief–Systems in Early Industrial England." In *The Church and Healing*, edited by W. J. Shiels. Oxford: Basil Blackwell.

Pierre-Deschênes, Claudine. 1981. "Santé publique et organisation de la profession médicale au Québec 1870–1918." *Revue d'histoire de l'Amérique Française* 35(3): 355–75.

Pinell, Patrice, and Monika Steffen. 1994. "Les médecins français: Genèse historique d'une profession divisée." In *Les politiques de santé en France et en Allemagne*, edited by Bruno Jobert and Monika Steffen. Paris: Observatoire Européen de la Protection Sociale.

Popham, G. T. 1981. "Government and Smoking: Policy Making and Pressure Groups." *Policy and Politics* 9(3): 331–47.

Porter, Roy. 1997. *The Greatest Benefit to Mankind*. New York: W. W. Norton.

———. 1998. "Concluding Remarks." In *Ashes to Ashes: The History of Smoking and Health*, edited by S. Lock, L. A. Reynolds, and E. M. Tansey. Amsterdam: Editions Rodopi.

Prasad, Monica. 2005. "Why Is France So French? Culture, Institutions, and Neoliberalism, 1974–1981." *American Journal of Sociology* 111(2): 357–407.

Preston, Samuel H. 1975. "The Changing Relation Between Mortality and Level of Economic Development." *Population Studies* 29: 231–48.

———. 1985. "Mortality and Development Revisited." *Population Bulletin of the United Nations* 18: 34–40.

———. 1996. "American Longevity: Past, Present, and Future." Syracuse, N.Y.: Center for Policy Research, Syracuse University.

Preston, Samuel H., and Michael R. Haines. 1991. *Fatal Years: Child Mortality in Late Nineteenth-Century America*. Princeton, N.J.: Princeton University Press.

Preston, Samuel H., and Etienne van de Walle. 1978. "Urban French Mortality in the Nineteenth Century." *Population Studies* 32(2): 275–97.

Price, Jacob M. 1995. "Tobacco Use and Tobacco Taxation: A Battle of Interests in Early Modern Europe." In *Consuming Habits: Drugs in History and Anthropology*, edited by Jordan Goodman, Paul E. Lovejoy, and Andrew Sherratt. London: Routledge.

Price, Roger. 1991. *A Concise History of France*. Cambridge: Cambridge University Press.

Quadagno, Jill. 1994. *The Color of Welfare: How Racism Undermined the War on Poverty*. New York: Oxford University Press.

———. 2004. "Why the United States Has No National Health Insurance: Stakeholder Mobilization Against the Welfare State, 1945–1996." *Journal of Health and Social Behavior* 45 (Extra Issue): 25–44.

Quadagno, Jill, and Debra Street. 2005. "Ideology and Public Policy: Antistatism in American Welfare State Transformation." *The Journal of Policy History* 17(1): 52–71

Radin, Beryl L., and Joan P. Boase. 2000. "Federalism, Political Structure, and Public Policy in the United States and Canada." *Journal of Comparative Policy Analysis: Research and Practice* 2: 65–89.

Ragin, Charles C. 1987. *The Comparative Case Method: Moving beyond Qualitative and Quantitative Strategies.* Berkeley: University of California Press.

Ragin, Charles C., and Howard S. Becker, eds. 1992. *What Is a Case: Exploring the Foundations of Social Inquiry.* Cambridge: Cambridge University Press.

Ramsey, Matthew. 1994. "Public Health in France." In *The History of Public Health and the Modern State,* edited by Dorothy Porter. Amsterdam: Editions Rodopi.

Rathjen, Heidi, and Charles Montpetit. 1999. *December 6: From the Montreal Massacre to Gun Control, the Inside Story.* Toronto: McClelland & Stewart.

Rayside, David. 1998. *On the Fringe: Gays and Lesbians in Politics.* Ithaca, N.Y.: Cornell University Press.

Rayside, David M., and Evert A. Lindquist. 1992. "Canada: Community Activism, Federalism, and the New Politics of Disease." In *AIDS in the Industrialized Democracies: Passions, Politics, and Policies,* edited by David L. Kirp and Ronald Bayer. New Brunswick, N.J.: Rutgers University Press.

Read, Melvyn D. 1992. "Policy Networks and Issue Networks: The Politics of Smoking." In *Policy Networks in British Government,* edited by D. Marsh and R. A. W. Rhodes. Oxford: Clarendon Press.

Reid, Roddy. 2005. *Globalizing Tobacco Control: Anti-Smoking Campaigns in California, France, and Japan.* Bloomington: Indiana University Press.

Rigotti, Nancy A. 2001. "Reducing the Supply of Tobacco to Youths." In *Regulating Tobacco,* edited by Robert L. Rabin and Stephen D. Sugarman. New York: Oxford University Press.

Riley, Diane. 1998. *Drugs and Drug Policy in Canada: A Brief Review and Commentary.* Ottawa: Canadian Foundation for Drug Policy.

Rinehart, Sue T. 1987. "Maternal Health Care Policy: Britain and the United States." *Comparative Politics* 19(2): 193–211.

RJR-MacDonald v. Canada (Attorney-General). 1995. 3 S.C.R. 199.

Rocher, François, and Miriam Smith. 2002. *Federalism and Health Care: The Impact of Political–Institutional Dynamics on the Canadian Health Care System.* Discussion Paper No. 18. Ottawa: Commission on the Future of Health Care in Canada.

Rollet, Catherine. 1997. "The Fight against Infant Mortality in the Past: An International Comparison." In *Infant and Child Mortality in the Past,* edited by Alain Bideau, Bertrand Desjardins, and Hector P. Brignoli. Oxford: Clarendon Press.

Rollet, Catherine, and Patrice Bourdelais. 1993. "Infant Mortality in France, 1750–1950. Evaluation and Perspectives." In *The Decline of Infant Mortality in Europe, 1800–1950: Four National Case Studies,* edited by Carlo A. Corsini and Pier P. Viazzo. Florence: UNICEF Innocenti Research Centre.

Rollet–Echalier, Catherine. 1990. *La politique à l'égard de la petite enfance sous la IIIe Republique.* Paris: Institut national d'études démographiques.

Rosen, George. 1993. *A History of Public Health.* Baltimore, Md.: Johns Hopkins University Press.

Rosenberg, Charles E. 1962/1987. *The Cholera Years,* 2nd. ed. Chicago: The University of Chicago Press.

———. 1988. "Disease and Social Order in America: Perceptions and Expectations." In *AIDS and the Burdens of History,* edited by Elizabeth Fee and Daniel M. Fox. Berkeley: University of California Press.

Rosman, Sophia. 1994. "Entre engagement militant et efficacité professionelle: Naissance et développement d'une association d'aide aux malades de sida." *Sciences Sociales et Santé* 12(2): 113–39.

Rothman, Sheila M. 1978. *Women's Proper Place: A History of Changing Ideals and Practices, 1870 to the Present.* New York: Basic Books.

———. 1994. *Living in the Shadow of Death: Tuberculosis and the Social Experience of Illness in American History.* New York: Basic Books.

Rouchy, Jean C., ed. 1996. *La double rencontre: Toxicomanie et sida.* Ramonville-Saint Agne: Editions Erés.

Royal College of Physicians of London. 1971. *Smoking and Health Now.* London: Pitman.

Santora, Marc. 2006. "Overhaul Urged for Laws on AIDS Tests and Data." *The New York Times.*, February 2, 2006.

Schecter, Martin T., Steffanie A. Strathdee, Peter G. A. Cornelisse, Sue Currie, David M. Patrick, Michael l. Rekart, and Michael V. O'Shaugnessy. 1999. "Do Needle Exchange Programmes Increase the Spread of HIV Among Injection Drug Users?: An Investigation of the Vancouver Outbreak." *AIDS* 13: F45–F51.

Scott, Anne F. 2004. "Introduction." In *My Friend Julia Lathrop*, by Jane Addams. Urbana: University of Illinois Press.

Scottish Home and Health Department. 1986. *HIV Infection in Scotland: Report of the Scottish Committee on HIV Infection and Intravenous Drug Misuse.* Edinburgh: Scottish Home and Health Department.

Serfaty, Annie. 1996. *Politique de reduction des risques envers les usagers de drogues.* Paris: Direction régionale des affaires sanitaires et sociale d'Ile-de-France.

Setbon, Michel. 1993. *Pouvoirs contre sida.* Paris: Seuil.

Shafey, O., S. Dolwick, and G. E. Guindon, eds. 2003. *Tobacco Control Country Profiles, 2003.* Atlanta, Ga.: American Cancer Society.

Shilts, Randy. 1987. *And the Band Played On: Politics, People, and the AIDS Epidemic.* New York: Penguin Books.

Shryock, Richard H. 1957. *National Tuberculosis Association, 1904–1954: A Study of the Voluntary Health Movement in the United States.* New York: National Tuberculosis Association.

Simpson, David. 1998. "ASH: Witness on Smoking." In *Ashes to Ashes: The History of Smoking and Health*, edited by S. Lock, L. A. Reynolds, and E. M. Tansey. Amsterdam: Editions Rodopi.

Sklar, Kathryn K. 1993. "The Historical Foundations of Women's Power in the Creation of the American Welfare State, 1830–1930." In *Mothers of a New World: Maternalist Politics and the Origins of Welfare States*, edited by Seth Koven and Sonya Michel. New York: Routledge.

Skocpol, Theda. 1979. *States and Social Revolutions: A Comparative Analysis of France, Russia, and China.* Cambridge: Cambridge University Press.

———. 1985. "Bringing the State Back In: Strategies of Analysis in Current Research." In *Bringing the State Back In*, edited by Peter B. Evans, Dietrich Rueschemeyer, and Theda Skocpol. Cambridge: Cambridge University Press.

———. 1992. *Protecting Soldiers and Mothers: The Political Origins of Social Policy in the United States.* Cambridge, Mass.: Harvard University Press.

———. 1995a. *Social Policy in the United States: Future Possibilities in Historical Perspective.* Princeton, N.J.: Princeton University Press.

———. 1995b. "Gender and the Origins of Modern Social Policies in Britain and the United States." In collaboration with Gretchen Ritter. In *Social Policy in the United States: Future Possibilities in Historical Perspective.* Princeton, N.J: Princeton University Press.

Skocpol, Theda, and Edwin Amenta. 1986. "States and Social Policies." *Annual Review of Sociology* 12: 131–57.

Skowronek, Stephen. 1982. *Building a New American State: The Expansion of National Administrative Capacities, 1877–1920.* Cambridge: Cambridge University Press.

Smith, Francis B. 1988. *The Retreat of Tuberculosis 1850–1919.* London: Croom-Helm.

Smith, Susan L. 1995. *Sick and Tired of Being Sick and Tired: Black Women's Health Activism in America, 1890–1950.* Philadelphia: University of Pennsylvania Press.

Snow, David A., E. B. Rochford, Jr., Steven K. Worden, and Robert D. Benford. 1986. "Frame Alignment Process, Micromobilization, and Movement Participation." *American Sociological Review* 51: 464–81.

Solomon, Robert M., and Sydney J. Usprich. 1991. "Canada's Drug Laws." *The Journal of Drug Issues* 21(1): 17–40.

Speck, W. A. 1993. *A Concise History of Britain, 1707–1975.* Cambridge: Cambridge University Press.

Starr, Paul. 1982. *The Social Transformation of American Medicine.* New York: Basic Books.

Steele, James H. 2000. " History, Trends, and Extent of Pasteurization." *Journal of the American Veterinary Medical Association* 217(2): 175–78.

Steffen, Monika. 1992. "France: Social Solidarity and Scientific Expertise." In *AIDS in the Industrialized Democracies: Passions, Politics, and Policies,* edited by David L. Kirp and Ronald Bayer. New Brunswick, N.J.: Rutgers University Press.

———. 1996. *The Fight against AIDS.* Grenoble: Presses Universitaires de Grenoble.

———. 1999. "The Nation's Blood: Medicine, Justice, and the State in France." In *Blood Feuds: AIDS, Blood, and the Politics of Medical Disaster,* edited by Eric A. Feldman and Ronald Bayer. New York: Oxford University Press.

Steffenhagen, Janet. 1997. "City Backs Addict Safe Houses as Eastside AIDS Rate Soars: Mayor Philip Owen Backs the Plan, but Health Minister Joy MacPhail Objects." *The Vancouver Sun,* September 27, 1997, p. A1.

Steinfeld, Jesse L. 1983. "Women and Children Last? Attitudes Toward Cigarette Smoking and Nonsmokers' Rights, 1971." *New York State Journal of Medicine* 83(13): 1257–58.

Stimson, Gerry V. 1995. "AIDS and Injecting Drug Use in the United Kingdom, 1987–1993: The Policy Response and the Prevention of the Epidemic." *Social Science and Medicine* 41(5): 699–716.

———. 2000. " 'Blair Declares War': The Unhealthy State of British Drug Policy." *International Journal of Drug Policy* 11: 259–64.

Stimson, Gerry V., and Rachel Lart. 1991. "HIV, Drugs, and Public Health in England: New Words, Old Tunes." *The International Journal of the Addictions* 26(12): 1263–77.

———. 1994. "The Relationship Between the State and Local Practice in the Development of National Policy on Drugs Between 1920 and 1990." In *Heroin Addiction and Drug Policy: The British System,* edited by J. Strang and M. Gossop. Oxford: Oxford University Press.

Stone, Judith F. 1985. *The Search for Social Peace: Reform Legislation in France, 1890–1914.* Albany: State University of New York Press.

———. 1997. " The Republican Brotherhood: Gender and Ideology." In *Gender and the Politics of Social Reform in France, 1870–1914,* edited by Elinor Accampo, Rachel G. Fuchs, and Mary L. Stewart. Baltimore, Md.: Johns Hopkins University Press.

Strathdee, Steffanie A. 1998. "Senate Staff Briefing on the Vancouver HIV Outbreak Among Injection Drug Users." Invited presentation (July 21, 1998).

Strathdee, Steffanie A., David M. Patrick, Sue L. Currie, Peter G. A. Cornelisse, Michael L. Rekart, Julio S. G. Montaner, Martin T. Schechter, and Michael V. O'Shaughnessy. 1997. "Needle Exchange Is Not Enough: Lessons from the Vancouver Injecting Drug Use Study." *AIDS* 11(8): 59–65.

Stratton, Kathleen, Padma Shetty, Robert Wallace, and Stuart Bondurant, eds. 2001. *Clearing the Smoke: Assessing the Science Base for Tobacco Harm Reduction.* Washington, D.C.: National Academy Press.

Street, John, and Albert Weale. 1992. "Britain: Policy–Making in a Hermetically Sealed System." In *AIDS in the Industrialized Democracies: Passions, Politics, and Policies*, edited by David L. Kirp and Ronald Bayer. New Brunswick, N.J.: Rutgers University Press.

Studlar, Donley T. 2002. *Tobacco Control: Comparative Politics in the United States and Canada.* Peterborough, Ont.: Broadview Press.

Sussman, George D. 1982. *Selling Mothers' Milk: The Wet–Nursing Business in France, 1715–1914.* Urbana: University of Illinois Press.

Szreter, Simon. 1988. "The Importance of Social Intervention in Britain's Mortality Decline c.1850–1914: A Reinterpretation of the Role of Public Health." *Social History of Medicine* 1: 1–37.

———. 1997. "Economic Growth, Disruption, Deprivation, Disease, and Death: on the Importance of the Politics of Public Health for Development." *Population and Development Review* 23(4): 693–728.

Tarrow, Sidney. 1998. *Power in Movement: Social Movements and Contentious Politics,* 2nd ed. Cambridge: Cambridge University Press.

Taylor, Peter. 1984. *Smoke Ring: The Politics of Tobacco.* London: The Bodley Head.

Teller, Michael E. 1988. *The Tuberculosis Movement: A Public Health Campaign in the Progressive Era.* New York: Greenwood Press.

Tempalski, Barbara. 2005. "The Uneven Geography of Syringe Exchange Programs in the United States: Need, Politics and Place." Ph.D. diss. University of Washington, Seattle.

Tétreault, Martin. 1983. "Les Maladies de la Misère: Aspects de la Santé Publique à Montréal, 1880–1914." *Revue D'Histoire De L'Amérique Française* 36(4): 507–26.

Thane, Pat. 1990. "Government and Society in England and Wales, 1750–1914." In *The Cambridge Social History of Britain 1750–1950,* vol. 3, edited by P. L. Thompson. Cambridge: Cambridge University Press.

———. 1991. "Visions of Gender in the Making of the British Welfare State: The Case of Women in the British Labour Party and Social Policy, 1906–1945." In *Maternity & Gender Policies: Women and the Rise of the European Welfare States, 1880s–1950s,* edited by Gisela Bock and Pat Thane. London: Routledge.

———. 1993. "Women in the British Labour Party and the Construction of State Welfare, 1906–1939." In *Mothers of a New World: Maternalist Politics and the Origins of Welfare States,* edited by Seth Koven and Sonya Michel. New York: Routledge.

Thom, Thomas J., and Frederick H. Epstein. 1994. "Heart Disease, Cancer, and Stroke Mortality Trends and Their Interrelations: An International Perspective." *Circulation* 90:574–82.

Thompson, Barbara. 1984. "Infant Mortality in Nineteenth Century Bradford." In *Urban Disease and Mortality in Nineteenth-Century England,* edited by Robert

Woods and John Woodward. London: Batsford Academic and Educational Press.

Thompson, Michael. 1983. "Postscript: A Cultural Basis for Comparison." In *Risk Analysis and Decision Processes: The Siting of Liquified Energy Gas Facilities in Four Countries*, edited by Howard C. Kunreuther and Joanne Linerooth. Berlin: Springer-Verlag.

Tilly, Charles. 1984. *Big Structures Large Processes Huge Comparisons*. New York: Russell Sage Foundation.

Tilly, Charles, Louise Tilly, and Richard Tilly. 1975. *The Rebellious Century. 1830–1930*. Cambridge, Mass.: Harvard University Press.

Tomes, Nancy. 1990. "The Private Side of Public Health: Sanitary Science, Domestic Hygiene, and the Germ Theory, 1870–1900." *Bulletin of the History of Medicine* 64: 509–39.

———. 1998. *The Gospel of Germs: Men, Women, and the Microbe in American Life*. Cambridge, Mass.: Harvard University Press.

Townsend, Joy. 1987a. "Economic and Health Consequences of Reduced Smoking." In *Health and Economics*, edited by Alan Williams. London: Macmillan.

———. 1987b. "Tobacco Price and the Smoking Epidemic." *Smoke-Free Europe-9*. Copenhagen: WHO Regional Office for Europe.

———. 1993. "Policies to Halve Smoking Deaths." *Addiction* 88: 43–52.

Townsend, Joy, Paul Roderick, and Jacqueline Cooper. 1994. "Cigarette Smoking by Socioeconomic Group, Sex, and Age: Effects of Price, Income, and Health Publicity." *British Medical Journal* 309: 924–27.

Trades Union Congress [TUC]. 2006. "Smoking Vote on 14 February." *Risks Newsletter* 243 (11 February): 1–2. http://www.tuc.org.uk/h_and_s/tuc-11362-f0. cfm#tuc-11362-2.

Trebach, Arnold S. 1982. *The Heroin Solution*. New Haven, Conn.: Yale University Press.

Troesken, Walter. 2004. *Water, Race, and Disease*. Cambridge, Mass.: The MIT Press.

Troyer, Ronald J. 1984. "From Prohibition to Regulation: Comparing Two Antismoking Movements." *Research in Social Movements: Conflict and Change* 7: 53–69.

Troyer, Ronald J., and Gerald E. Markle. 1983. *Cigarettes: The Battle Over Smoking*. New Brunswick, N.J.: Rutgers University Press.

Tubiana, Maurice. 1997. "Tabagisme passif. rapport et voeu de l'Académie Nationale de Médecine." *Bulletin de l'Académie Nationale de Médecine* 181(4): 3–43.

Turmel, André, and Louise Hamelin. 1995. "La grande facheuse d'enfants: La mortalité infantile depuis le tournant du siècle." *CRSA/RCSA* 32(4): 439–63.

UK Department of Health. 1993. Government Response to the Second Report from the Health Committee, Session 1992–93, "The European Commission's Proposed Directive on the Advertising of Tobacco Products." London: Her Majesty's Stationery Office.

———. 1998. *Smoking Kills: A White Paper on Tobacco*. Cm. 4177. London: Her Majesty's Stationery Office.

Union-Tribune. 2000. "Social Nihilism: City Council Considers Needle Exchange." *Union–Tribune* (San Diego), September 11, 2000, Editorial.

UK Department of Health and Social Security. 1988. *AIDS and Drug Misuse: Report by the Advisory Council on the Misuse of Drugs*. London: Her Majesty's Stationery Office.

———. 1993. *AIDS and Drug Misuse Update: Report by the Advisory Council on the Misuse of Drugs*. London: Her Majesty's Stationery Office.

UK Health Protection Agency. 2005. *Shooting Up: Infections Among Injecting Drug Users in the United Kingdom 2004*. London: Health Protection Agency.

United Kingdom. 1976. "Smoking and Health." *Parliamentary Debates*, Commons, vol. 903, cols. 785–887 (16 January 1976).

———. 1986. "Acquired Immune Deficiency Syndrome." *Parliamentary Debates*, Commons, vol. 105, cols. 799–864 (21 November 1986).

———. 1987a. "AIDS (Control) Etc. Bill." *Parliamentary Debates*, Commons, vol. 108, 1168–95 (23 January 1987).

———. 1987b. "AIDS (Control) Etc. Bill." *Parliamentary Debates*, Commons, vol. 113, 679–708 (27 March 1987).

———. 1994. "Tobacco Advertising Bill." *Parliamentary Debates*, Commons, vol. 243, cols. 445–525 (13 May 1994). http://www.publications.parliament.uk/pa/cm199394/cmhansrd/1994-05-13/Debate-1.html.

———. 1995. "Tobacco Products Labelling Bill." *Parliamentary Debates*, Commons, vol. 254, cols. 1240–73 (17 February 1995). http://www.publications.parliament.uk/pa/cm199495/cmhansrd/1995-02-17/Debate-1.html.

———. 2002. "Tobacco Advertising and Promotion Bill [Lords]." *Parliamentary Debates*, Commons, vol. 384, cols. 683–775 (29 April 2002). http://www.publications.parliament.uk/pa/cm200102/cmhansrd/vo020429/debindx/20429-x.htm.

U.S. Bureau of the Census. 1975. *Historical Statistics of the United States: Colonial Times to 1970*. Washington: U.S. Government Printing Office.

U.S. Bureau of the Census, Population Division, and International Programs Center. 2005. "International data base" [Web Page]. April 26. Available at: http://www.census.gov/ipc/www/idbprint.html.

U.S. Center for Disease Control [CDC]. 1981a. "Pneumocystis Pneumonia—Los Angeles." *Morbidity and Mortality Weekly Report* 30: 250–52.

———. 1981b. "Kaposi's Sarcoma and Pneumocystis Pneumonia among Homosexual Men—New York City and California." *Morbidity and Mortality Weekly Report* 30: 305–8.

U.S. Centers for Disease Control and Prevention [CDC]. 1996. *HIV/AIDS Surveillance Report, 1996*. Atlanta: U.S. Department of Health and Human Services.

———. 1998. "Commentary." *HIV/AIDS Surveillance Report*. Atlanta: U.S. Department of Health and Human Services.

———. 1999. "CDC on Infant and Maternal Mortality in the United States: 1900–99." *Population and Development Review* 25(4): 821–26.

———. 2001. *HIV/AIDS Surveillance Report, 2001*, vol. 13. Atlanta: U.S. Department of Health and Human Services.

———. 2004. "AIDS Public Information Dataset, CDC Wonder On-Line Database, U.S. Surveillance Data for 1981–2001." Atlanta: U.S. Department of Health and Human Services.

———. 2005a. *HIV/AIDS Surveillance Report, 2004*, vol. 16. Atlanta: U.S. Department of Health and Human Services, Centers for Disease Control and Prevention. Available at: http://www.cdc.gov/hiv/stats/hasrlink.htm.

———. 2005b. "Update: Syringe Exchange Programs—United States, 2002." *Morbidity and Mortality Weekly Report* 54(27): 673–76. http://www.cdc.gov/mmwr/PDF/wk/mm5427.pdf.

—————. 2005c. "Access to Sterile Syringes" Fact Sheet Series. Atlanta: Centers for Disease Control and Academy for Educational Development. http://www.cdc.gov/idu/facts/aed_idu_acc.htm.

—————. 2005d. "AIDS Public Information Data Set (APIDS), U.S. Surveillance Data for 1981–1999." Atlanta: Centers for Disease Control and Prevention, National Center for HIV, STD, and TB Prevention.

U.S. Department of Health and Human Services [HHS]. 1989. *Reducing the Health Consequences of Smoking: Twenty-Five Years of Progress. A Report of the Surgeon General.* HHS Publication No. (CDC) 89-8411. Rockville, Md.: U.S. Government Printing Office.

—————. 1990. "Methadone Interim Maintenance Hearing." Rockville, Maryland (February 28, 1990).

—————. 1991. *Strategies to Control Tobacco Use in the United States: A Blueprint for Public Health in the 1990s.* NIH Publication No. 92-3316 (October). Rockville, Md.: U.S. Government Printing Office.

—————. 1995. "Analysis Regarding FDA's Jurisdiction over Nicotine-Containing Cigarettes and Smokeless Tobacco Products: Notice." *Federal Register* 60(155): 41454–59.

—————. 2006. *The Health Consequences of Involuntary Exposure to Tobacco Smoke: A Report of the Surgeon General.* Atlanta: U.S. Department of Health and Human Services, Centers for Disease Control and Prevention, Coordinating Center for Health Promotion, National Center for Chronic Disease Prevention and Health Promotion, Office on Smoking and Health.

U.S. Department of Health, Education, and Welfare. 1964. *Smoking and Health: Report of the Advisory Committee to the Surgeon General of the Public Health Service.* Public Health Service Publication No. 1103. Washington: U.S. Government Printing Office.

U.S. Department of Health and Human Services, Food and Drug Administration. 1989. "Drugs Used for Treatment of Narcotic Addicts." *Federal Register,* Vol. 54, No. 40, March 2, 1989, 221 CFR Part 291.

U.S. Food and Drug Administration and the National Institute on Drug Abuse [FDA-NIDA]. 1989. "Use of Methadone in Maintenance and Detoxification Treatment of Narcotic Addicts." *Federal Register* 54: 8973.

U.S. National Commission on AIDS. 1991. *America Living With AIDS.* Washington: U.S. Government Printing Office.

U.S. National Institute on Drug Abuse. 2006. "Statement from the Director." NIH Publication No. 06-5760. Rockville, Md.: U.S. Department of Health and Human Services. http://www.drugabuse.gov/ResearchReports/HIV/hiv.html.

U.S. Office of National Drug Control Policy [ONDCP]. 2002. *National Drug Control Strategy: FY2003 Budget Summary.* Washington: Executive Office of the President.

—————. 2004. *National Drug Control Strategy: FY2005 Budget Summary.* Washington: Executive Office of the President.

U.S. Substance Abuse and Mental Health Services Administration. 2001. "New Federal Regulations Issued to Improve Methadone Treatment." News Release. Rockville, Md.: U.S. Department of Health and Human Services. http://www.samhsa.gov/news/newsreleases/010117nrmeth.htm.

Vancouver Sun. 1998. "Methadone Has to Be Part of Solution to Drug Crisis." *The Vancouver Sun,* January 28, 1998, p. A18.

Ventilator, The. 1971. Newsletter of the Group Against Smokers' Pollution, College Park, Md., v.I (1).

Verney, Douglas V. 1986. *Three Civilizations, Two Cultures, One State: Canada's Political Tradition.* Durham, N.C.: Duke University Press.

Vlahov, David, Don C. Des Jarlais, Eric Goosby, Paula C. Hollinger, Peter G. Lurie, Michael D. Shriver, and Steffanie A. Strathdee. 2001. "Needle Exchange Programs for the Prevention of Human Immunodeficiency Virus Infection: Epidemiology and Policy." *American Journal of Epidemiology* 154(12): S70–S77.

Vogel, David. 1986. *National Styles of Regulation: Environmental Policy in Great Britain and the United States.* Ithaca, N.Y.: Cornell University Press.

Walker, Jack L., Jr. 1991. *Mobilizing Interest Groups in America: Patrons, Professions, and Social Movements.* Ann Arbor: University of Michigan Press.

Walton, John. 1992. "Making the Theoretical Case." In *What Is a Case: Exploring the Foundations of Social Inquiry,* edited by Charles C. Ragin and Howard S. Becker. Cambridge: Cambridge University Press.

Warner, Kenneth E. 1979. "Clearing the Airwaves: The Cigarette Broadcast Ad Ban Revisited." *Policy Analysis* 5: 435–50.

———. 1981. "Cigarette Smoking in the 1970s: The Impact of the Antismoking Campaign." *Science* 211(4483): 729–31.

Waserman, Manfred. 1975. "The Quest for a National Health Department in the Progressive Era." *Bulletin of the History of Medicine* 49: 353–80.

Weber, Max. 1949. *The Methodology of the Social Sciences.* Glencoe, Ill.: The Free Press.

Weeks, Jeffrey. 1985. *Sexuality and Its Discontents: Meanings, Myths, and Modern Sexualities.* London: Routledge.

Weisz, George. 2003. "The Emergence of Medical Specialization in the Nineteenth Century." *Bulletin of the History of Medicine* 77(3): 536–75.

Wherrett, George. 1977. *The Miracle of the Empty Beds: A History of Tuberculosis in Canada.* Toronto: University of Toronto Press.

White, Michael. 2006. "MPs Vote to Stub Out Smoking in Public." *The Guardian* (London), February 24, 2006.

Wiebe, Robert H. 1967. *The Search for Order, 1877–1920.* New York: Hill and Wang.

Wills, Terence. 1997. "Reformers Take on Bloc in Defence of Anti–Tobacco Bill." *The Gazette* (Montreal), February 22, 1997, p. A15.

Wilsford, David. 2001. "Paradoxes of Health Care Reform in France: State Autonomy and Policy Paralysis." In *Success and Failure in Public Governance: A Comparative Analysis,* edited by Mark Bovens, Paul Hart, and B. G. Peters. Cheltenham, Gloucestershire: Edward Elgar.

Wilson, Leonard G. 1990. "The Historical Decline of Tuberculosis in Europe and America: Its Causes and Significance." *Journal of the History of Medicine and Allied Sciences* 45:366–96.

Winslow, C. E. A. 1929. *The Life of Hermann Biggs.* Philadelphia, Pa.: Lea and Febiger.

Winter, Greg.2001. "Philip Morris Seeks Backers for Tobacco Legislation." *New York Times,* June 7, 2001, p. C2, 4.

Wohl, Anthony. 1983. *Endangered Lives: Public Health in Victorian Britain.* Cambridge, Mass.: Harvard University Press.

Wolfson, Mark. 2001. *The Fight Against Big Tobacco: The Movement, the State, and the Public's Health.* New York: Aldine de Gruyter.

Wood, Evan, Mark Tyndall, Patricia M. Spittal, Kathy Li, Aslam H. Anis, Robert S. Hogg, Julio S. G. Montaner, Michael V. O'Shaugnessy, and Martin T. Schecter. 2003. "Impact of Supply-Side Policies for Control of Illicit Drugs in the Face of the AIDS and Overdose Epidemics: Investigation of a Massive Heroin Seizure." *Canadian Medical Association Journal* 168(2): 165–69.

Woods, Robert. 1997. "Infant Mortality in Britain: A Survey of Current Knowledge on Historical Trends and Variations." In *Infant and Child Mortality in the Past*, edited by Alain Bideau, Bertrand Desjardins, and Hector P. Brignoli. Oxford: Clarendon Press.

———. 2000. *The Demography of Victorian England and Wales*. Cambridge: Cambridge University Press.

Woods, Robert, P. A. Watterson, and J. H. Woodward. 1988. "The Causes of the Rapid Decline of Infant Mortality in England and Wales, 1821–1921, Part I." *Population Studies* 42:343–66.

———. 1989. "The Causes of the Rapid Decline of Infant Mortality in England and Wales, 1821–1921, Part II." *Population Studies* 43:113–32.

World Health Organization. 2005. "WHO Mortality Database: Tables" Geneva: World Health Organization. http://www.who.int/healthinfo/morttables/en/print.html.

Wynder, Ernest L., and Evarts A. Graham. 1950. "Tobacco Smoking as a Possible Etiologic Factor in Bronchogenic Carcinoma." *Journal of the American Medical Association* 143: 329–36.

Wynne, Brian. 1987. *Risk Management and Hazardous Waste: Implementation and the Dialectics of Credibility*. Berlin: Springer-Verlag.

Young, Michael P. 2002. "Confessional Protest: The Religious Birth of U.S. National Social Movements." *American Sociological Review* 67(October): 660–88.

Index